Medical Ventilator System Basics

Medical Ventilator System Basics
A Clinical Guide

Yuan Lei
Senior e-learning manager, Hamilton Medical AG, Switzerland
Formerly Surgeon, University Hospital of Zurich, Switzerland, and Xinhua Hospital, Shanghai Second Medical University, China

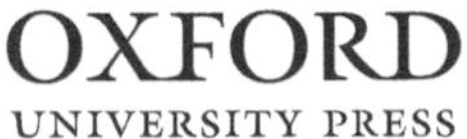
OXFORD
UNIVERSITY PRESS

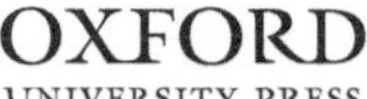

Great Clarendon Street, Oxford, OX2 6DP,
United Kingdom

Oxford University Press is a department of the University of Oxford. It furthers the University's objective of excellence in research, scholarship, and education by publishing worldwide. Oxford is a registered trade mark of Oxford University Press in the UK and in certain other countries

Impression: 2

Published in the United States of America by Oxford University Press
198 Madison Avenue, New York, NY 10016, United States of America

British Library Cataloguing in Publication Data
Data available

Library of Congress Control Number: 2016960950

ISBN 978-0-19-878497-5

Printed in Great Britain by Ashford Colour Press Ltd, Gosport, Hampshire

Foreword by Peter Rimensberger

From the development of positive pressure ventilators in the 1940s—ventilators that offered only non-synchronized volume-controlled ventilation—technical development has continued, resulting in today's sophisticated ventilatory systems. These systems can provide patient-triggered mechanical ventilation and a wide array of ventilator modes.

At the same time, we observe a clear trend towards 'smart' or 'intelligent' ventilation concepts and algorithms that provide decision support and even automation of mechanical ventilation. This involves integrating physiological data which has been acquired directly from the ventilator's built-in monitoring or indirectly through other bedside technologies.

However, these sophisticated control systems, while exploiting many of the advantages of today's microprocessor technology, do not eliminate the responsibility of the critical care team to optimize mechanical ventilation for each patient. To be able to carry out this responsibility and to provide mechanical ventilation in the best possible way, the care provider not only has to have a good understanding of mechanical ventilation, physiology, and respiratory mechanics, but also of the device's operating principles, essential variables, and control parameters.

Unfortunately, in the clinical setting we observe that a basic understanding of how a ventilator works and how to apply the information it provides, is increasingly lost to the younger generation of health care providers. In parallel, the knowledge of what might be detrimental to a ventilated patient is increasing—although there is often a tendency to generalize and even oversimplify the best ventilator strategies and concepts to be applied in a patient. The increasing number of sophisticated algorithm-based ventilator modes on which we quickly come to rely further supports this trend.

So the question arises whether we, as care providers, still know how to 'drive' the ventilator and to 'troubleshoot' in an appropriate and rapid way without putting the patient at risk.

A good understanding of the technical equipment, including its operating principles and safety backup systems, seems to be crucial to maintain this knowledge.

This has been recognized by Yuan Lei, the author of this book, who, like me, can look back on about 45 years of progress in the development of ventilator technology for intensive care. Over these years we have seen, either from the standpoint of a product manager or of a clinician, many ICU ventilators of various brands. We have also read their user manuals. Although the manuals should provide all the necessary information on how to use the devices, they mainly explain the details of their ventilator modes and provide some information on the alarms that may occur, along with some troubleshooting advice. This information often does not really help one to understand how the ventilator interacts with the patient and how the data provided by the ventilator can be used to assure its proper functioning and settings.

In short, there is generally little education offered to help one understand first, the ventilator equipment, including its operating principle and technical limitations, and second, how the device's respiratory mechanics information can be used to set basic ventilator parameters appropriately.

Based on his extensive personal experience in this field and many lessons learned from direct contact with ventilator users, as well as the recognition that those who design and manufacture devices have to take some responsibility in the process of education and training of users, the author has, for many years, had a dream to help. His goal, that we, the clinical users, gain a greater understanding of a properly functioning ventilator system and its proper use—this will be a key determinant in the successful application of specific ventilator strategies.

With the realization of this book for clinical ventilator users, he not only fulfils his own dream, but also gives us a comprehensive educational tool to improve our understanding of the essential basic principles for the use of a mechanical ventilator—a highly dangerous medical device, when inappropriately used.

Peter Rimensberger, MD
Professor of Intensive Care Medicine
Professor of Neonatology and Pediatrics
Service of Neonatology and Pediatric Intensive Care
Department of Pediatrics
University Hospital of Geneva
Switzerland

Foreword by Giorgio A. Iotti

In his preface, the author recommends reading the chapters of his book in sequence. I also recommend the reader start the sequence from the preface, reading his story of the young physician faced with the challenge of introducing intensive care and modern mechanical ventilation in China in the 1980s.

Although at that time intensive care was well established in Europe, our problems in understanding and implementing modern mechanical ventilation were not so different from those experienced by the author in China. We were leaving the old established way, using simple and robust machines that provided just volume control ventilation, with PEEP generated by water-seal or spring valves, and monitoring based simply on a mechanical manometer and spirometer. We were starting to use the new electronic machines, which provided a number of ventilation modes (each one with a number of controls), without a clear knowledge of their indications and benefits.

Also, monitoring of mechanical ventilation was changing from the pure technical control of the ventilator to functional assessment of the patient with respiratory failure. Finally, the new technology included extensive alarming; the new ventilator alarms were sounding a lot, sometimes with bells and whistles upsetting both clinicians and patients, especially during the night! Considering all these issues, the sources of information available to guide our use of mechanical ventilators were limited.

Since then, education in the field of mechanical ventilation has become a complex matter indeed. The science of mechanical ventilation has greatly advanced and several important principles are now consolidated. However, driving a mechanical ventilator is not just a matter of understanding principles that can be found in the scientific literature; it also requires a deep knowledge of the actual machine that we are using. And here comes one major difficulty: unlike vehicles, that are necessarily designed to respond homogeneously to approved standards, mechanical ventilators are frequently designed to look different from each other, even more different than they actually are. The difficulty in 'driving' a mechanical ventilator could be overcome by reading and studying the user's manual, usually a great source of accurate and useful information. Unfortunately, this simple solution fails to consider a common professional disease of clinicians: a severe allergy to reading user's manuals! On the other hand, the language and approach of user's manuals, usually written by engineers, do not help.

Medical Ventilator System Basics: A Clinical Guide stems from the recognition of all these difficulties. It is indeed a book conceived to answer a need for education, with simplicity and completeness being the evident bywords that inspired the author's work. The book deals with technology, but it is not written by an engineer: it is written by a physician for the needs of clinicians. It intends to provide practical information for the proper use of mechanical ventilators, but it is not focused on a specific machine; rather, the book aims to help the reader to obtain the best from his own ventilator.

Very interestingly, the book is based on an original concept: the 'ventilator system', which is not just the 'mechanical ventilator', but the unit composed of all the elements, both natural and artificial, that make up the functional respiratory system of a mechanically ventilated patient. Thus, the 'ventilator system' also includes the patient's airways, lungs, chest wall, and respiratory muscles, as essential components contributing to and affecting the physiological result of gas exchange. Similarly, the artificial components include not just the high technology ventilator, but also humble but essential parts such as the external circuit (that might be leaking, for instance) and the endotracheal tube (that might be clogged). The analytical view provided by the 'ventilator system' concept can be extremely useful for fast troubleshooting when mechanical ventilation becomes ineffective. This kind of concept may be profitably translated to other kinds of artificial support of organs, such as extracorporeal membrane oxygenation.

I am confident that *Medical Ventilator System Basics: A Clinical Guide* will become a classic of medical literature on mechanical ventilation, mostly appreciated by those clinicians aware of the importance of integrating a strong theoretical background with a deep understanding of the instruments used to provide mechanical ventilation.

Giorgio A. Iotti, MD
Anesthesia and Intensive Care, 2nd Dpt
Fondazione IRCCS Policlinico San Matteo
Pavia, Italy

Preface

In the late 1980s, as a young surgical resident at a teaching hospital in Shanghai, I experienced first-hand the introduction of the intensive care unit (ICU) and mechanical ventilation to mainland China. Medical professionals then perceived an ICU and ventilator to be a cure-all, although few had the knowledge to back up their beliefs. 'We must have our own ICUs', the head of my hospital declared. So a new surgical ICU was set up in two large, air-conditioned rooms. It was equipped with three Siemens SERVO 900C ventilators, a few patient monitors, and other basic equipment. The first ICU crew included a group of young physicians and nurses. I was a crew member.

A big challenge we faced was that none of us knew about mechanical ventilation or the ventilator and its operation; something I was then assigned to learn. I delved into the operator's manual, which was, at the time, the only source of information available. I quickly discovered that the manual was written by technical people, for technical people, and that my medical education was of little use in this particular area. And so the nightmare began as I was called around the clock to resolve various problems with mechanical ventilation. In a typical scenario, I would find the ventilated patient clearly in trouble, the ventilator was alarming persistently, and I hadn't a clue what had gone wrong. I was forced to learn in a tough way, through trial and error.

Ironically, around a decade later I became product manager for a ventilator manufacturer. In this position, I had the opportunity for the comprehensive study of mechanical ventilation and equipment. I also became deeply involved in ventilator development, marketing, and customer training. From this experience I made several interesting discoveries:

a. The current mechanical ventilation education in medical or nursing schools is neither adequate nor structured. Meaningful learning often begins after a graduate starts clinical practice.
b. The equipment required for mechanical ventilation is a ventilator system with six essential components. A ventilator is just one of them.
c. All positive pressure ventilator systems have the same or highly similar operating principles and system composition, and all require the same conditions for operation. They may differ here and there in technical implementation. Interestingly, their differences are often exaggerated and the similarities unmentioned.
d. The clinical outcome of mechanical ventilation relies much more on the user's knowledge of this therapy than it does on the equipment in use.
e. The knowledge specific to mechanical ventilation has two dimensions: its clinical application and its equipment. The second dimension is often ignored in the related education.
f. Today, ample information about clinical application is widely available, but little exists about the equipment.
g. Clinicians often feel responsible for the clinical application of mechanical ventilation, but hold technicians responsible for the equipment.

Mechanical ventilation can be described as the clinical application of a ventilator system. Clinicians who conduct this therapy need to understand both the application and the equipment for three reasons. First, equipment knowledge is required to set up and maintain a properly functioning ventilator system. Second, equipment knowledge is required to understand the real meaning of a ventilator's functions and features. Third, equipment knowledge is required to determine the source of, and to resolve, problems that can stem from the equipment, the ventilated patient, or the operator's commands or settings.

Recognizing this need, I wrote this book, mainly for the clinician involved in mechanical ventilation therapy, to clearly and systematically explain the operating principles, composition, required operating conditions, and major functions of positive pressure ventilator systems, regardless of brand and model. The book is based on my own knowledge, experience, and the information I have collected.

The information in this book is organized into 13 chapters. Chapters 1 through 3 lay the groundwork for understanding the ventilator system; Chapters 4 through 6 deal primarily with the 'anatomy' of a ventilator system; Chapters 7 through 10 detail how the ventilator system performs mechanical ventilation; Chapters 11 and 12 describe ventilator monitoring and alarms; and Chapter 13 tells you how to troubleshoot common ventilator problems, and how to report adverse events to authorities.

I tried to make the content easy to understand, with plain English text and plentiful graphics. Reading the chapters in sequence is recommended. It is helpful, but not required, that the reader has experience in mechanical ventilation and/or a technical background.

After reading through the entire book, you should have a clear and thorough understanding of positive pressure ventilator systems, independent of brand and model. This knowledge can help pave the way for further study of advanced features and functions.

This project was a great challenge because I did it solely in my spare time. The writing occupied over half of my weekends and holidays over the last five years, and proved difficult, because, in many cases, there was little or no reference material to be found. Some concepts I set forth are original, for instance, the concept of a ventilator system.

I would like to thank Sandy Miller for her valuable encouragement, constructive discussions, and excellent editing. I would also like to thank my wife, Zhiping, and children, Mathias and Andrea, for their understanding and patience. This book would not have seen the light of day without their support.

Yuan Lei, MD

Contents

Abbreviations

A/C	assist/control
AARC	American Association of Respiratory Care
AC	alternating current
AH	absolute humidity
ALI	acute lung injury
APRV	airway pressure release ventilation
ARDS	acute respiratory distress syndrome
ASV	adaptive support ventilation
ATC	automatic tube compensation
ATP	adenosine triphosphate
BCT	breath cycle time
BiPAP	bilevel positive airway pressure
CMV	continuous mandatory ventilation
COPD	chronic obstructive pulmonary disease
CPAP	continuous positive airways pressure
DISS	diameter indexed safety system
EPAP	expiratory positive airway pressure
ETS	expiratory trigger sensitivity
ETT	endotracheal tube
EVA	ethylene-vinyl acetate
F_iO_2	fraction of inspired oxygen
FRC	functional residual capacity
GUI	geographical user interface
Hb	haemoglobin
HFOV	high-frequency oscillatory ventilation
HFPV	high-frequency percussive ventilation
HFV	high-frequency ventilation
HIS	hospital information system
HME	heat and moisture exchanger
I:E	inspiratory:expiratory ratio
ICU	intensive care unit
IMV	intermittent mandatory ventilation
INPV	intermittent negative pressure ventilation
IPAP	inspiratory positive airway pressure
IPPV	intermittent positive pressure ventilation
IRV	inverse ratio ventilation
LCD	liquid crystal display
LED	light-emitting diode
MAP	mean airway pressure
MVexp	expiratory minute volume
NAVA	neurally adjusted ventilatory assist
NIST	non-interchangeable screw thread
NIV	non-invasive ventilation
$PaCO_2$	partial pressure of CO_2 in arterial blood
P_{alv}	alveolar pressure
P_{ao}	airway opening pressure
PaO_2	partial pressure of oxygen in arterial blood
PAO_2	partial pressure of O_2 in alveoli
PAV	proportional assist ventilation
P_{AW}	airway pressure
$P_{control}$	pressure control
PDMS	patient data management system
PEEP	positive end-expiratory pressure
$P_{et}CO_2$	partial pressure of CO_2 (end-tidal)
P_{insp}	inspiratory pressure
PIP	peak inspiratory pressure
PLV	pressure-limited ventilation
Pmean	mean airway pressure
PO_2	partial pressure of oxygen
Ppeak	peak airway pressure
P_{ramp}	pressure ramp

$P_{support}$	pressure support
PSV	pressure support ventilation
PVC	polyvinyl chloride
PvO_2	partial pressure of O_2 in venous blood
RC	time constant
RDS	respiratory distress syndrome
RH	relative humidity
SAAS	severe acute respiratory syndrome
SIMV	synchronized intermittent mandatory ventilation
SpO_2	oxygen saturation
SSRD	sudden and severe respiratory distress
T_e	expiratory time
TF	technical fault/failure
T_i	inspiratory time
TRC	tube resistance compensation
TT	tracheostomy tube
VAPS	volume-assured pressure support
V_T	tidal volume
VTE	expiratory tidal volume
VTI	inspiratory tidal volume
WOB	work of breathing
ZEEP	zero PEEP

Chapter 1

Introduction

1.1 What is mechanical ventilation?

Mechanical ventilation can be realized with one of three operating principles: *intermittent positive pressure ventilation (IPPV), intermittent negative pressure ventilation (INPV)*, and *high-frequency ventilation (HFV)*. Of these, IPPV is currently the most popular and is the basis for most commercially available ventilators. Unless otherwise noted, 'mechanical ventilation' in this book means mechanical ventilation using the IPPV principle.

Mechanical ventilation is a respiratory care therapy to treat serious respiratory failure or respiratory deficiency resulting from a wide variety of clinical causes. If performed appropriately, this therapy can temporarily and artificially support or replace seriously damaged pulmonary functions, maintaining normal or nearly normal ventilation and oxygenation. This gives the clinician time to treat primary diseases and to improve the patient's general clinical condition. If performed appropriately, mechanical ventilation is a powerful and effective life-saving tool. If performed inappropriately, however, mechanical ventilation may be equally powerful and effective in harming the ventilated patient.

A set of specialized medical equipment is essential to perform this therapy (see Box 1.1). This equipment is a *ventilator system*, which typically has six essential components: (1) compressed gas (oxygen and air) supplies, (2) an electrical power supply, (3) a ventilator, (4) a breathing circuit, (5) an artificial airway, and (6) the patient's pulmonary system. A ventilator, therefore, is just one part of a ventilator system. We will discuss the concept of the ventilator system in greater depth in Chapter 4.

Mechanical ventilation is highly risky, not only because respiration is vital for survival, but also because, with IPPV a ventilated patient breathes exclusively through a gas-tight ventilator system. If the therapy goes awry clinically or technically, the patient's safety may be immediately endangered.

Mechanical ventilation is highly complicated, because it requires a clinician to have two types of specialized expertise in addition to their knowledge and skills in general clinical medicine. The clinical outcome of this therapy depends heavily on this specialized knowledge. Thus, a clinician who is good at clinical medicine is not automatically qualified to perform mechanical ventilation.

Mechanical ventilation is labour intensive. In addition to the clinician's typical routines, mechanical ventilation requires therapy-specific work. This includes defining and modifying the therapeutic strategy, assembling and maintaining the ventilator system, checking and adjusting ventilator settings, responding to alarms and troubleshooting, managing the airway, and managing nebulization and humidification, not to mention taking care of documentation.

Mechanical ventilation is error prone. Because it is complex and labour intensive, mechanical ventilation invites human error. Errors occur far more frequently than we would like to believe; some, with very serious consequences.

Box 1.1 Primary characteristics of mechanical ventilation

1. It is a life-supporting respiratory therapy;
2. It requires a ventilator system;
3. It is powerful and effective;
4. It is highly risky;
5. It is highly complicated;
6. It is labour intensive;
7. It is error prone;
8. It is typically applied by a group of clinicians on different shifts;
9. It is extraordinarily costly;
10. It is widely applied the world over.

Typically, a patient is ventilated for a period ranging from several hours to several days, although this period can be much longer. So, several clinicians on different shifts—experts and novices alike—perform the therapy jointly. The quality of the therapy on a single patient may vary, depending on the expertise of the clinicians on duty and how well they communicate with one another.

Mechanical ventilation therapy is very expensive. To a great extent it defines the length of stay in the intensive care unit (ICU). A large-scale investigation discovered that in the US, the mean incremental cost of mechanical ventilation was $1522 per patient per day (Dasta et al., 2005). In theory, if the therapy could be shortened by even one hour for every ventilated patient, enormous savings would result.

The application of mechanical ventilation has accelerated the world over. This is particularly the case in developing countries.

1.2 What knowledge is required for mechanical ventilation?

Many hospitals are eager to perform mechanical ventilation, knowing that it is an effective life-supporting and sustaining therapy. Their directors may believe that a mere investment in first-class ventilators along with a strong medical and nursing staff and infrastructure will guarantee the therapy's success. In truth, the results may be very disappointing, if not catastrophic.

What can go wrong? Unwanted consequences can occur for a number of reasons. The primary one is that clinicians do not have adequate knowledge to perform this therapy.

What types of knowledge are required for mechanical ventilation therapy, then?

Well, to achieve the best possible outcome from mechanical ventilation, clinicians must have two types of expertise: clinical knowledge and therapy-specific knowledge (Fig. 1.1).

Obviously, any clinician involved in mechanical ventilation must be sufficiently qualified in the related branches of clinical medicine, e.g. intensive care medicine, anaesthesiology, pulmonology, intensive care nursing, and emergency medicine. Less obvious is the need for therapy-specific knowledge. Mechanical ventilation can become a nightmare for a clinician—even an excellent one—with little therapy-specific knowledge. Without this knowledge, they cannot understand what the problem is, why it occurred, and how to correct it. Even the most determined clinician cannot help the patient in trouble. Blind trials often make the situation even worse. This happened to the author, as described in the preface.

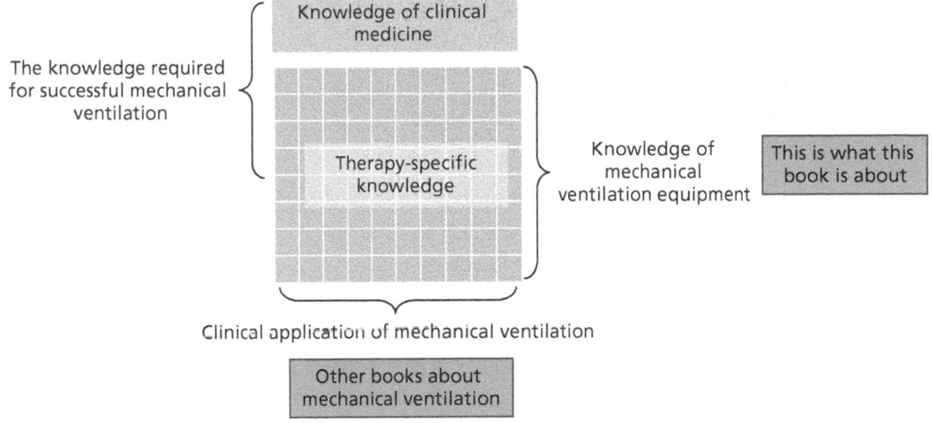

Fig. 1.1 The knowledge required for successful mechanical ventilation.

And what few may recognize is that there are two dimensions to therapy-specific knowledge. The first pertains to the *clinical application of mechanical ventilation*, while the second pertains to the required *therapeutic equipment*.

1.2.1 Dimension 1: Clinical application of mechanical ventilation

The first dimension of therapy-specific knowledge belongs to the domain of respiratory care and clinical medicine. It focuses on how to carry out this therapy correctly, effectively, and safely. It answers questions like these:

- Is mechanical ventilation necessary for this patient?
- Should the patient be ventilated invasively or noninvasively?
- Must this patient be intubated now?
- Which ventilation mode is optimal for this patient now?
- What are the optimal control settings for this patient, such as respiratory rate, tidal volume, inspiratory pressure, positive end-expiratory pressure (PEEP), and fraction of inspired oxygen (F_iO_2)?
- How can I optimize the patient-ventilator interaction?
- Is sedation necessary?
- What can I do to minimize ventilator-induced lung injury?
- How should I wean the patient from the ventilator?

Having been administered for over a half century, mechanical ventilation is a relatively mature respiratory therapy. However, it keeps evolving, and there are controversies about how best to perform it. Today a substantial body of information exists in the public domain, in the form of monographs, published articles, workshops, training courses, symposiums, and congresses, although the quality of the information from these sources varies considerably.

1.2.2 Dimension 2: The therapeutic equipment

The second dimension of therapy-specific knowledge focuses on the equipment required for mechanical ventilation, that is, the ventilator system. It answers questions like these:

- What therapeutic equipment is needed for mechanical ventilation?
- What are the essential components of a ventilator system?
- How is a ventilator system assembled?

- How is intermittent positive airway pressure generated?
- What are the required conditions for a ventilator system to function?
- How does a ventilator control delivery of inspiratory gas?
- What are the differences between volume modes, pressure modes, and adaptive modes?
- What do the various ventilator controls mean and how do they work?
- What do the ventilator monitoring parameters mean?
- What do the ventilator alarms mean and how do they work?
- How can I prevent and troubleshoot equipment problems during mechanical ventilation?
- How can I warm and humidify the inspiratory air properly?

Unlike the first dimension, the second dimension of therapy-specific knowledge has been all but ignored in mechanical ventilation education. Educational materials may touch on it, but so superficially and in such a fragmented manner that it is impossible to see the big picture.

Consequently, ventilator users may share some common yet unspoken perceptions. For instance:

- A ventilator is the equipment needed for mechanical ventilation. Other parts such as breathing circuits, artificial airways, humidifying devices, and gas and electrical supplies, are inconsequential.
- The ventilator should function properly under all possible conditions of use.
- If mechanical ventilation goes awry, the ventilator must be malfunctioning.
- Technicians are responsible for the equipment. Clinicians just need to operate it.

Do you agree with these points? Why or why not?

1.3 Why does the clinician need to know the equipment?

There are four important reasons why the clinician needs to know the equipment.

1.3.1 The functioning of the equipment is the foundation of the therapy

The clinical application of mechanical ventilation depends entirely on the functional status of the therapeutic equipment. If the equipment malfunctions, mechanical ventilation theory and strategy become merely hypothetical.

1.3.2 Clinicians need to assemble the equipment

Typically, ventilator system assembly is a clinician's task. It should include:

a. Acquiring the ventilator system components;
b. Assembling these components correctly and securely into a complete ventilator system;
c. Ensuring that all required conditions are satisfied (refer to Box 1.2);
d. Verifying the critical functions of the assembled system through pre-operational checks and calibration;
e. Maintaining the system during mechanical ventilation.

Obviously, these tasks require equipment knowledge. Otherwise, the probability of incorrect equipment preparation is high. In fact, failure to meet one or more required conditions is a common source of mechanical ventilation issues.

1.3.3 Clinicians need to understand the ventilator settings they make

By design, a ventilator system is an unintelligent machine that carries out the task (mechanical ventilation) exactly according to the operator's commands in the form of ventilator settings. Proper settings lead to good results, while improper ones lead to bad results.

Box 1.2 The prerequisites for mechanical ventilation

1. All required components are present, functioning, and compatible;
2. The components are assembled correctly and securely;
3. The electrical supply is continuous and appropriate;
4. Compressed air and oxygen supplies are continuous and appropriate;
5. The entire system is gas tight and free from occlusion;
6. The lung volume can respond to changes in applied airway pressure;
7. The operator adapts the ventilator settings to changes in the patient's clinical condition.

The ventilator operator requires equipment knowledge to understand the meaning and functions of ventilator settings, such as ventilation modes, control parameters, and alarm limits. A lack of this knowledge greatly increases the probability of errors. Inappropriate ventilator settings are a significant source of mechanical ventilation issues.

1.3.4 Clinicians need to troubleshoot the equipment

Numerous problems can occur during mechanical ventilation. We can divide their root causes roughly into three categories: those of patient or clinical origin, those of equipment origin, and those of operation origin (Fig. 1.2). Despite the very different causes, the clinical consequence of these problems is typically nonspecific respiratory distress.

The problems of each type of origin must be resolved correspondingly, that is, a clinical problem must be resolved clinically, a technical problem must be resolved technically, and an operational problem must be resolved by optimizing ventilator settings.

We require equipment knowledge to quickly and correctly identify and remove the true cause of problems that we encounter. For example, if the respiratory distress is caused by occlusion

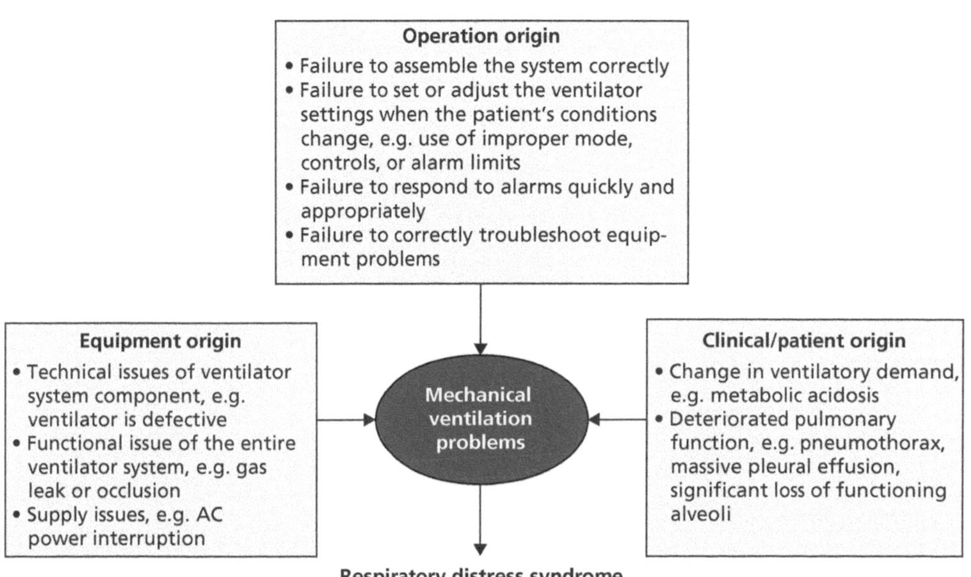

Fig. 1.2 Three major origins of mechanical ventilation problems

of the expiratory valve, an equipment function problem, then attempts to modify the ventilator settings or to sedate the patient are inappropriate.

1.4 About this book

This is not just another book on the clinical application of mechanical ventilation, but a book on the *equipment* of mechanical ventilation. The general operating principle, composition, and major functions of ventilator systems are explained in a systematic and comprehensive way. The description of the equipment applies to all *positive pressure ventilator systems*.

The book contains 13 chapters. Chapters 1 and 2 introduce the ventilator system and its basic pneumatic concepts. Chapters 3 through 5 describe the concept and composition of the ventilator system. Two special topics, humidification and in-line nebulization, are explained in Chapter 6. Chapters 7 through 10 cover various aspects of ventilation functions. Chapters 11 and 12 cover ventilator monitoring and alarms. The last chapter covers the all-important topic of troubleshooting.

The intended readers of this book include:

- Healthcare providers involved with mechanical ventilation therapy. They may be respiratory therapists, physicians, and nurses in intensive care medicine, anaesthesiology, respiratory care, pulmonology, emergency medicine, and long-term nursing stations;
- Hospital technical (biomed) staff members;
- Senior medical and nursing students;
- Research fellows involved with mechanical ventilation therapy and equipment;
- Staff members in ventilator manufacturing and distribution companies.

To facilitate its reading and understanding, the book is written in plain English and includes numerous illustrations. Having technical background and experience in mechanical ventilation is advantageous, but not required.

It is the author's sincere hope that all readers will gain practically useful equipment knowledge, making mechanical ventilation easier and better.

Reference

Dasta JF, McLaughlin TP, Mody SH, Piech CT. Daily cost of an intensive care unit day: the contribution of mechanical ventilation. *Crit Care Med* 2005: **33**; 1266–71.

Chapter 2

Basic Concepts

2.1 Introduction

Some basic concepts of *pneumatics*, a branch of physics, are required to understand the operating principle, composition, and functions of a ventilator system. These basic concepts are the common foundation of all ventilator systems, simple or sophisticated.

2.2 Pressure (P) and pressure gradient (ΔP)

pressure (P): A force exerted against resistance or a force applied uniformly over a unit area of surface. Atmospheric pressure and peak airway pressure are two typical examples.

pressure gradient (ΔP): The pressure difference between two connected areas.

Let's assume that two areas, A and B, are connected so that gas can move freely in either direction (Fig. 2.1). Gas moves only when two conditions are satisfied. First, there must be a difference between the pressures in areas A and B. The pressure gradient drives the gas to move from the area of high pressure to the area of low pressure. Second, the connection must be open.

A ventilator system has a defined gas passageway. Along the passageway, the pressure differs at different points, generating several regional pressure gradients. For a ventilator system to function properly, it is critically important to keep the pressures within their specified (normal) ranges, because ultimately these pressure gradients provide the driving forces to move gas in a controlled manner.

Fig. 2.2 shows the gas passageway and the normal pressure ranges in the Hamilton Medical GALILEO ventilator system.

Understandably, if the gas passageway has a hole anywhere, the positive internal pressure pushes the gas out.

Inspiratory pressure, peak pressure, plateau pressure, mean airway pressure, and PEEP (positive end-expiratory pressure) are common terms to describe the pressures encountered in mechanical ventilation.

Gas pressure is expressed in various units. The common ones include bars and pounds per square inch (psi) for high pressures, and millibars (mbar), centimetres of water (cmH_2O), kilopascals (kPa), and hectopascals (hPa) for low pressures. Pressure units may be converted back and forth as shown in Table 2.1.

2.3 Volume (V)

volume (V): A measure of the space occupied by an amount of gas at a given pressure level.

Tidal volume, minute volume, and leak volume are common volume-related terms used in mechanical ventilation. Gas volume is typically expressed in millilitres (ml) or litres (L or l). One litre equals 1000 millilitres.

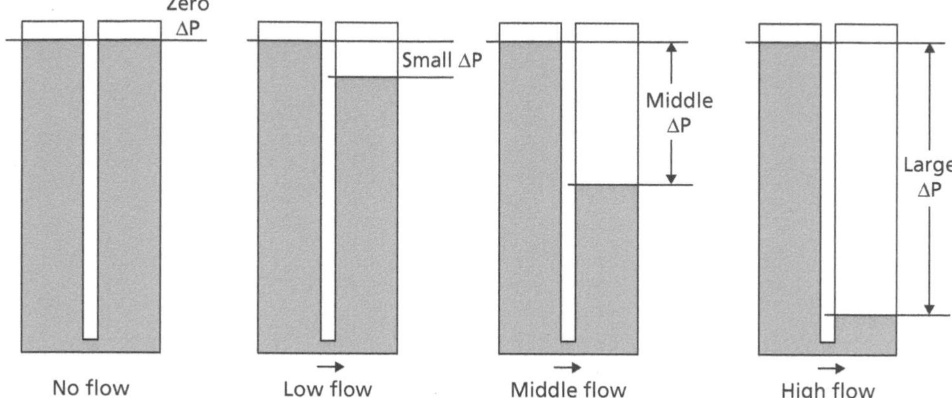

Fig. 2.1 A pressure gradient drives gas to move from an area of high pressure to an area of low pressure.

Gas is compressible. The volume of a given amount of gas decreases when the applied pressure increases, and vice versa. Therefore, a large amount of medical gas at atmospheric pressure (e.g. oxygen) may be compressed into a small gas cylinder at a very high pressure.

The pressure inside the gas passageway of a ventilator system fluctuates regularly during mechanical ventilation. In a passive patient, the circuit, airway, and alveolar pressures typically range between zero and 40 cmH_2O. The pressure variation causes corresponding gas compression. For a pressure-based mechanical breath where volume is not directly controlled, the small gas compression is not an issue. However, for a volume-based mechanical breath where the volume of delivered gas is controlled, the compression is the major cause of a phenomenon called 'lost volume', which will be described in Chapter 5.

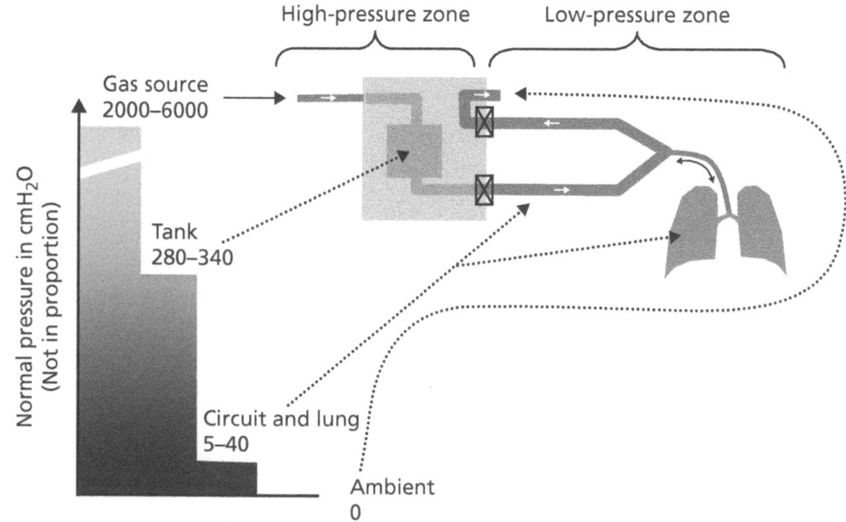

Fig. 2.2 Pressure decreases in steps along the gas passageway of the GALILEO ventilator system.

Table 2.1 Conversion of common pressure units

1 bar = 1000 mbar	
1 psi = 68.9 mbar	1 mbar = 0.0145 psi and 1 bar = 14.5 psi
1 cmH_2O = 0.98 mbar	1 mbar = 1.02 cmH_2O*
1 kPa = 10 hPa = 10 mbar	
1 hPa = 1 mbar	

*For convenience, 1 mbar is rounded to 1 cmH_2O.

2.4 **Time (t)**

time (t): The duration of a process or event.

Time is important because mechanical ventilation is essentially the regular alteration of airway pressure over time.

In the vocabulary of mechanical ventilation, you find many terms directly or indirectly related to time, including triggering, cycling, inspiratory or expiratory time, *I:E ratio*, rate, %T_i, and time constant.

Time is expressed in minutes (min), seconds (s), or milliseconds (ms).

1 hour = 60 minutes
1 minute = 60 seconds
1 second = 1000 milliseconds

2.5 **Flow**

flow ($\acute{V}$ or $\dot{V}$): The motion of *gas volume* over *time*. Flow = volume/time.

Gas moves between two connected areas when there is a pressure gradient between the two areas and the connection is open (Fig 2.3). Flow is the movement of gas over time. The consequence of flow is volume change.

Gas flow has two essential properties: direction and rate. Flow direction is determined by the pressure gradient alone. Flow rate, defined as the amount of gas that flows in a given time, is determined by both the pressure gradient and resistance encountered (refer to the next section). So, gas does not flow if there is a zero pressure gradient or if the resistance is infinite.

In mechanical ventilation, we use positive and negative values to indicate the direction of airway gas flow. Inspiratory flow, expressed in positive values, refers to the gas movement towards the patient. Expiratory flow, expressed in negative values, refers to the gas movement away from the patient.

The rate of gas flow is usually expressed in litres per minute (L/min) or millilitres per second (ml/s). One litre per minute is equal to 16.7 millilitres per second.

At a low flow rate, gas tends to move smoothly. The resultant pattern is called *laminar flow*. At a high flow rate, gas tends to move unevenly. The resultant pattern is called *turbulent flow*.

2.6 **Resistance (R)**

resistance (R): A force that tends to oppose or retard gas movement.

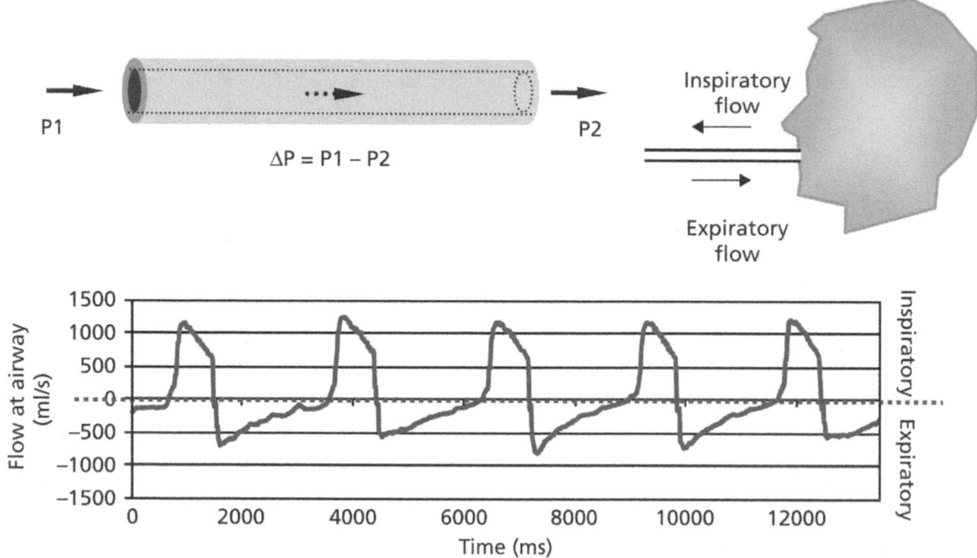

Fig. 2.3 Flow refers to gas movement, which is driven by a pressure gradient and restricted by resistance. Positive and negative values indicate the direction of airway gas flow.

Resistance is flow dependent. Whenever a gas flows through a tube, a given resistance is generated. It is usually expressed in millibars per litre per minute (mbar/L/min) or centimetres of water per litre per minute ($cmH_2O/L/min$).

The following factors determine the magnitude of resistance:

- Flow rate. The higher the flow rate, the greater the resistance, and vice versa. If the flow rate drops to zero, resistance disappears.
- Physical properties of the tube, such as length, internal diameter, inner surface, and curvature.
- Physical properties of the gas, such as density and viscosity. *Heliox* is a mixture of helium and oxygen. It is sometimes used as a supply gas in mechanical ventilation. The density of heliox is lower than that of air, which is a mixture of nitrogen and oxygen. At the same flow rate, heliox generates less resistance than air. This may be clinically beneficial in patients with abnormally high airway resistance. This fact is the foundation of heliox therapy.

The relationship between pressure gradient, flow, and resistance is described by Ohm's law. Flow equals the pressure gradient divided by resistance:

$$Flow = \Delta P/R$$

So, flow increases when the pressure gradient increases and/or resistance decreases, and vice versa.

To better understand this concept, let's take a look at some examples we see routinely in clinical practice:

- Intubation decreases the effective cross section of the airway, resulting in a higher airway resistance. A larger pressure gradient is required to achieve the same airway flow. This is particularly important for a ventilated patient who is actively breathing.

- A partial occlusion of the gas passageway results in higher resistance to gas flow. Typical examples include a kinked endotracheal tube (ETT), a bent or compressed patient circuit tube, and a blocked air filter.
- An arbitrary change in length or inner diameter of a tube causes a corresponding change in resistance.
- Asthma and bronchial spasm are well known clinical examples of excessive airway resistance.

2.7 **Compliance (C)**

compliance (C): A parameter to describe the pressure–volume relationship in a balloon-like structure.

A balloon and human lungs have the following in common: they are elastic, hollow, and gas-tight structures. Their volumes change when their internal pressures vary. Compliance is a parameter used to describe the pressure–volume relationship of such structures. A simple physical model can help our understanding (Fig 2.4).

Imagine that we have two balloons made of the same elastic material. The wall of one balloon is slightly thicker than the other. Using a T-piece equipped with a valve, we connect the two balloons to a source of high-pressure gas. In this arrangement, the pressure in both balloons always remains the same.

Now we gradually open the valve, causing gas to flow into both balloons and increasing their internal pressure. As a result, both balloons begin to expand. Not surprisingly, the balloon with the thin wall 'grows' faster than that with the thick wall.

If we measure the internal pressure and balloon volumes simultaneously and then plot the readings on a two-dimensional chart, we get two pressure–volume curves with different angles to the horizontal. The angles represent the compliances of the two balloons.

By nature, compliance is a static property, and should be measured under conditions of zero flow.

Compliance is usually expressed in millilitres per centimetre of water (ml/cmH_2O).

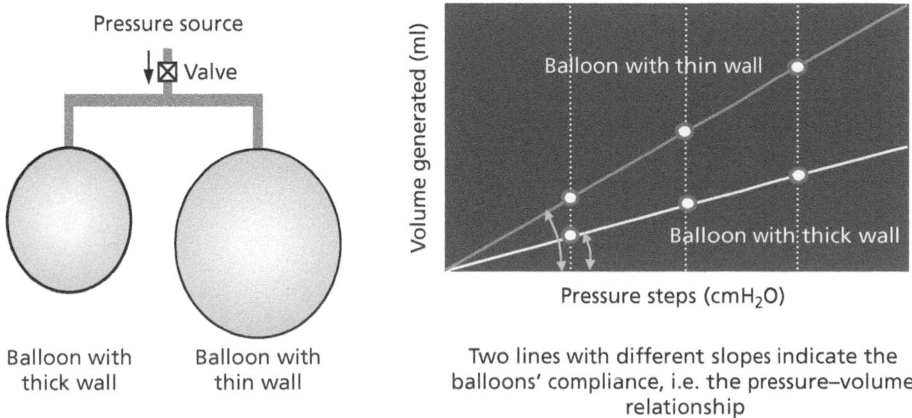

Fig. 2.4 Compliance describes the pressure–volume relationship in a balloon-like structure.

Normal respiratory compliance is approximately 150–200 ml/cmH_2O in adults and 6–8 ml/cmH_2O in newborns. This means that an increase in alveolar pressure of 1 cmH_2O causes an increase in the lung volume by 150–200 ml in an adult or 6–8 ml in a newborn. Respiratory compliance is the sum of lung compliance and chest wall compliance.

Both overly high and overly low compliances are abnormal. '*Soft lung*' refers to the situation where lung compliance is abnormally high. Even a small pressure gradient results in a sizeable lung volume change. Typical clinical examples are chronic obstructive pulmonary disease (COPD) and emphysema patients. '*Stiff lung*' refers to the situation where the lung compliance is abnormally low. Even a large pressure gradient results in a small lung volume change. Typical clinical examples are *acute respiratory distress syndrome (ARDS)*, acute lung injury (ALI), and respiratory distress syndrome (RDS) in newborns.

2.8 Time constant (RC)

time constant (RC): An estimation of the time needed to complete the process of lung inflation or deflation.

Flow is defined as the change in volume over time. It takes time to complete lung inflation or lung deflation. If the defined time is shorter than required, the process is incomplete.

If the permitted inspiratory time (T_i) in a pressure-based breath is shorter than required, the resultant tidal volume may be substantially reduced. Perhaps surprisingly, you can increase tidal volume by increasing T_i.

If the permitted expiratory time (T_e) is shorter than required, a part of the gas volume that should be expired is trapped in the lungs. This results in higher alveolar pressure at the end of

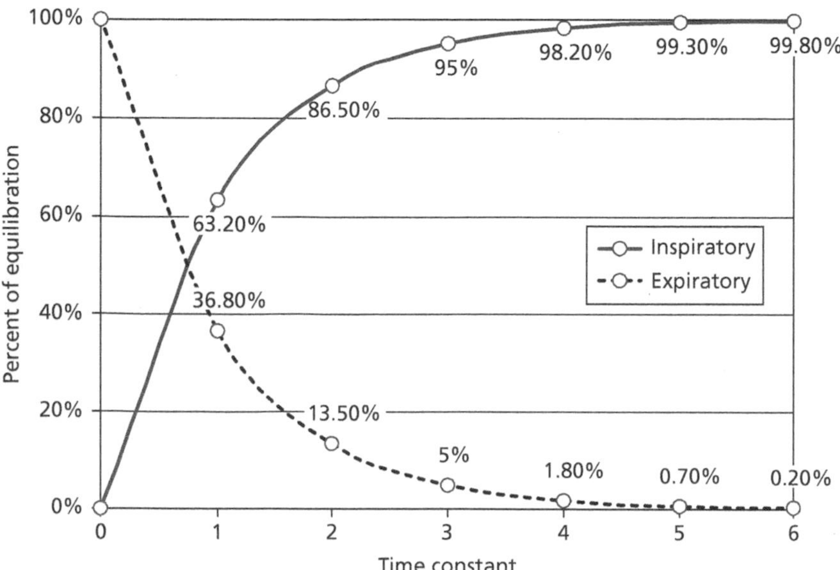

Fig. 2.5 The time constant is used to estimate the time required to complete a flow process (e.g. expiration) with the current compliance and resistance in a passive model.

expiration than would otherwise be the case. This abnormal phenomenon is called *autoPEEP* or *intrinsic PEEP*.

The length of time required to complete a volume change varies in individual patients, depending on their clinical condition. Is there any way to objectively estimate the time required to complete a volume change for a specific patient, you may wonder. Yes—the tool is the time constant. (Fig 2.5).

The *time constant* is the product of the monitored compliance (C) and resistance (R) of the respiratory system:

$$\textit{Time constant (RC)} = \textit{airway resistance (R)} \times \textit{lung compliance (C)}$$

Therefore, the time constant increases when resistance and/or compliance increases, and vice versa. In a *passive* lung model, the volume change is exponential over the course of inspiration or expiration, being highest at the beginning and then slowing down.

The time constant is expressed in seconds. In theory:

- After one time constant (1 × RC), 63% of the volume change is complete;
- After two time constants (2 × RC), 86.5% is complete;
- After three time constants (3 × RC), 95% is complete;
- After four time constants (4 × RC), 98% is complete; and
- After five time constants (5 × RC), 99% is complete.

It is generally agreed that, to be adequate, inspiratory time should be at least three inspiratory time constants long, while expiratory time should be at least three expiratory time constants long. For instance, if the estimated expiratory RC is 1 second, T_e should be at least 3 seconds.

The time constant is clinically significant, as it is how we can estimate the minimal T_i and T_e required for a given patient.

In most clinical cases, there may be sufficient room for T_i and T_e to complete lung inflation and deflation. In COPD patients, characterized by high R and high C, the time constant is often very long. To ensure complete lung inflation and deflation, we may need a low rate for a very long T_e and a corresponding large tidal volume. In this case, the acceptable ranges for the T_i and T_e settings are very limited.

Chapter 3

Lung Ventilation: Natural and Mechanical

3.1 Introduction

This chapter describes the processes of respiration and lung ventilation. It focuses on the issues directly related to mechanical ventilation, especially its pneumatic process. It touches just briefly on general respiratory anatomy and physiology; please refer to relevant text or reference books for more details.

3.2 An overview of respiration

3.2.1 Anatomy of the respiratory system

The *respiratory system* refers to the six functional parts required to complete the vital process of gas exchange: the *airway, lungs, chest wall, respiratory muscles, phrenic nerve*, and *respiratory centre*. These parts can be divided roughly into two groups: (a) the anatomic foundation for gas exchange, and (b) the driving force and regulation of that gas exchange (Fig. 3.1).

Airway

The airway, also known as the *pulmonary airway* or *respiratory tract*, refers to those parts of the respiratory system through which air flows, beginning at the nose and mouth, and ending at the alveoli (Fig. 3.2). As these names imply, the airway is the gas passageway between the atmosphere and alveoli. It is not involved in gas exchange between the alveoli and blood.

The airway consists of the *upper airway* and the *lower airway*. Typically, we think of the upper airway as including the nose, nasal cavity, mouth, pharynx, and larynx. The lower airway includes everything from the trachea to the small bronchioles.

The airway poses resistance to gas flow in both directions. Airway resistance is one of the most important properties in lung mechanics. Several respiratory diseases, such as asthma, upper airway obstruction, and bronchospasm, result from abnormally high airway resistance.

The airway normally contains a certain amount of gas, which is always an inevitable part of tidal volume. This volume is called *dead space* or *anatomical dead space* because the volume is not involved in gas exchange. We need to pay particular attention to dead space, particularly when the tidal volume is tiny.

Lungs

Humans have two *lungs* located in the rib cage. They are sponge-like organs. The *trachea* divides into two main stem *bronchi* for the respective lungs. Each main stem bronchus then branches into smaller and smaller bronchi like a tree. The tiniest branch is called a *bronchiole*. At the end of each bronchiole is a cluster of tiny air sacs called *alveoli*.

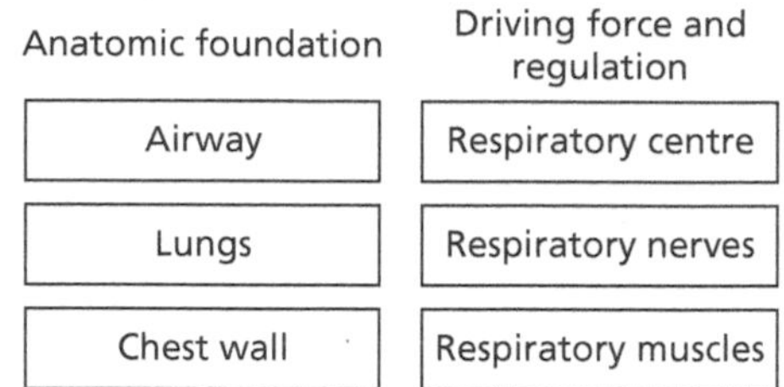

Fig. 3.1 Six key parts of the respiratory system.

Each alveolus has a mesh of tiny blood vessels called *capillaries*. The very thin walls of the alveoli and bronchioles provide a moist, extremely thin, and large surface for gas exchange to occur. The gradients of partial pressure of O_2 and CO_2 drive the gases to diffuse (Fig. 3.3). Inhaled O_2 diffuses *from* the alveoli into the capillaries, while CO_2 from the blood diffuses *into* the alveoli. The waste CO_2 in the alveoli is then expired through lung ventilation.

Because energy demand for all living cells and tissues is continuous, respiration must also be continuous. For an individual cell as well as for the whole body, death is inevitable if respiration stops for a certain length of time.

The lungs and the chest wall are elastic. During quiet breathing, inspiration is an active process, meaning that contraction of respiratory muscles, especially the diaphragm, causes the total lung volume to increase from when the lungs were in their resting position. Expiration is normally a passive process, meaning that the inspiratory muscles relax, and the loaded *elastic recoil force* of the chest wall and lungs brings the lungs back to their resting position. This is similar to a stretched rubber band retracting when the applied force is removed. The elasticity of the lungs and chest wall is the basis of *lung compliance*, which is another key property of respiratory

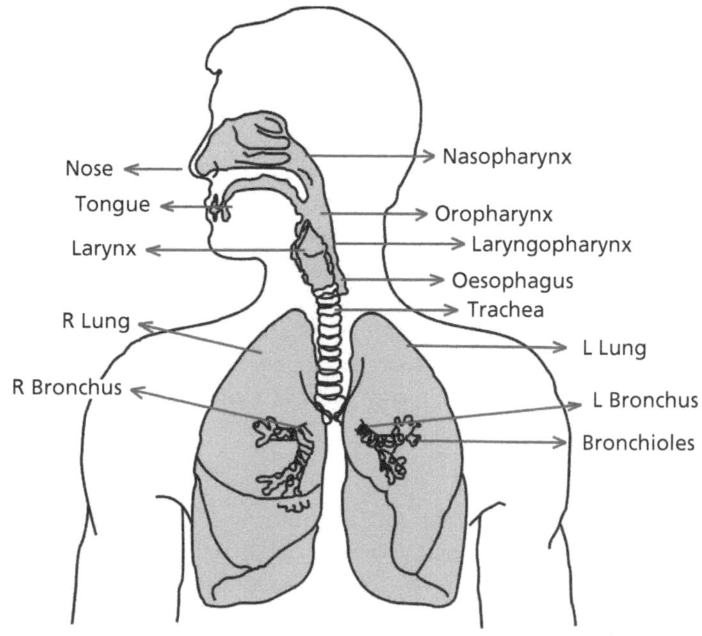

Fig. 3.2 Airway and the lungs.

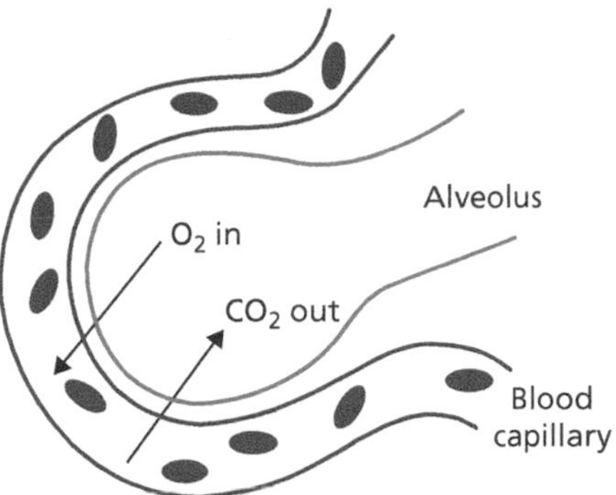

Fig. 3.3 Gas exchange at alveolar wall.

mechanics. The elasticity may be higher than normal (causing 'stiff lungs', as in patients with acute respiratory distress syndrome (ARDS)), or lower than normal (causing 'soft lungs', as in patients with chronic obstructive pulmonary disease (COPD)). In the case of pneumothorax, the elasticity causes the affected lung to collapse partially or completely.

The effectiveness of alveolar gas exchange is determined by: (a) the total area and thickness of the diffusion membrane, (b) alveolar ventilation, and (c) pulmonary capillary circulation. We will discuss these further in section 3.2.2.

Chest wall

The *chest* or *thorax* is a part of the human trunk between the neck and the abdomen (Fig. 3.4). The chest wall is made up of bones and muscles. The bones (primarily ribs, sternum, and vertebrae) form a protective cage for the internal structures of the thorax. The main muscles of the chest wall are the *external and internal intercostals.* The contraction of external intercostals enlarge the thoracic cavity by drawing the ribs together and elevating the rib cage, while the internal intercostals decrease the dimensions of the thoracic cavity.

There are three subdivisions inside the thorax. The two lateral subdivisions hold the lungs. Between the lungs is the *mediastinum*, which contains the heart, the great vessels, parts of the trachea and oesophagus, and other structures.

The lung surface and the inner wall of the chest cage are actually not attached directly to each other. Instead, the lung literally floats in the thoracic cavity, surrounded by a very thin layer

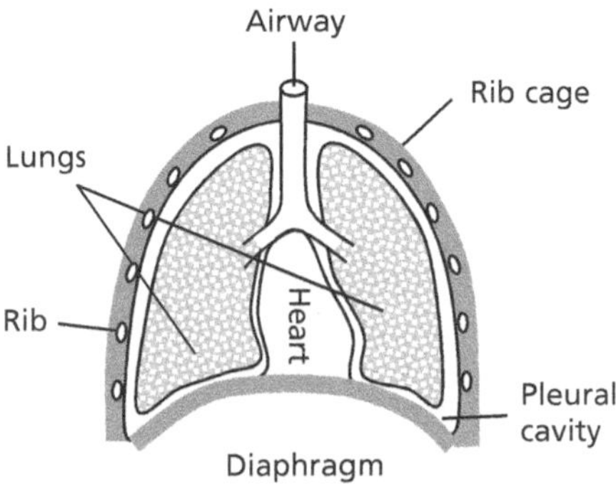

Fig. 3.4 Anatomic structure of the chest wall and the organs inside.

of pleural fluid. This potential space is called the *pleural cavity*. The cavity normally contains a small amount of serous liquid for lubrication of lung movement during breathing. Although normally the pleural cavity is a potential space, under abnormal conditions it can contain a large amount of air (pneumothorax) or liquid (pleural effusion). If so, the affected lung collapses partially or totally, preventing it from performing its function.

The thorax contains several vital soft organs, including the heart, lungs, and large blood vessels. A high positive end-expiratory pressure (PEEP) to expand the lungs compresses the neighbouring organs, and disturbs haemodynamics to a certain extent.

As we mentioned earlier, lung compliance is a key property of a pulmonary system. It is the measurement of elasticity of the lungs and chest wall together. Sometimes *respiratory compliance* is used to indicate the total or sum of lung compliance and chest wall compliance.

The chest and abdomen are separated by the soft *diaphragm*, which permits thoracic pressure to be easily transmitted to the abdomen, and vice versa. For this reason, a high PEEP can lead to high abdominal tension. On the other hand, a high abdominal tension can decrease respiratory compliance.

Respiratory muscles

The contraction and relaxation of respiratory muscles increases or decreases the volume of the thoracic cavity, resulting in corresponding changes in alveolar pressure. Air is sucked into the lungs when alveolar pressure is lower than ambient pressure. Gas is pushed out of the lungs when alveolar pressure is higher than ambient pressure.

During inspiration The principal muscles involved in inspiration are the diaphragm and the external intercostal muscles. The thoracic cavity is enlarged in two ways: (a) contraction of the diaphragm increases the vertical dimensions of the thoracic cavity, or (b) contraction of the external intercostal muscle increases the width of the thoracic cavity. During intensive breathing, accessory respiratory muscles also participate in inspiration. Typical accessory muscles are the sternocleidomastoid and the scalene muscles.

During expiration During peaceful breathing, expiration is a passive process. When the inspiratory muscles relax, the elastic recoil force of lungs and chest wall brings the lung volume to its resting position, generating a positive alveolar pressure. The resultant pressure gradient pushes out a certain amount of the gas inside the lungs. When expiration is active, the abdominal muscles and the internal and innermost intercostal muscles help expel the gas.

Alternating contraction and relaxation of respiratory muscles provide the ultimate driving force for lung ventilation. If the muscle activities are weakened or suppressed by disease, fatigue, general anaesthesia, or trauma, lung ventilation deteriorates. In this case, mechanical ventilation is indicated.

The activation of accessory respiratory muscles is a strong indication of respiratory distress or 'air hunger'.

Respiratory nerves

The diaphragm is innervated by the left and right phrenic nerves, which arise from the cervical spinal cord (C3–C5) in humans. Innervation of respiratory intercostal and abdominal muscles comes from the thoracolumbar spinal cord, T1–T11 and T7–L2, respectively.

Drawing on this fact, Swedish ventilator manufacturer Maquet developed a technical feature called NAVA (neurally adjusted ventilatory assist). Neurally adjusted ventilatory assist uses a special catheter *sensor* positioned at the lower oesophagus to detect phrenic nerve impulses. The detected signals in turn are used to guide the ventilator operation.

Spinal cord injury at C4 or higher can disrupt nerve impulses from the brain to the phrenic nerve. Such injuries can paralyse the diaphragm, requiring the injured person to be on a ventilator. A spinal cord injury below C5 does not involve the phrenic nerve; thus, a person with such an injury can still breathe despite possible paralysis of the lower limbs.

Respiratory centre

The *respiratory centre* refers to a group of nerve cells in the medulla oblongata and pons of the brain that: (a) receive sensory signals about the level of O_2, CO_2, and pH in the blood and cerebrospinal fluid; (b) determine whether and how to change the breathing pattern; and (c) send the signals to the respiratory muscles to execute this change in breathing pattern.

The functioning of the respiratory centre is critical to proper respiration. In most ventilated patients, the respiratory centre is intact, that is, an active patient has a normal respiratory response to changes in blood O_2, CO_2, and pH. A normal respiratory centre is required for several newer ventilator features, such as the proportional assist ventilation (PAV) mode, *tube resistance compensation* (TRC, or automatic tube compensation (ATC)), and NAVA. Nevertheless, the respiratory centre may not function properly in neurological or neurosurgical patients.

3.2.2 Physiology of respiration

Two essential questions about respiration

Why is respiration necessary? All living cells need an energy supply to survive and execute their physiological functions. Energy is produced in the cells through the biochemical process of metabolism (Fig. 3.5). The metabolic chemical process consumes oxygen (O_2) and glucose, and produces water, carbon dioxide (CO_2), and adenosine triphosphate (ATP), which is the major 'currency' of energy in the body.

Metabolism is a continuous process, continuously consuming O_2 and producing CO_2. To keep local O_2 and CO_2 concentrations within proper ranges, new O_2 must be continuously brought to the cells and the waste CO_2 removed. This is the task of respiration.

What is respiration? In short, respiration is the process of transporting O_2 from atmospheric air to the cells within tissues, and transporting CO_2 from the cells to the air. In general, respiration has three major parts: gas exchange in the lungs, blood circulation, and gas exchange in tissues and cells (Fig. 3.6).

Oxygen and CO_2 are transported in blood as it circulates. If the blood supply to a tissue is drastically reduced or even stopped, the local O_2 concentration falls, and the CO_2 concentration rises rapidly. The tissue will die if the normal blood supply does not resume quickly. A typical example is a heart infarct.

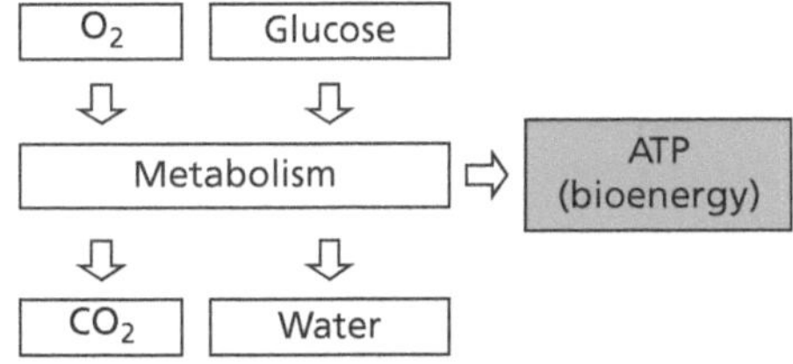

Fig. 3.5 Diagram of metabolic process.

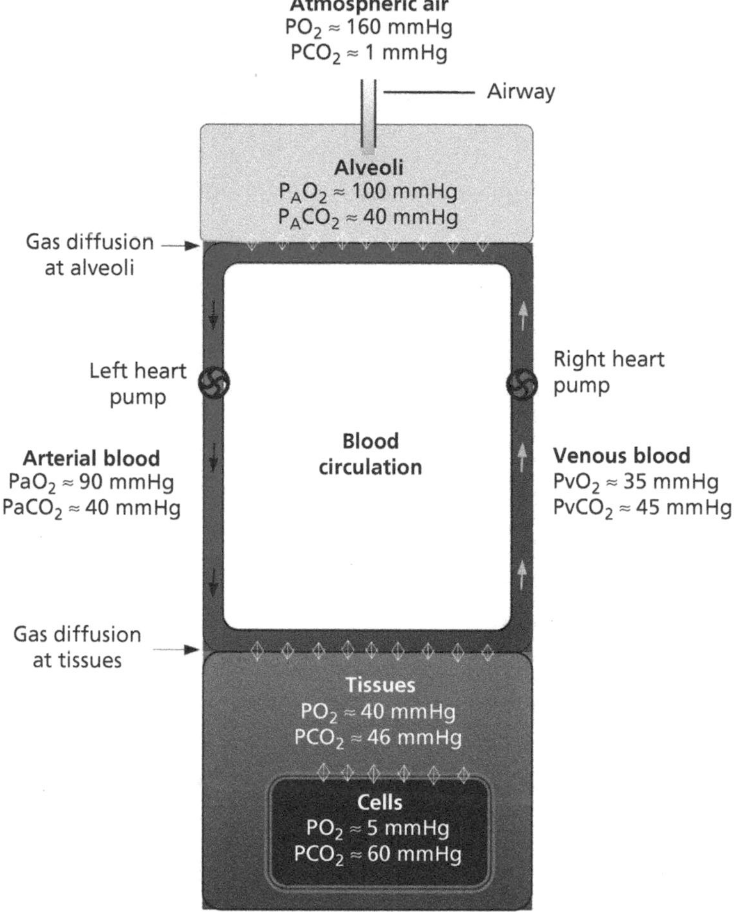

Fig. 3.6 Diagram of the entire respiration process.

Gas transport

Oxygen and CO_2 are transported in three ways: (1) gas diffusion, (2) lung ventilation, and (3) blood circulation.

Gas diffusion *Gas diffusion* is a natural process in which gas molecules move from an area of high concentration to a neighbouring area of low concentration. The two areas share a common diffusion membrane. Such gas diffusion takes place mainly in three areas: (a) alveolar walls, (b) blood capillary walls, and (c) tissues and cell membranes.

The speed of gas diffusion depends on: (a) the difference in gas molecular concentrations, (b) properties of the diffusion membrane, including its total area and thickness, and (c) the solubility and molecular weight of the gas involved. Carbon dioxide diffuses 20 times as fast as O_2.

Blood transport of O_2 and CO_2 Oxygen is transported in two ways within the blood. *Red blood cells* or *erythrocytes* carry 97% of all O_2 molecules in chemical combination with haemoglobin. The remaining 3% are dissolved in plasma.

Haemoglobin (Hb), a globular protein, is the primary vehicle for O_2 transport in blood. At the alveolar capillary where the O_2 concentration is high, O_2 binds readily to the haemoglobin

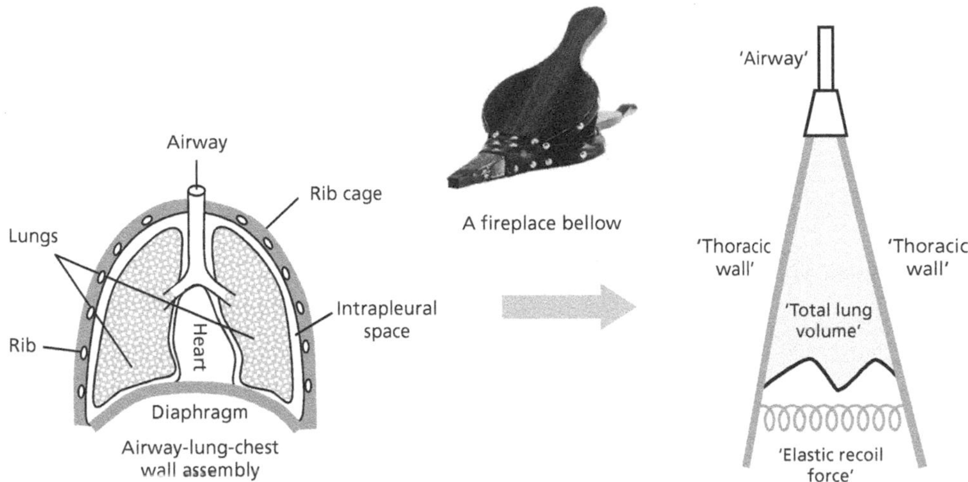

Fig. 3.7 The airway-lung-chest wall assembly can be mimicked by modified fireplace bellows.

present. At tissue blood capillaries where the O_2 concentration is low, the haemoglobin releases the O_2 into the tissue. The oxygen-haemoglobin dissociation curve is used to express the relationship between the O_2 concentration and whether the haemoglobin is acquiring or releasing O_2 molecules.

CO_2 is transported in blood in three ways. Most CO_2 molecules are transported in the form of bicarbonate ions (HCO_3-), about 10% are bound to haemoglobin and plasma proteins, and the remaining 5% are dissolved in plasma.

Lung ventilation *Lung ventilation* is an essential part of respiration, responsible for the gas exchange between alveoli and the atmospheric air. It involves regularly replacing stale gases in the lungs with fresh gases from the atmosphere.

A simple physical model can help us better understand lung ventilation (Fig. 3.7). A suitable one is a modified pair of fireplace bellows with 'extendable thoracic walls,' an 'airway,' and a 'total lung volume.' A spring is added between the two handles of the bellow to mimic 'elastic recoil force'. Another modification is that the model does not have a one-way valve, so the air enters and exits exclusively through the nozzle.

The respiratory system always has two opposite forces, one for lung expansion and the other for lung retraction. The lung volume is determined by the balance of the two forces. The lungs are inflated if the expansion force is greater than the retraction force, and they are deflated if the opposite occurs. The lung volume is unchanged if both forces are equal. At the end of expiration, the lung volume is stable at the resting position. This volume is called the *functional residual capacity (FRC)* (Fig. 3.8). FRC is critical for alveolar gas exchange.

During natural inspiration, the contraction of respiratory muscles (mainly the diaphragm) increases the chest volume, generating a temporary negative *alveolar pressure* (P_{alv}). Air is sucked into the lungs, and is mixed with the gases present there. This inhaled gas volume is called the *inspiratory tidal volume*. During inspiration the elastic recoil force (shown as the stretched spring) is loaded.

During expiration, the respiratory muscles relax, and the elastic recoil force pulls the chest and lungs back to their resting position, generating a temporary positive P_{alv}. A certain amount of gas is pushed out of the lungs. This expelled gas volume is called *expiratory tidal volume*.

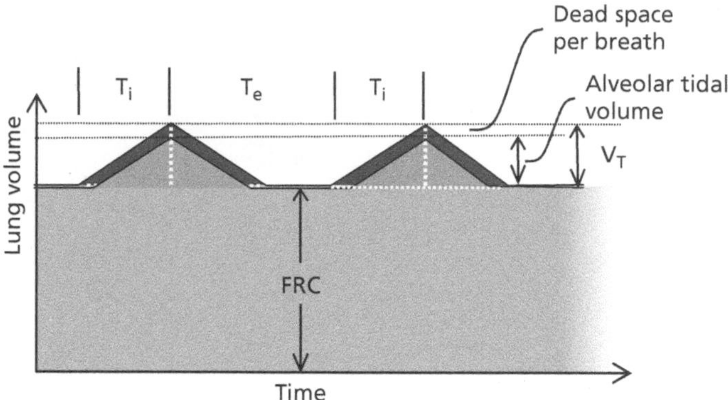

Fig. 3.8 Functional residual capacity (FRC), tidal volume, and dead space.
T_e: expiratory time: T_i; inspiratory time: V_T; tidal volume.

A breath must include both an inspiratory action and an expiratory action. Inspiratory and expiratory tidal volumes are roughly equal.

The tidal volume of every breath contains two parts. The part that participates in alveolar gas exchange is *alveolar tidal volume*. The other part that does not participate in the gas exchange is *(anatomical) dead space*. Dead space volume is always moved in or out first.

Dead space is inevitable. Do not forget it when setting and interpreting tidal volume or minute volume. During mechanical ventilation, the dead space usually increases due to the presence of the artificial airway. The effective alveolar ventilation is determined by the difference between the tidal volume and the total dead space. If the tidal volume is very close to, or equal to, the dead space volume, the alveolar ventilation is (nearly) zero, i.e. CO_2 removal is (nearly) zero. This unwanted situation is known as *dead space ventilation*.

Note that after every breath, only a part of the alveolar gas is replaced.

In addition to defining ventilation in terms of a single breath, we can also define it over a minute interval (Fig. 3.9). When we talk about *minute ventilation* or *minute volume*, we need to define a few common respiratory terms:

- *Respiratory rate*: The number of breaths occurring per minute;
- *Minute volume*: The sum of the tidal volume (inspiratory or expiratory) of all breaths occurring per minute;

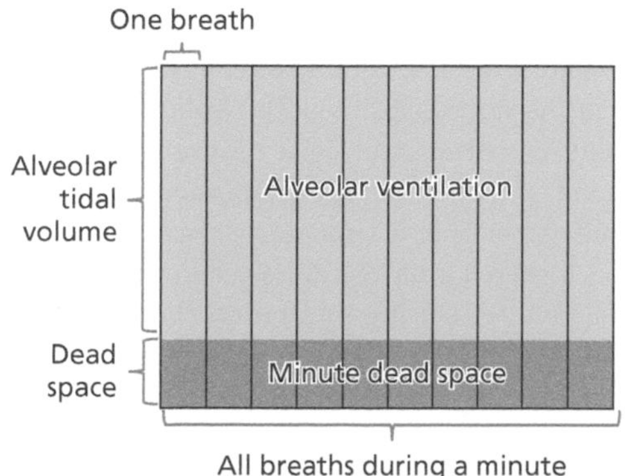

Fig. 3.9 The relationship between minute volume, tidal volume, rate, and dead space.

- *Alveolar ventilation:* The sum of the alveolar tidal volume (inspiratory or expiratory) of all breaths occurring per minute.

The relationship can be expressed with a simple equation:

$$Alveolar\ minute\ volume = Rate \times (Tidal\ volume - Dead\ space)$$

Regulation of respiration Even under normal conditions, a human's energy demand varies widely. Think about how much energy you need during sleep compared to during physical exercise. Biochemically these activities differ greatly in metabolic rate, O_2 consumption, and *CO_2 production*. There is no such thing as a normal value for energy demand.

On the other hand, it is physiologically important to maintain the arterial partial pressure of oxygen and carbon dioxide (PaO_2, $PaCO_2$), and pH within relatively narrow normal ranges even when energy demand changes. This is achieved through a control mechanism that automatically and precisely adapts the breathing pattern (i.e. rate and depth of breathing) to the current levels of PaO_2, $PaCO_2$, and pH. To a limited extent, we can freely change our breathing pattern.

This control mechanism uses a three-part sequence:

a. Central and peripheral chemoreceptors detect the current O_2, CO_2, and pH in the blood and cerebrospinal fluid.
b. The controller (respiratory centre) at the medulla and pons receives signals from the receptors, decides how to respond, and then sends the instruction to the effectors.
c. The effectors (respiratory muscles) execute the commands received.

The mechanism responds to changes in $PaCO_2$, PaO_2, and arterial pH. Of these, $PaCO_2$ is the primary stimulant. As Fig. 3.10 shows, increased $PaCO_2$ results in sharply increased alveolar ventilation, and vice versa. In this manner, all three stimulants are normally maintained within their normal ranges even when O_2 consumption and/or CO_2 production changes drastically.

In most ventilated patients, this respiratory control mechanism remains intact. The mechanism plays a key role in respiratory distress syndrome, patient-ventilator asynchrony, and weaning. It may be abnormal in some neurological and neurosurgical patients.

3.2.3 Respiratory failure

In summary, respiration is a mechanism to maintain PaO_2 and $PaCO_2$ within their normal ranges even when energy demand fluctuates.

Respiratory failure refers to the syndrome where the respiratory system fails to maintain PaO_2 or $PaCO_2$ within normal ranges, that is PaO_2 = 80–100 mmHg and $PaCO_2$ = 35–45 mmHg (Table 3.1). Respiratory failure can occur due to severe functional impairment of the airway, lungs, chest wall, respiratory centre, respiratory nerves, and respiratory muscles for a variety of clinical reasons.

At this point, it is necessary to introduce two key terms. *Hypoxia* means that PaO_2 is below 80 mmHg, while *hypercapnia* means that $PaCO_2$ is above 45 mmHg.

Respiratory failure can be classified roughly into two types, type 1 and type 2.

Type 1 respiratory failure is also known as *hypoxic respiratory failure* or *lung failure.* Its primary feature is abnormally low PaO_2 (<60 mmHg) but nearly normal $PaCO_2$. Type 1 respiratory failure is typically caused by inadequate oxygenation when blood passes through the lungs due to: (a) ventilation/perfusion mismatch, (b) arteriovenous shunt, or (c) gas diffusion impairment.

Type 2 respiratory failure is also known as *hypercapnic respiratory failure* or *pump failure.* Its primary feature is abnormally high $PaCO_2$ (>50 mmHg) and abnormally low PaO_2 (<60 mmHg). Type 2 respiratory failure is typically caused by inadequate lung ventilation due to: (a) excessive

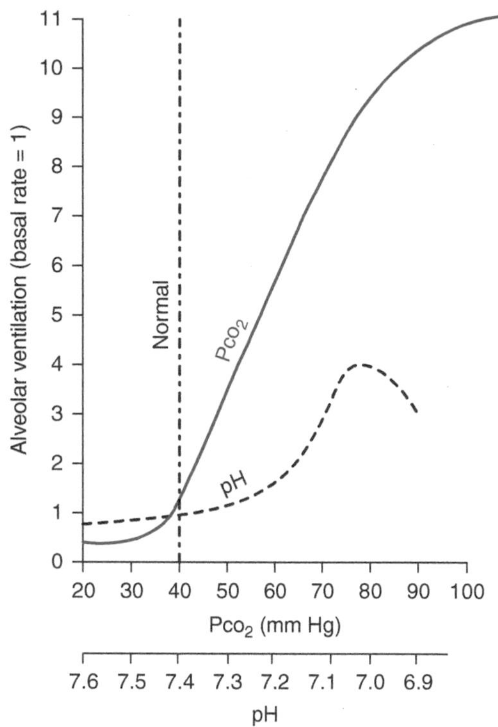

Fig. 3.10 Effect of increased arterial PCO_2 and decreased arterial pH on the rate of alveolar ventilation.

Reprinted with permission from *Textbook of Medical Physiology*, 8th edition, Guyton A.C., p447. Copyright (1990) with permission from Harcourt College Publishers and Elsevier Inc.

airway resistance, (b) decreased respiratory drive, (c) respiratory muscle fatigue or failure, or (d) abnormal status of the lungs and chest wall.

The clinical signs of respiratory failure include tachypnoea, tachycardia, cyanosis, sweating, intercostal retractions, grunting, and nose flaring. Pulse oximetry and blood gas analysis can help diagnose respiratory failure. Note that these clinical signs are non-specific.

For simplicity, we can think of the pathophysiologic process of respiratory failure as having several steps (Fig. 3.11):

a. The underlying diseases lead to deterioration in the efficiency and effectiveness of respiratory function.
b. PaO_2 tends to decrease and/or $PaCO_2$ tends to increase.

Table 3.1 Definition of normal and abnormal pH, PaO_2, and $PaCO_2$

Below normal	Normal ranges	Above normal
pH < 7.35 Acidosis	pH 7.35–7.45	pH > 7.45 Alkalosis
PaO_2 < 80 mmHg Hypoxaemia	PaO_2 80–100 mmHg	PaO_2 > 100 mmHg Hyperoxaemia
$PaCO_2$ < 35 mmHg Hypocapnia	$PaCO_2$ 35–45 mmHg	$PaCO_2$ > 45 mmHg Hypercapnia

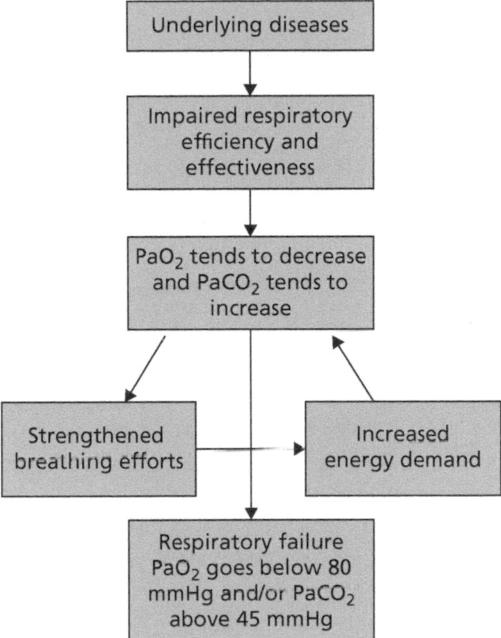

Fig. 3.11 Respiratory failure is a downward spiral.

c. The patient strengthens their breathing efforts with the intention to maintain normal PaO_2 and/or $PaCO_2$.
d. Increased breathing efforts further increase the energy demand.

If the patient can maintain normal PaO_2 and $PaCO_2$ with these intensified breathing efforts, the compensation is successful. If not, however, respiratory failure is inevitable.

Depending on the underlying diseases, both types of respiratory failure can be acute, with symptoms occurring rapidly; as in near drowning, asthma attack, respiratory arrest, drug overdose, upper airway obstruction, or chest and lung injury. Respiratory failure can also be progressive (chronic), as in emphysema, chronic bronchitis, or neuromuscular disease. For purposes of clinical treatment, it is important to differentiate between types 1 and 2, as shown in Table 3.2.

The treatment of respiratory failure typically involves: (a) oxygen therapy, (b) ventilatory support with a ventilator system or a continuous positive airway pressure (CPAP) system, (c) treatment of the underlying cause, and (d) other supporting measures, such as administration of fluids and nutrition. Acute respiratory failure is usually treated in an intensive care unit, while chronic respiratory failure is usually treated at home or in a long-term care facility.

3.3 **Mechanical ventilation**

3.3.1 **What is mechanical ventilation?**

Today, mechanical ventilation is the principal therapy used to treat severe respiratory failure caused by a serious disease or injury of any of the six key parts of respiratory system (i.e. the lungs, chest wall, airway, respiratory centre, respiratory nerves, and respiratory muscles).

If applied appropriately, this therapy effectively assists, supports, or replaces compromised natural lung ventilation, artificially satisfying the vital demands of respiration. This gives the clinician valuable time to treat the underlying diseases and improve the general condition of the patient.

Table 3.2 Summary of respiratory failure

Classification	Type 1 respiratory failure	Type 2 respiratory failure
Other names	◆ Hypoxic respiratory failure ◆ Lung failure	◆ Hypercapnic respiratory failure ◆ Pump failure
Main feature	Hypoxia and normal $PaCO_2$	Hypercapnia and hypoxia
Typical causes	◆ Ventilation/perfusion mismatch ◆ Arteriovenous shunt ◆ Gas diffusion impairment	◆ Excessive airway resistance ◆ Decreased ventilator drive ◆ Respiratory muscle fatigue or failure ◆ Abnormal status of the lungs and chest wall

In most cases, mechanical ventilation therapy is temporary, lasting several hours, days, or weeks. The therapy should be terminated as soon as the patient can breathe adequately on their own. The only exception is the patient with permanently damaged pulmonary function, who may be ventilator dependent for their entire life.

Is there a limit to what mechanical ventilation can accomplish?

This is a critical but seldom asked question. The answer is yes. Mechanical ventilation depends entirely on the residual functioning of the patient's injured lungs. When the functionality of a patient's lungs falls below a certain threshold, mechanical ventilation cannot help. In this case, *ECMO (extracorporeal membrane oxygenation)* should be used.

3.3.2 Three operating principles

As we noted in Chapter 1, mechanical ventilation can be realized with one of three principles: intermittent positive pressure ventilation (IPPV), intermittent negative pressure ventilation (INPV), and high-frequency ventilation (HFV). Let's take a close look at each of these operating principles.

Intermittent positive pressure ventilation (IPPV)

With the IPPV principle, the patient's respiratory system is integrated into the ventilator system. A positive pressure is applied intermittently to the patient's airway. When the airway pressure is temporarily higher than the alveolar pressure, fresh gas is pushed into the lungs, the process of *inspiration*. When the airway pressure is lower than alveolar pressure, the gas is expelled out of the lungs, the process of *expiration*. Both inspiration and expiration are regulated by the operator's settings. Fig. 3.12 shows a typical pressure waveform in IPPV.

IPPV is the common principle of most modern ventilators, whether invasive or non-invasive. Some popular IPPV ventilator models are shown in Fig 3.13.

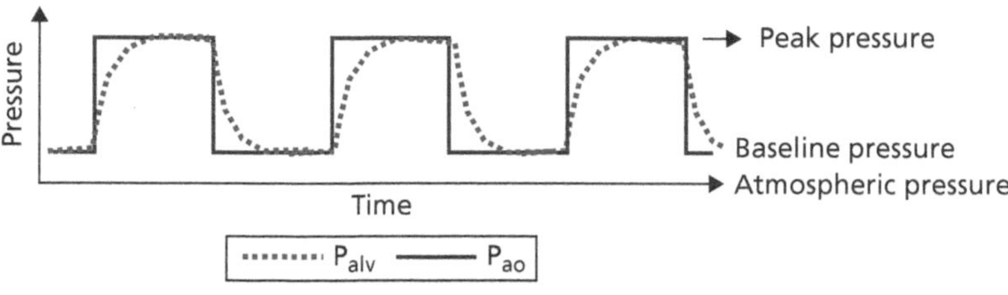

Fig. 3.12 Pressure waveform in intermittent positive pressure ventilation (IPPV).

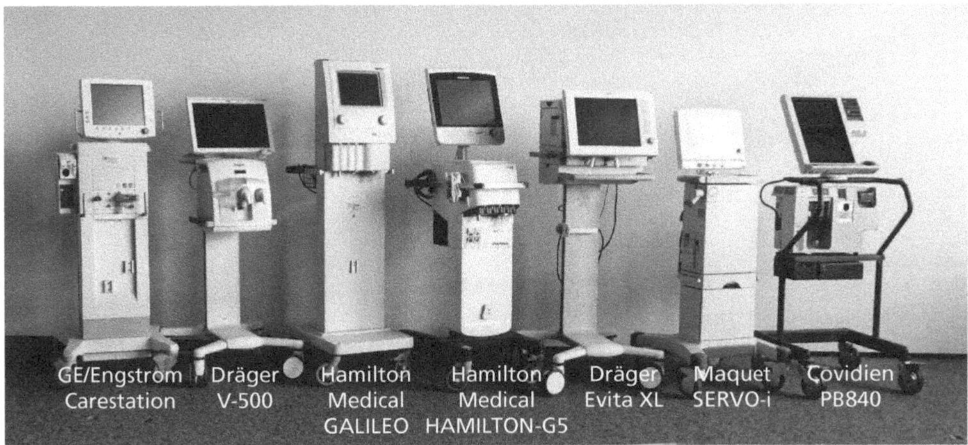

Fig. 3.13 Some popular ICU ventilators based on the intermittent positive pressure ventilation (IPPV) principle.

Intermittent negative pressure ventilation (INPV)

With the INPV principle, the ventilated patient's mouth and nose are open to the atmosphere so that gas can move in or out when alveolar pressure changes relative to atmospheric pressure. During inspiration, a negative pressure is applied to the surface of the chest wall, temporarily reducing the alveolar pressure. Fresh air is now sucked into the lungs. During expiration, the applied negative pressure is removed. The elastic recoil force temporarily generates a positive alveolar pressure, squeezing the stale gas out of the lungs. The driving pressure changes opposite to the way it does in IPPV. Fig. 3.14 shows a typical pressure waveform in INPV.

Two common ventilator designs are based on INPV (Fig. 3.15). The first is the famous *iron lung*, where a patient's body, except for the head, is placed in a sealed gas container with rigid walls. A negative pressure is generated intermittently inside the container, resulting in inspiration and expiration. Different variations of the iron lung were developed during the 1920s and 1930s. They were used widely during the polio outbreaks in the 1940s and 1950s. The second type is the cuirass ventilator, in which a rigid shell or cuirass fits over the thoracic area only. An intermittent negative pressure is applied locally to change the thoracic volume.

Today, INPV ventilators are used primarily for non-invasive ventilatory assistance.

High-frequency ventilation (HFV)

Both IPPV and INPV are regarded as 'conventional', because the tidal volume and respiratory rate are similar to physiological ones.

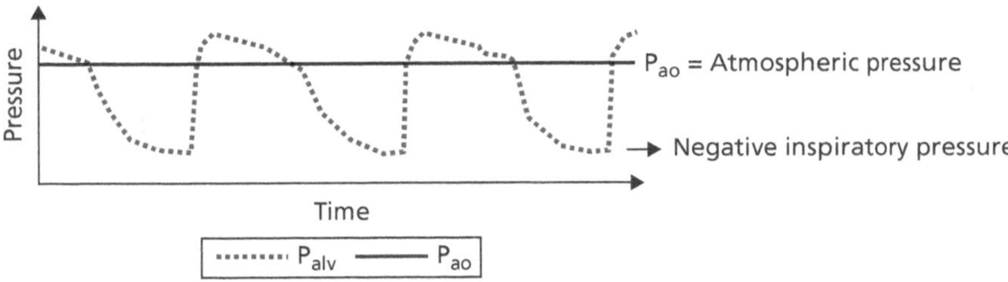

Fig. 3.14 Pressure waveform in intermittent negative pressure ventilation (INPV).

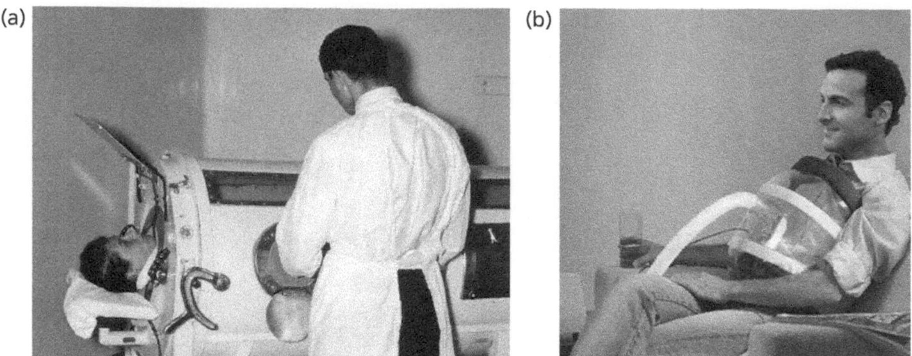

Fig. 3.15 a) An iron lung, b) A cuirass ventilator.
(a) Poumon artificiel, Wikimedia Commons, accessed 6 October 2016, https://commons.wikimedia.org/wiki/File:Poumon_artificiel.jpg This image is in the public domain and thus free of any copyright restrictions. This media comes from the Centers for Disease Control and Prevention's Public Health Image Library.

The third principle of mechanical ventilation is high-frequency ventilation. HFV uses a much higher respiratory rate (150 b/min or higher) than we see with the other types (Fig. 3.16). The tidal volume is much smaller than the physiological range, often smaller than dead space.

The mechanisms of gas transport and exchange in HFV are very different from IPPV and INPV, and are not well understood.

Due to the differences in deployed technologies, respiratory rate, ranges of pressure swings, and baseline pressure, HFV has evolved into five forms: (a) *high-frequency positive pressure ventilation (HFPPV)*, (b) *high-frequency jet ventilation (HFJV)*, (c) *high-frequency flow interruption (HFFI)*, (d) *high-frequency percussive ventilation (HFPV)*, and (e) *high-frequency oscillatory ventilation (HFOV)*. HFJV and HFOV are the commonly used forms.

Clinically HFV is often applied in neonates. Sometimes it is also used to treat patients with ARDS, especially those who require very high positive airway pressures. HFV can be combined with conventional IPPV as well as surfactant therapy. Fig. 3.17 shows a typical high-frequency ventilator.

Of all the three principles, IPPV currently dominates. Unless otherwise specified, the term 'mechanical ventilator' in this book refers to a ventilator based on the IPPV principle.

3.3.3 IPPV pneumatic process

To recap, the objective of mechanical ventilation is to restore or maintain adequate lung ventilation by using artificial means to intermittently change lung volume. Mechanical ventilation requires a ventilator system, which will be described in depth in Chapters 4 and 5.

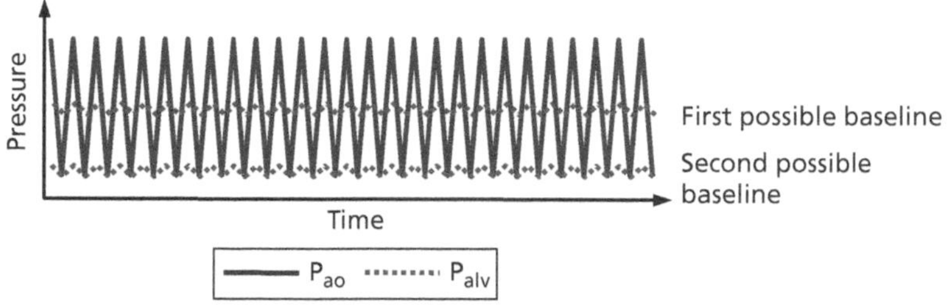

Fig. 3.16 During high-frequency ventilation (HFV), positive pressure or positive-negative pressure is applied to the airway opening at a very high rate.

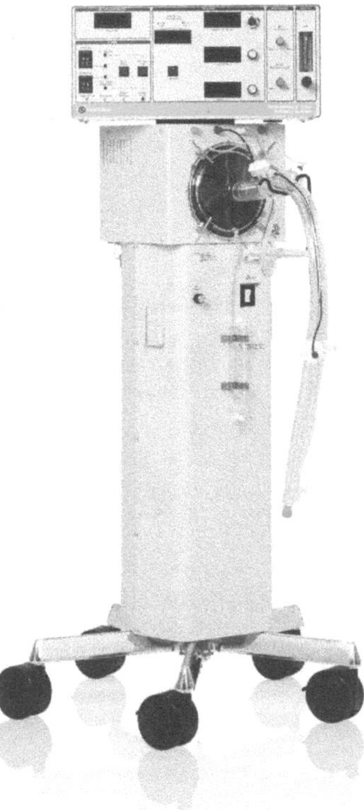

Fig. 3.17 3000A high-frequency oscillatory ventilator from CareFusion.
Image of 3100A Ventilator © 2014, CareFusion Corporation; Used with permission.

Pneumatically, a ventilator system can be regarded as having two pressure areas connected by an airway (Fig. 3.18). The pressure on the device side is called the airway opening pressure (P_{ao}), and the pressure on the lung side is called the alveolar pressure (P_{alv}). Both P_{ao} and P_{alv} fluctuate regularly during mechanical ventilation. If the ventilated patient is passive, P_{ao} is actively changed, while P_{alv} follows. If the patient is active, both P_{ao} and P_{alv} can change actively.

It is necessary to mention that a patient's lungs are a dead-end structure. During inspiration, alveolar pressure rises as more and more gas enters the lungs. In a pressure-based breath, *inspiratory flow* drops to zero if P_{ao} and P_{alv} are equal at any level.

Under normal conditions of mechanical ventilation, at any time point P_{ao}, P_{alv}, and lung volume are determined by these forces (Fig. 3.19):

- The inherent force to keep the lungs open, including that contributed by the chest wall, pleural negative pressure, and surfactant;
- The inherent force to retract the lungs, mainly the elastic recoil force of the lungs and chest wall;
- The external force to inflate the lungs, including contraction of inspiratory muscles and the application of a positive P_{ao};
- Additional recoil force, which is generated when the lungs and chest wall are stretched. This is the force to pull the lung and chest wall back to the resting position. This situation is comparable to a stretched rubber band. Whenever the stretching force is removed, the recoil force causes the band to retract.

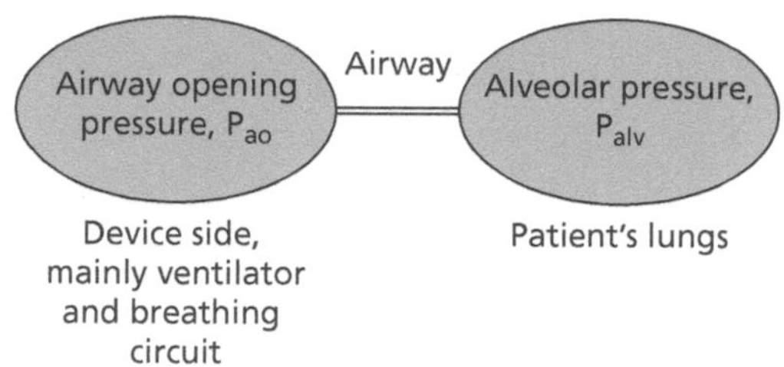

Fig. 3.18 A ventilator system has two pressure areas that are connected by an airway.

The lungs at their resting position

The lungs are at their resting position typically at the end of an adequate expiration. This is a static state with zero airway flow, because the inherent forces to open and retract the lungs are equal and there is no externally applied force. Note that in this position, the lungs are not totally empty, but instead contain a volume of gas known as the FRC. The FRC is physiologically important. Some lung diseases can cause FRC to abnormally increase (e.g. COPD) or decrease (e.g. ARDS).

The lungs at their inflated position

The inflated position of the lungs represents another static state with zero airway flow. Here the forces to inflate the lungs and the forces to deflate the lungs are equal. The lungs are at their inflated position in these two cases: (a) at the end of an adequate inspiration in a pressure-based breath, and (b) at the end of inspiration in a volume breath with inspiratory pause.

Inspiration

Inspiration is the process to increase lung volume. Typically it begins at the resting position and may or may not end at the inflated position. The process differs in pressure breaths and volume breaths.

In a pressure breath, P_{ao} rises quickly to and stays at a preset level (Fig. 3.20). The pressure gradient is the greatest at the beginning, resulting in the maximum inspiratory flow. Over time, P_{alv} increases as more and more gas enters the lungs. The pressure gradient diminishes, causing

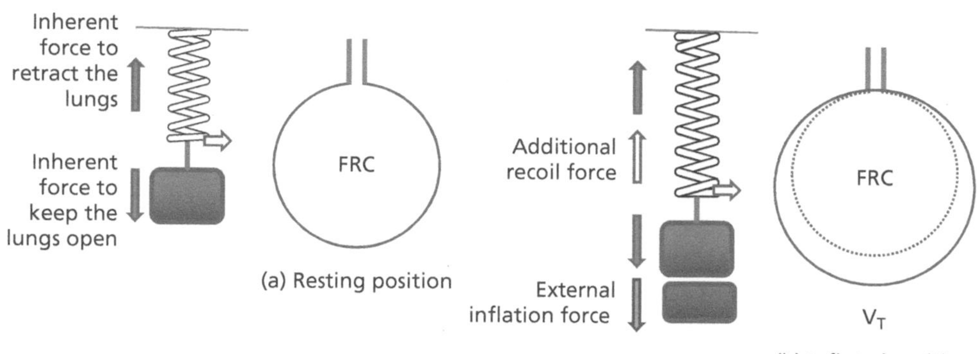

Fig. 3.19 The forces to inflate and deflate the lungs.

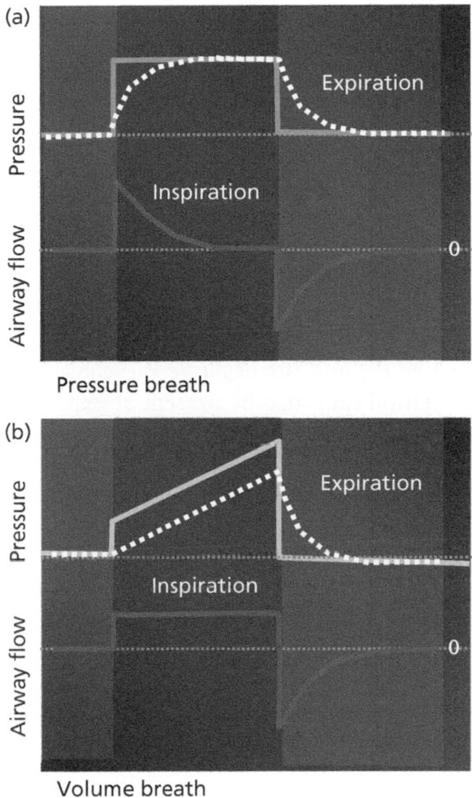

Fig. 3.20 Typical P_{ao} (orange), P_{alv} (dotted white), and airway flow change during a pressure breath (a), and volume breath (b), in a passive patient.

a corresponding drop in inspiratory flow. If the inspiration is sufficiently long, the lungs reach the inflated position.

In a volume breath with constant flow, the most common inspiratory flow pattern, the applied positive P_{ao} pushes gas into the lungs at a constant, defined inspiratory flow. The applied P_{ao} must increase steadily to maintain the required pressure gradient. At the end of inspiration, the lungs do not reach their inflated position unless an inspiratory pause is imposed.

Expiration

Expiration is the process to decrease lung volume. The applied positive P_{ao} drops suddenly to the baseline. The additional recoil force causes the lungs to retract. The pressure gradient (P_{alv} > P_{ao}) pushes the gas out. Over time, P_{alv} and the resultant *expiratory flow* decrease. The lungs return to their resting position if sufficient expiratory time is allowed. The expiration process is the same in both pressure and volume breaths.

In spontaneously breathing patients

So far, we have discussed the four driving forces, the lung resting and inflated positions, and the inspiration and expiration processes. All of them share the same condition: the patient is passive. In reality, however, many ventilated patients are actively breathing. But the situation is more complicated than that. We know there are two external forces to inflate

Table 3.3 The six physical forces involved in mechanical ventilation

Situation	Lung inflating forces	Lung deflating forces
Lung at resting position (with FRC)	Inherent force to keep the lungs open	Inherent recoil force to retract the lungs
Lung tidal volume change	Applied positive P_{ao} to expand the lungs	Additional recoil force to bring the lungs back to the resting position
Active patients only	Contraction of inspiratory muscles to enlarge the chest cavity and lower P_{alv}	Contraction of expiratory muscles to reduce the chest cavity and raise P_{alv}

the lungs, the applied positive P_{ao} and the negative P_{alv} caused by contraction of inspiratory muscles. A similar situation may also be present at expiration, as the contraction of expiratory muscles generates additional positive P_{alv}. This gives us six forces altogether (Table 3.3).

Ideally, the patient's breathing efforts synchronize with the intermittently applied positive P_{ao} for inspiration and expiration. If not, a troubling phenomenon called patient-ventilator asynchrony or 'patient-ventilator fight' is inevitable.

3.3.4 Comparison of natural and mechanical ventilation (IPPV)

Similarities

The ultimate goal of lung ventilation, for both natural and mechanical ventilation, is to alternately increase and decrease the lung volume.

Both natural and mechanical ventilation are realized through the natural pulmonary system, although the functioning of this system is often deteriorated in mechanically ventilated patients. The direction of gas movement during inspiration and expiration is the same for both forms of lung ventilation.

Natural and mechanical expiration are similar. In both cases, the elastic recoil force generates a positive P_{alv}, and the gradient ($P_{alv} > P_{ao}$) drives the gas out of lungs.

Differences

With natural ventilation, gas exchange occurs directly between the human's lungs and the atmosphere. With mechanical ventilation, the patient's airway and lungs are integrated into a ventilator system. The patient breathes exclusively through the connected ventilator, isolated from atmospheric air.

With natural inspiration, the contraction of inspiratory muscles generates a negative P_{alv}. The pressure gradient ($P_{alv} < P_{ao}$) sucks air into the lungs. With mechanical inspiration, a positive P_{ao} is applied, and the pressure gradient ($P_{ao} > P_{alv}$) pushes the gas into the lungs.

Normally, the FRC is related to the balance of the inherent lung inflation/deflation forces. During mechanical ventilation, a moderate level of PEEP (3–5 cmH_2O) is frequently used. It can be regarded as an addition to the inherent force to inflate the lungs, leading to an increased FRC.

With natural ventilation, the respiratory centre automatically and precisely regulates respiratory rate and breath intensity to satisfy current physiological demand. With mechanical ventilation, however, an operator must set the mechanical breath rate and intensity. Ventilator settings often require readjustment to meet the patient's changing metabolic demands and lung conditions. Actively breathing patients may refuse to accept the imposed ventilation, including the rate, tidal volume, and inspiratory pressure, causing patient-ventilator asynchrony.

Chapter 4

Ventilator System Concept

4.1 Introduction

In Chapter 3, we learned that artificial lung ventilation (intermittent positive pressure ventilation or IPPV) is accomplished by intermittently alternating the airway opening pressure (P_{ao}) between a baseline level and a defined peak level.

In this chapter, we will discuss:

- How variable P_{ao} is generated;
- The concept of the ventilator system;
- The conditions required for a ventilator system to function properly.

4.2 How is variable P_{ao} generated?

To answer this question, let's start by inflating a balloon (Fig 4.1).

Coloured balloons are often used to decorate parties or ceremonies. We all have had the experience of blowing up a balloon. If we need to inflate many balloons, we often use a simple device that includes:

- A pressurized gas reservoir;
- A hand (A) to control gas flow through the connecting tube;
- A blue connecting tube;
- A balloon to be inflated.

There is clearly a huge pressure difference between the gas reservoir and the balloon. If both are connected and hand A opens, then gas is pushed into the balloon. The balloon is 'growing'.

Now, let's modify the balloon inflating device by adding three more parts and assembling them as shown. We add:

- A Y-piece;
- A pink side tube with one end connected to the Y-piece and the other end open to the atmosphere;
- A hand (B) to control gas flow through the side tube.

After the modification is completed, can you see that we have built the simplest working model of an IPPV ventilator system?

4.2.1 Balloon inflation

If hand A opens the connecting tube and hand B closes the side tube simultaneously, the tube pressure is much higher than the balloon pressure. The pressure gradient drives the gas toward the balloon, inflating it.

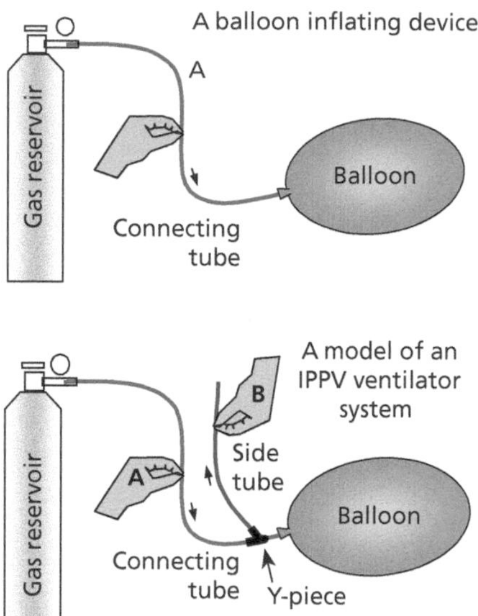

Fig. 4.1 The foundation of intermittent positive pressure ventilation (IPPV) is the alternation of P_{ao}. The desired P_{ao} change is created by opening and closing the two tubes with hands A and B in the balloon model.

4.2.2 **Balloon deflation**

If hand A closes the connecting tube and hand B opens the side tube simultaneously, the tube pressure is lower than the balloon pressure due to the elastic recoil force. The pressure gradient drives the gas out of the balloon, deflating it.

In an actual ventilator system, hand A is replaced with an *inspiratory valve*, and hand B, with an *expiratory valve* (Fig 4.2). The tube pressure is comparable to P_{ao}, while the balloon pressure is comparable to P_{alv}.

4.2.3 **Inspiration**

During inspiration, the inspiratory valve opens and the expiratory valve closes. P_{ao} becomes higher than P_{alv}. The pressure gradient generated pushes the gas into lungs, increasing the lung volume.

4.2.4 **Expiration**

During expiration, the inspiratory valve closes and the expiratory valve opens. P_{ao} becomes lower than P_{alv}. The opposite pressure gradient pushes gas out of lungs, decreasing the lung volume.

Two technical details are worth mentioning here. In late expiration, a ventilator system opens the inspiratory valve slightly to generate a constant base flow, which is required for flow triggering. It also regulates the expiratory valve to generate the positive end-expiratory pressure (PEEP). In other words, the expiratory valve is not completely closed during expiration.

If the 'inflation' and 'expiration' alternate, the balloon is 'mechanically ventilated', like lungs. This is how variable P_{ao} is generated.

This simple balloon model is highly comparable to a real IPPV system (Fig 4.3). The gas cylinder corresponds to the high-pressure gas supply. Hand A corresponds to the inspiratory valve,

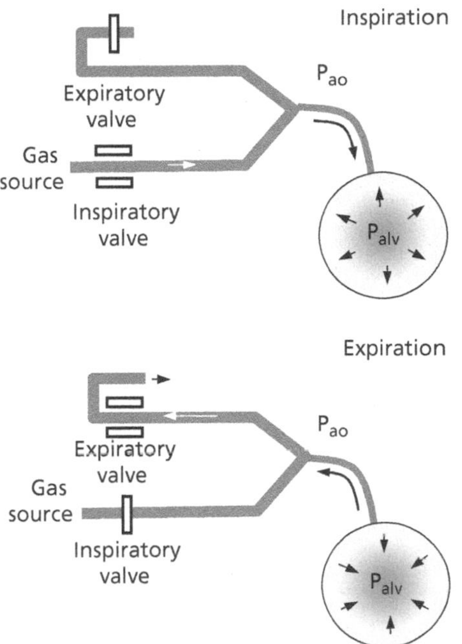

Fig. 4.2 A simplified ventilator system to create the desired P_{ao} alternation.

while hand B corresponds to the expiratory valve. The blue and pink tubes between the Y-piece and the two hands correspond to a breathing circuit. The blue tube piece between the Y-piece and the balloon corresponds to the airway. Finally, the balloon itself corresponds to the lungs of a ventilated patient.

4.3 **Ventilator system concept**

Perhaps you have noticed that we are using the term *ventilator system* instead of *ventilator*.

What is the therapeutic tool for mechanical ventilation?

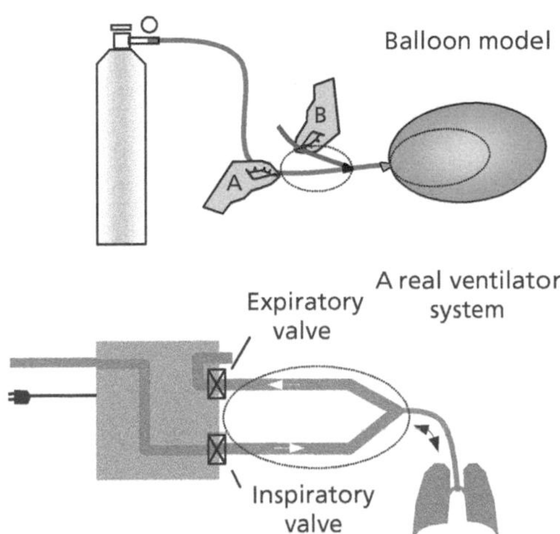

Fig. 4.3 The balloon model and a real ventilator system have a very similar structure.

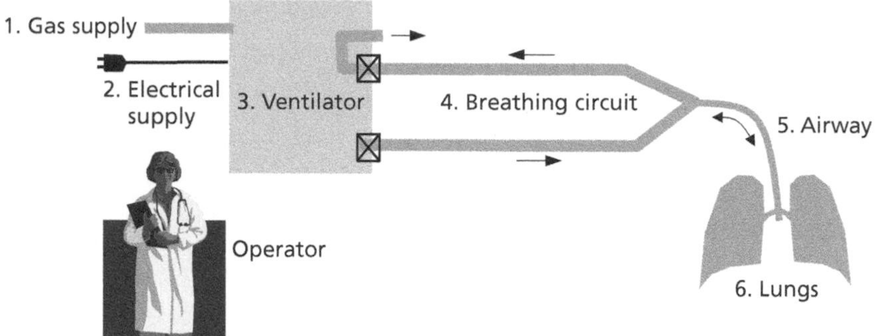

Fig. 4.4 A complete ventilator system and its operator.

The balloon model has already given us a clue to the correct answer: the therapeutic tool required for mechanical ventilation is a ventilator system, which is typically composed of six essential parts (Fig 4.4):

1. Pressurized O_2 and air supplies;
2. An electrical supply;
3. A ventilator;
4. A breathing circuit;
5. An airway;
6. A patient's lungs or a test lung to mimic the lungs.

So, the ventilator is not *the* tool, but just a *part* of it. In a ventilator system, all six required parts—whether a $40,000 ventilator or a $10 breathing circuit set—are equally important, because the system does not function at all if any of these parts is missing. We will discuss the individual parts in Chapter 5.

The relationship between a ventilator system and a ventilator is comparable to the relationship between a car and its engine. A car must *have* an engine, but an engine *is not* a car. The ventilator alone can provide no mechanical ventilation unless it is integrated into a ventilator system.

Understanding the ventilator system concept is critical to our understanding of the therapeutic equipment for mechanical ventilation. It is one of the key concepts in this book.

4.4 **The required conditions**

A modern ventilator is sophisticated and expensive.

Many clinicians assume that a 'good', high-priced ventilator will work under all possible clinical conditions. They often blame the ventilator, believing it is technically faulty if the therapy goes awry. In many cases, this assumption is not valid.

We have learned that the therapeutic tool for mechanical ventilation is an entire ventilator system. We must now add that the tool will work as expected only when all required conditions are met. In other words, the proper functioning of a ventilator system is conditional, based on these eight requirements being met:

1. All required parts are present and functioning properly;
2. The system is assembled correctly and securely;
3. The supplies of compressed air and oxygen are continuous and appropriate in pressure and flow;
4. The electrical supply is continuous and appropriate in voltage and frequency;

5. The entire system is gas tight;
6. The entire system is free from occlusion;
7. The patient's lung volume is capable of changing normally as the applied airway pressure changes;
8. The operator has sufficient expertise to define and adjust the ventilator mode, controls, and alarm limits when the patient's condition changes during mechanical ventilation.

Even when the ventilator is functioning perfectly, mechanical ventilation can still fail unless *all required conditions are fully satisfied.*

The list of the required conditions serves as the top-level guideline for systematic trouble-shooting of mechanical ventilation. We will return to these conditions in Chapter 13.

Ventilator designers and producers assume that all these conditions are fully satisfied and that operators are sufficiently trained. Unfortunately, this assumption is not always valid.

Chapter 5

Ventilator System Composition

5.1 Introduction

In Chapter 4 we learned that a ventilator system is the therapeutic tool for mechanical ventilation based on the intermittent positive pressure ventilation (IPPV) principle. The system is composed of six essential parts, the ventilator being just one of them. The system works properly only when all required conditions are fully satisfied. This chapter opens by discussing the composition of a ventilator system and it continues with in-depth descriptions of each of the required parts.

Humidification devices, in-line nebulization devices, and gas filters are not among the required parts of a ventilator system. They are added to the system to meet specific clinical needs; yet these devices are important, as they reshape the composition of a ventilator system and pose additional challenges to the system. We will discuss these devices in Chapter 6.

5.2 The gas passageway inside a ventilator system

As Fig. 5.1 shows, at the core of a ventilator system is a gas passageway, which begins at the gas supply hoses and ends with the exhaust of expired gas. By design, gas moves in one direction throughout the gas passageway, with the exception of the airway, where the gas moves in both directions.

The gas passageway must be gas tight and free from occlusion. If the gas passageway has a hole, the internal positive pressure pushes the gas out. The magnitude of the gas leak depends on the difference in pressure inside and out, as well as the size of the 'hole'. Disconnection gives rise to the maximum possible leak. An excessive gas leak can cause the system to fail totally. For example, a massive gas leak at the mask is the most common cause of failure of non-invasive ventilation.

Occlusion refers to the condition where gas movement along the passageway is hindered due to abnormally high resistance. Infinite resistance stops gas movement completely. For instance, an airway HME (heat and moisture exchanger) may suddenly clog up with excessive secretions or blood from the trachea—a real emergency.

We will discuss both leak and occlusion in greater depth in Chapter 13.

As we already know, gas movement between two neighbouring areas is driven by the pressure gradient between the two. A ventilator system has a series of invisible pressure 'waterfalls' along the gas passageway. As an example, let's look at the GALILEO ventilator from Hamilton Medical (Fig. 5.2):

- The gas supply pressure is between 2000 and 6000 cmH_2O.
- The tank pressure is between 280 and 340 cmH_2O (Note that not all IPPV ventilators have a tank).
- The circuit pressure, equivalent to airway opening pressure (P_{ao}), is between 5 and 40 cmH_2O in most clinical cases.

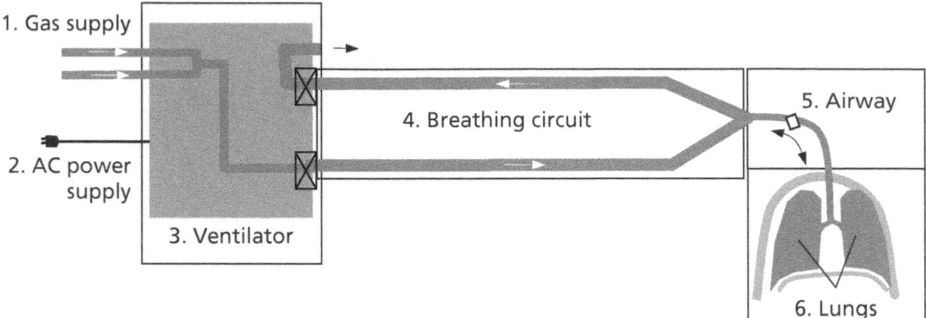

Fig. 5.1 The gas passageway of a ventilator system.

- The lung or alveolar pressure (P_{alv}) is also between 5 and 40 cmH_2O.
- The ambient pressure is 0 cmH_2O.

5.3 A close look at the individual parts

Now let's look at each of the parts required for a functional ventilator system.

5.3.1 Compressed gas supplies

Dual-gas supply

A ventilator system requires supplies of both compressed air and compressed oxygen. The gas supplies serve not only as the source of the fresh gas delivered to a ventilated patient, but also as the ultimate force to propel the gas throughout the gas passageway.

Compressed oxygen supply The oxygen concentration of inspiratory gas is defined as F_iO_2 or *fraction of inspired oxygen*. You can freely set and adjust F_iO_2 to between 21% and 100% in most ventilators.

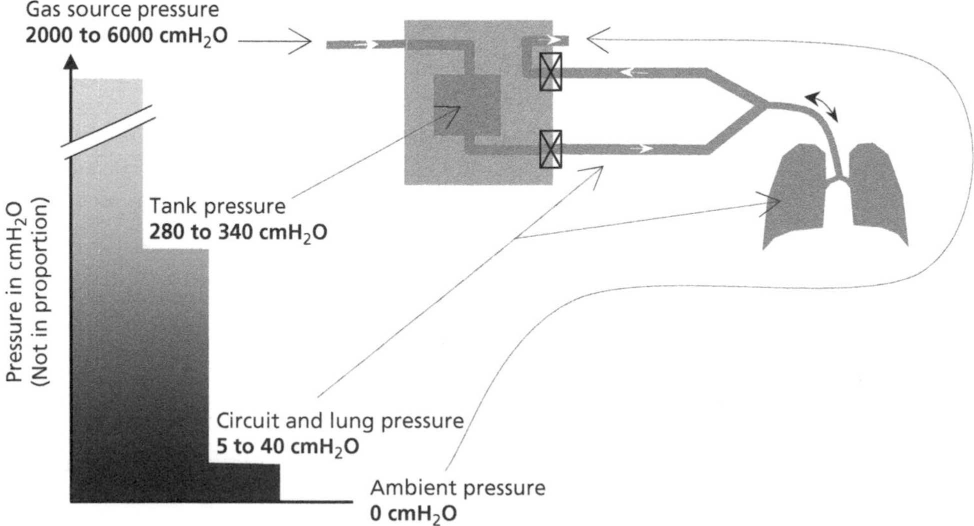

Fig. 5.2 Pressure waterfalls inside the GALILEO ventilator system. The diagram assumes an intubated, passively ventilated patient with a positive end-expiratory pressure (PEEP) of 5 cmH_2O.

If one gas supply fails, a ventilator typically continues mechanical ventilation with the remaining gas supply, and sets off an alarm to alert the clinician of the abnormal condition. In this case, the ventilated patient receives either pure air or pure oxygen only. Restore the non-functional gas supply as quickly as possible. If both supplies fail simultaneously, mechanical ventilation invariably stops.

The typical oxygen source is either the hospital's central oxygen supply delivered through a wall pipeline network, or oxygen cylinders. A newer oxygen source, for use in hospital, is a special oxygen concentrator. It is still in its testing phase.

Compressed air supply Compressed air is traditionally provided from a standalone air compressor, from air cylinders, or from a central supply delivered through a wall pipeline network. Some ventilators use internal turbines as the internal air supply. In this case, an external air supply is not required.

Requirements for gas supplies

Compressed air and oxygen to a ventilator system should meet the following general requirements:

- The gas pressure must meet the specifications for the applicable ventilator. For instance, Hamilton Medical ventilators require both air and oxygen in the range of 2 to 6 bars (or 29 to 87 psi). A supply pressure that is too low can cause the ventilator system to malfunction or fail. A supply pressure that is too high can damage the ventilator.
- Maximum flow capability is an important pneumatic property of a ventilator. It is defined as the maximum gas flow a ventilator can deliver instantaneously or continuously. This capability is, however, limited by the maximum flow delivery of the gas supply source. Obviously a ventilator cannot deliver more flow than the gas source can provide.
- The gas supply must be continuous and stable over the specified range. Reliability is an important factor to consider when deciding how the compressed gas should be supplied.

Gas hoses, fittings, and water trap

Two gas hoses are needed to connect the gas sources and a ventilator, one for compressed air and the other for compressed oxygen.

Gas hoses are special tubes with connecting parts or gas fittings at both ends. The fittings for different gases have different diameters and screw threads to prevent possible misconnection. It is physically impossible, for instance, to connect oxygen to the air inlet of a ventilator, and vice versa. However, there are different standards for gas fittings. *NIST* (non-interchangeable screw threaded) and *DISS* (diameter indexed safety system) are the most popular. Other gas fitting systems may also be used in hospitals. For more information, refer to standard EN ISO 5350, *Low-pressure hose assemblies for use with medical gases.*

The supplied air and oxygen should be clean, dry, and of medical grade; however, in reality the gases may not meet these requirements. For this reason, a ventilator *gas inlet*, particularly the air inlet, typically has a *water trap* with a microfilter (Fig. 5.3). The supplied gas passes through the water trap and filter before entering the ventilator. This captures moisture and particles.

While a ventilator is running, inspect the gas inlet water traps periodically. Before the container is half full, you should empty the trap by pressing the pin at the bottom or unscrewing the screw-type mechanism. To retain its efficacy, be sure to have the microfilter replaced by a qualified technician at the interval recommended by the ventilator manufacturer.

5.3.2 Electrical supply

Almost all key functions of a modern ventilator are electrically powered, including valves, microprocessors, sensors, alarms, and displays. Electricity to a ventilator is comparable to

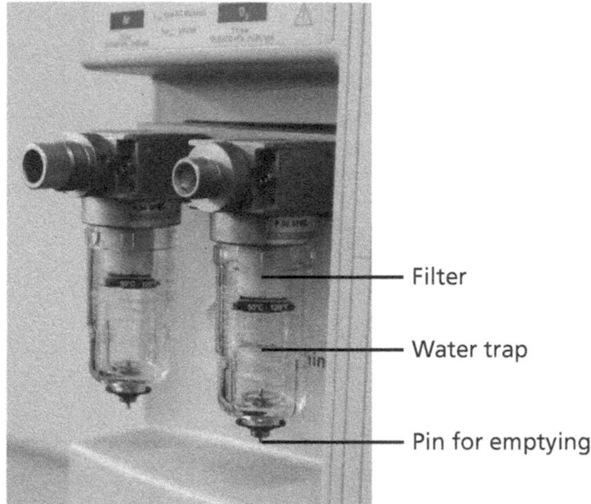

Fig. 5.3 Gas inlets with water traps and gas filters (GALILEO ventilator).

blood in a living body. If the electrical supply stops, the ventilator system is immediately paralysed.

Most ventilators have two electricity sources: AC (alternating current) power is the primary one, and an integrated battery is the secondary one (Fig. 5.4); while the ventilator is connected to AC power, this battery charges. If AC power is unexpectedly interrupted, the running ventilator should switch immediately and automatically to battery power so that mechanical ventilation continues. Typically the ventilator also alarms to alert the operator to the abnormal condition. If AC power resumes, the ventilator switches back to AC power and recharges the battery.

The internal battery is, however, just a temporary electrical source with limited capacity. Should a ventilator switch to its battery, it is important that the AC supply be restored as quickly as possible, because mechanical ventilation discontinues if the battery is depleted. The battery duration is listed in the ventilator's operating manual. Remember that the duration of battery power is noticeably shortened if the battery is aged or just partially charged.

AC voltages and frequencies

Globally, there are four common types of AC power supply in terms of nominal voltage and frequency (Fig. 5.5):

- 220–240 V/50 Hz
- 220–240 V/60 Hz

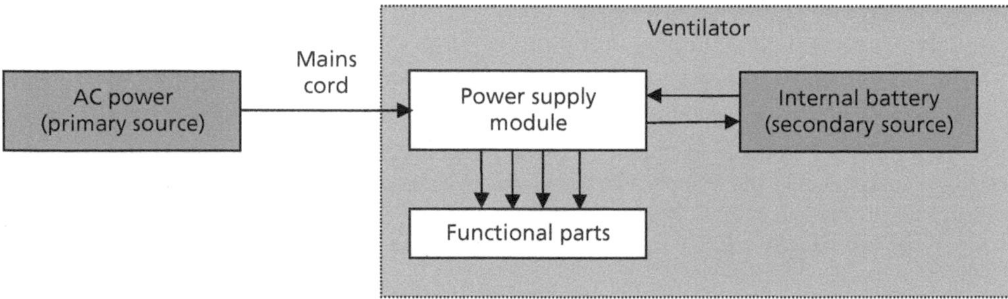

Fig. 5.4 Simplified diagram of ventilator electrical supply.

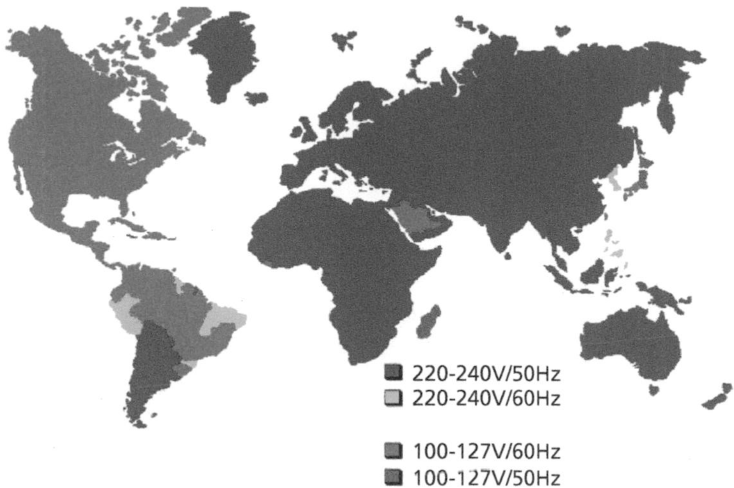

Fig. 5.5 AC power standards around the world.
Adapted from Map of the world coloured by voltage and frequency, Wikimedia Commons, accessed Nov 2016, http://wikitravel.org/shared/File:800px-Map_of_the_world_coloured_by_voltage_and_frequency.png This image is in public domain and free of any copyright restrictions; released by Shoestring.

- 100–127 V/60 Hz
- 100–127 V/50 Hz.

A ventilator requires that the AC supply have a specific voltage and frequency. These requirements are listed on the device label. The nominal voltage of an AC supply is what its output *should be*, while the actual voltage is what its output *is*. There is almost always a difference between the two. An electrically powered medical device typically continues to perform to specification if the actual AC voltage is within ±10% of the nominal level (Table 5.1).

In reality, however, the actual voltage of a local AC supply can fluctuate considerably, potentially causing ventilator malfunction or damage. For instance, if the local nominal AC voltage is 230 V, a ventilator can typically tolerate voltage fluctuations between 198 and 264 V. However, the actual AC voltage can drop to 180 V at peak power consumption. The ventilator may or may not function properly under this condition.

The opposite situation occurs when the actual AC voltage is far above the nominal one, in the form of electrical surges or spikes, which are sudden, instantaneous rises in voltage or current. These may damage the ventilator. For instance, in an area with an inadequate infrastructure, an electrical surge may occur when a hospital backup generator starts in response to an unexpected blackout.

Power or mains cord

A power (mains) cord connects a ventilator to AC power. A power cord has three parts: a plug for a wall socket, an insulated cable of varying length, and an instrument adapter to the ventilator.

Table 5.1 AC voltage ranges, nominal and with tolerances

Nominal AC voltage range	220 to 240 V	100 to 127 V
Practicable AC voltage range	198 V to 264 V	90 V to 139.7 V

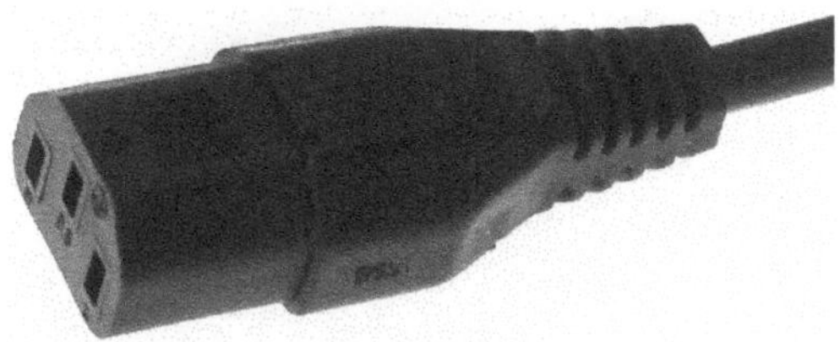

Fig. 5.6 Standard instrument adapter.

The plug of the power cord must match the local socket and make good contact. Make sure the socket in use is powered. Typically, a three-pole plug should be used so that the connected ventilator is well grounded.

The other end of a power cord is a standard instrument adapter. In most medical devices, it is the IEC 3-pin line socket, shown in Fig. 5.6.

Common AC supply problems

Common problems associated with the AC power supply include:

- Accidental unplugging at either end (e.g. during regular room cleaning);
- Unexpected blackout;
- Dead socket;
- Poor connection or broken cable;
- Substantial voltage fluctuation of the local AC supply;
- AC power surge;
- Mismatch between the specified and the actual AC voltage or frequency;
- Mismatch between the plug and wall socket;
- Mismatch between the adapter and ventilator socket.

To safeguard against AC power-related issues, ventilators incorporate preventive features including the internal battery, a cable security mechanism at the device side, as well as alarming. Periodic socket checks are also recommended as a preventive measure.

5.3.3 **Ventilator**

A ventilator is a key component of a ventilator system. Its importance is self-evident.

Physical parts of the ventilator

A modern ventilator typically has three basic physical parts: a main unit, a user interface, and a mobile stand. The main unit contains all the mechanical and electrical components. The *user interface*, which may include a display, a touchscreen, knobs, and a keypad, facilitates communication between the ventilator and the operator. The mobile stand (or trolley or cart) positions the ventilator at a convenient height for the user, and it provides mobility. On a ventilator, the three parts may be separate, or the main unit may be integrated with the user interface, or the stand, or both.

Categories of ventilator function

As we know already, a simple balloon model can be used to demonstrate how a real ventilator system functions. Over time, a number of non-ventilation features have been developed, including monitoring, alarming, and device interface. Modern ventilators require a lot of sophistication to be able to provide their full range of functionality. A modern ICU ventilator is so complex that its manual often contains hundreds of pages. Regrettably, ventilator users often do not read through the book before operating the ventilator, as they should.

To give us a clear overview of what a ventilator has and can do, it helps to group the features and functions:

- **Ventilation:** The principal function of a ventilator; this group includes all functions and features that directly contribute to mechanical ventilation. These include intended patient population, ventilation modes, control parameters, apnoea ventilation, and additional ventilation functions.
- **Monitoring:** Ventilator monitoring includes functions that continuously sense the status of the ventilator system. The monitoring results may be displayed numerically and graphically. Clinicians use this information to check and understand the status of mechanical ventilation. These monitoring signals also serve as the inputs to the alarm system and may be used for some automatic regulation mechanisms. Common sensed signals include pneumatic ones (pressure, flow, and volume), airway CO_2, F_iO_2, and oxygen saturation (SpO_2). If we think of ventilation functions as the 'doing'; the monitoring functions are the 'seeing' and 'knowing'. Monitoring functions should be totally independent from ventilation. Chapter 11 is devoted to ventilator monitoring.
- **Alarm and safety mechanisms:** Ventilator alarms use audible and visual signals to alert the clinician to predefined abnormal conditions that require special attention or corrective actions. Ventilator alarms are based on both monitoring inputs and the alarm criteria set by the manufacturer or operator. If designed and used appropriately, alarms are a major contributor to the safety of the ventilated patients. They may create difficulties of their own if they are not.Besides ventilator alarms, ventilators may also have automatic *safety mechanisms*. These include apnoea ventilation, an overpressure relief valve, and an emergency mode, the 'ambient state', where the patient can breathe unassisted through the ventilator in an emergency. Chapter 12 is devoted to ventilator alarms and safety mechanisms.
- **User interface or graphical user graphic interface, GUI:** The ventilator user interacts with the ventilator through the user interface. This allows the user to control and manipulate the ventilator operation as they desire. The user interface typically includes an operating panel with elements such as LCDs (liquid crystal displays), knobs, switches, and keypads. Touch screens are an increasingly popular means of input. The importance of the ventilator user interface is increasingly recognized. A poorly designed user interface confuses the operator, with possibly disastrous consequences.
- **Configuration:** When a ventilator is switched on, it starts operating with default settings, including patient population, language, mode, and controls. The default settings are initially defined by the manufacturer (*factory defaults*). Some ventilators allow the operator to change the default settings (customer defaults). Configuration refers to the process of changing the default so that the ventilator always starts up in a desired manner.
- **Power supply:** See section 5.3.2 for a discussion of the power supply.
- **Communication interface or connectivity:** A *communication interface* allows a ventilator to transmit data (monitoring data and alarms) to another medical device such as a patient monitor, or a patient data management system (PDMS), or a hospital information system (HIS). The transmitted ventilator data may be displayed or stored continuously as medical records. A nurse call or remote alarm system is a simple form of communication interface.

As an example, Fig. 5.7 shows the grouped functions of the GALILEO ventilator. Note that the groups may overlap one other.

Ventilation

- Adult, paediatric, and neonatal patient populations
- 11 conventional, adaptive, and biphasic ventilation modes
- Ventilation features including tube resistance compensation, sigh, manual trigger, 100% O_2 enrichment, standby, and nebulization
- Bidirectional apnoea ventilation

Monitoring

- Proximal flow sensing
- 26 monitoring parameters
- Display of numeric parameters, waveforms, and dynamic loops
- Trend curves of all monitoring parameters
- Hold and P/V tool manoeuvres
- Special ASV (adaptive support ventilation) window
- Event logger

Alarms and safety

- Adjustable, non-adjustable, information, and technical failure alarms
- Alarm prioritization
- Alarm silence
- Audible alarm volume adjustment
- Alarm information buffer
- Overpressure relief valve
- Emergency ambient mode
- Bidirectional apnoea ventilation

Communication interface

- To compatible patient monitors or a PDMS (patient data management system)
- To a remote alarm (nurse call) system

Power supply

- AC input, 100 V to 230 V, 50/60 Hz
- One-hour backup by internal battery power typical

Configuration

- Configurability of startup state, including enabling/disabling of alarms and oxygen monitoring, and selection of displayed parameters
- Additional configurable parameters and functionality

User interface

- Large colour display
- Two press-and-turn knobs and four membrane keys
- Display of current mode and key information
- Trigger indicator
- Support for various languages

Fig. 5.7 Feature/function categories in the GALILEO ventilator.

Ventilator pneumatic design

An IPPV ventilator typically has an *inspiratory channel* and an *expiratory channel* (Fig. 5.8). The inspiratory channel includes the inspiratory valve, and the expiratory channel includes the expiratory valve. Each channel precisely controls the flow of the passing gas. Both channels work in harmony to carry out the work of mechanical ventilation.

The inspiratory channel performs the following functions:

- Precisely mixes air and oxygen to produce the inspiratory gas, based on the F_iO_2 setting;
- Regulates the flow, pressure, and timing of the delivered inspiratory gas;
- Helps generate base flow, which facilitates flow triggering.

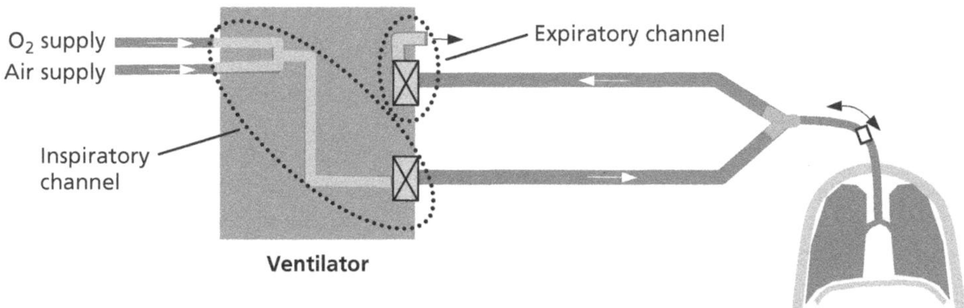

Fig. 5.8 Inspiratory and expiratory channels in a ventilator.

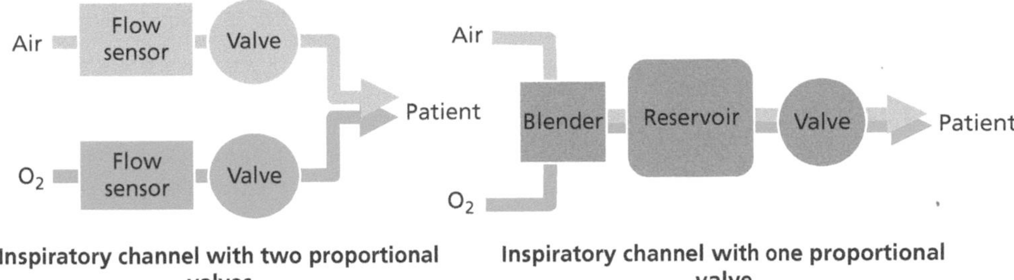

Fig. 5.9 Two typical inspiratory channel designs.

Ventilators typically use one of two inspiratory channel designs, characterized by the number of proportional valves (Fig. 5.9):

- Dual proportional valve design: This design uses two branches; one for air and one for oxygen. Each branch has its own solenoid valve, flow sensor, and pressure regulator. The valves are controlled by a microprocessor. This design is used in Puritan Bennett 840 (Covidien) and SERVO 300 (Maquet) ventilators.
- Single proportional valve design: In this design air and oxygen are mixed in a blender. The mixed gas is stored in a reservoir, and then passed through a single proportional valve. This design is used in the GALILEO and Bird 8600 (CareFusion) ventilators.

The expiratory channel controls gas exiting from the ventilator system. It performs the following functions:

- Regulates the expiratory flow and timing;
- Generates and maintains the desired PEEP;
- Helps generate base flow, which facilitates flow triggering.

The expiratory valve imposes controlled resistance to expiratory flow. The resistance must be truly minimal at the start of expiration, increasing later on to generate PEEP.

Depending on the design, the expiratory valve may be mounted either internally or externally (Fig. 5.10). Modern ICU ventilators have an internal expiratory valve for more precise valve control. When an external expiratory valve is used, the expiratory limb may be very short, or the valve may be a PEEP valve only.

Control module

The control module determines and coordinates the activities of all parts of the ventilator. In modern microprocessor-controlled ventilators, special software programs serve as the 'brain'.

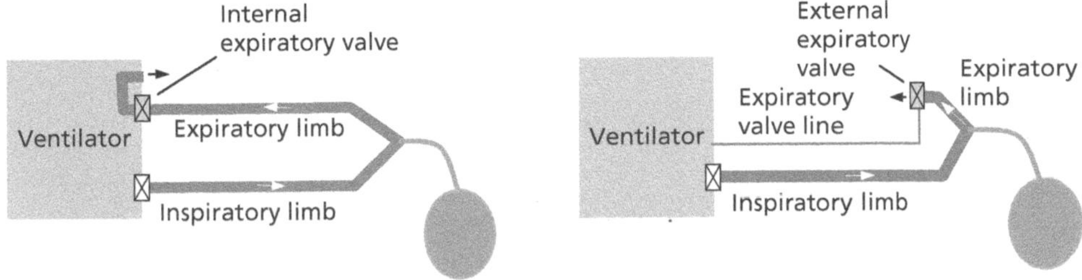

Fig. 5.10 Two typical expiratory channel designs.

The marriage of computer technology with ventilator design has permitted a marked increase in the functionality of today's ventilators.

5.3.4 Breathing circuit

The *breathing circuit* or *patient circuit* is another essential part of a ventilator system. Its primary function is to provide a flexible, gas-tight channel connecting the ventilator and the artificial airway. It is also the location where an active humidifier, in-line nebulizer, and gas filter can be mounted.

Do not underestimate the importance of the breathing circuit, because it is the source of many ventilation problems, including disconnection, leakage, occlusion, and circuit rainout.

Basic structure and variations

The breathing circuit and the artificial airway together are shaped like a large tuning fork (Fig. 5.11). This section focuses on the breathing circuit, excluding the artificial airway.

The breathing circuit has three parts: the *inspiratory limb*, the *expiratory limb*, and the *Y-piece* or *wye*.

Both the inspiratory and expiratory limbs are flexible tubes that connect the Y-piece to the inspiratory or expiratory port of a ventilator.

Under normal conditions, gas moves freely in the breathing circuit and airway, driven by the pressure gradient. In each of these limbs, gas moves in one direction only.

Various medical devices and accessories can be installed in the inspiratory and expiratory limbs. In the inspiratory limb we can insert an active humidifier, an in-line nebulizer jar, and an inspiratory filter. In the expiratory limb we can insert a water trap and expiratory filter. These additional items complicate the structure of the breathing circuit. In Chapter 6 we will discuss artificial humidification and in-line nebulization.

The structure of the breathing circuit varies, depending mainly on the humidification device in use. The four primary circuit variations are described in the following paragraph.

Type A circuit setup: non-heated. In the type A circuit, inspiratory gas is warmed and humidified when it passes through the humidifier's water chamber (Fig. 5.12). This chamber is heated and maintained at a set temperature. A thermometer is positioned at the Y-piece to indicate the airway gas temperature. Two water traps are needed, one at the inspiratory limb and the other at the expiratory limb, to drain the condensed water from the circuit. A typical example is the circuit used with the Fisher & Paykel MR410 humidifier set. A type A circuit includes one active humidifier heater with a chamber, two water traps, five tubes, a Y-piece, and an airway thermometer.

The type A circuit is designed for multi-patient use. The humidifier itself is relatively simple. The chamber is heated continuously, and the heating is independent from the airway gas

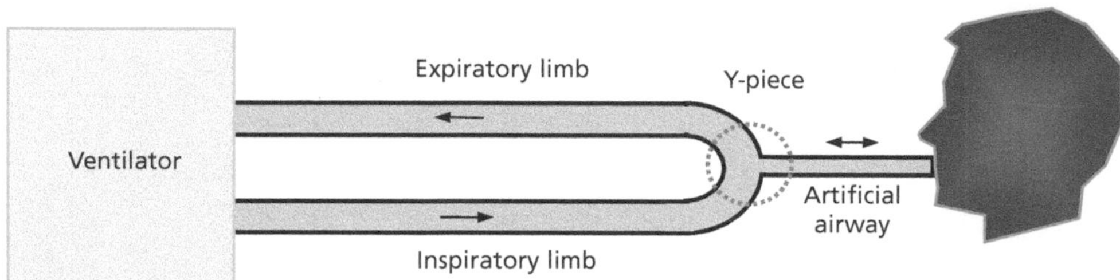

Fig. 5.11 The breathing circuit and artificial airway together are shaped like a large tuning fork.

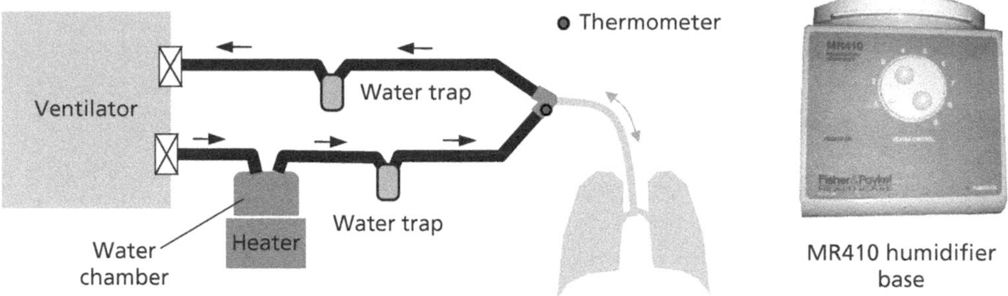

Fig. 5.12 Type A circuit setup with no heated limbs.

temperature monitoring. Use of this circuit is labour intensive and error prone. This type of circuit has been replaced by more advanced variations.

Type B circuit setup: single heated limb. The type B circuit represents the second milestone in circuit evolution (Fig. 5.13). It operates according to the same principles as type A, but it has two important design improvements. The first improvement is that the tube between the chamber outlet and the Y-piece is actively heated. In theory, the tube heating eliminates local condensation so that the inspiratory water trap can be omitted. The second improvement is that the chamber heating is servo-regulated with the feedback from a dual-temperature sensor. A typical example of the type B circuit is used with the Fisher & Paykel MR730 humidifier set. A type B circuit includes one active humidifier heater with chamber, one water trap, four tubes (one of which is heated), a Y-piece, and a dual-temperature sensor. The operator may set and adjust the chamber and wire heating.

The type B circuit may be either for multi-patient or single use. It once dominated the circuit market, but it has gradually lost ground to the type C circuit.

Type C circuit: dual heated limbs. The type C circuit represents the third milestone in circuit evolution (Fig. 5.14). It has two major improvements. The first is automation of heating regulation. This eliminates the need for manual operator setting, an improvement that is nevertheless not appreciated by all clinicians. The second is optional expiratory limb heating, which eliminates the need for the second water trap. This circuit is often referred to as a dual heated circuit. A typical example of the type C circuit is used with the Fisher & Paykel MR850 humidifier set. A type C circuit includes one active humidifier heater with a water chamber, three tubes, a Y-piece, and a dual-temperature sensor.

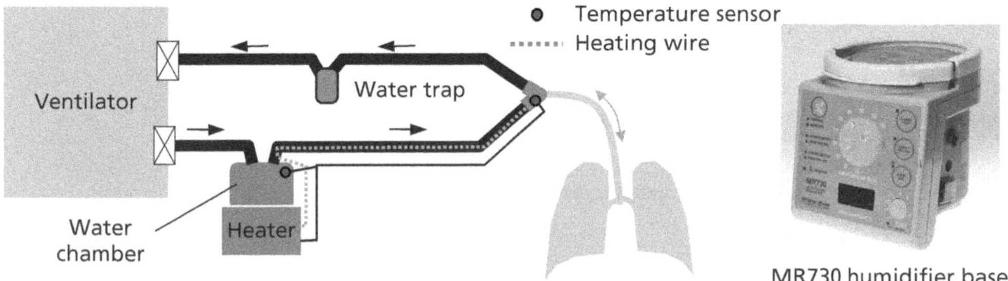

Fig. 5.13 Type B circuit setup with heated inspiratory limb.

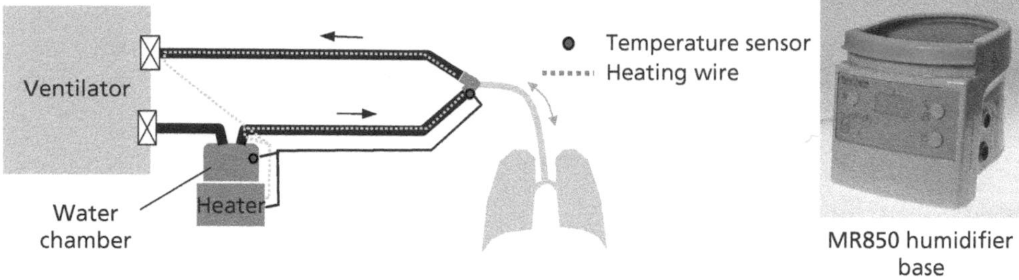

Fig. 5.14 Type C circuit setup with both limbs heated.

The type C circuit is exclusively for single use. This circuit appears to work well. In a few cases, the automatic heating regulation may not function as intended, and there is little the clinician can do to remedy this. The humidifier set may be expensive.

Type D circuit: HME. The type D circuit has the most basic breathing circuit structure, but with an HME installed at the artificial airway (Fig. 5.15). It includes just two long tubes and a Y-piece, eliminating all components needed for active humidification. This circuit type is mainly suitable for short-term mechanical ventilation therapy.

More about breathing circuits

Different circuit sizes for different populations. The basic circuit structure and variations generally work for all patient age groups. The tubing inner diameters, however, differ for adults, children/paediatric patients, and infants/neonates, as indicated in Table 5.2. The inner diameters are directly related to the circuit resistance and compliance.

It is important to be aware of these circuit sizes when you select a circuit for a particular population or reassemble reusable circuits after *reprocessing*, which is the process to prepare the used items for the next patient, typically through cleaning and disinfection or sterilization.

Reusable circuits versus single-use circuits Breathing circuits may be designed for *multi-patient use* (*reusable* circuits) or for single use only (*single-use* or *disposable*) circuits. The main difference between the two is the materials used.

Reusable circuits typically are made of silicone rubber and polysulfone, which is a medical plastic that resists the heat of autoclaving as well as the chemicals used in chemical disinfection or sterilization (Fig. 5.16).

Single-use circuits typically are made of medical plastics, including polyvinyl chloride (PVC), polyethylene (PE), polypropylene (PP), polycarbonate (PC), or ethylene-vinyl acetate (EVA) (Fig. 5.17). They are preassembled and stored in sealed packages, ready for use.

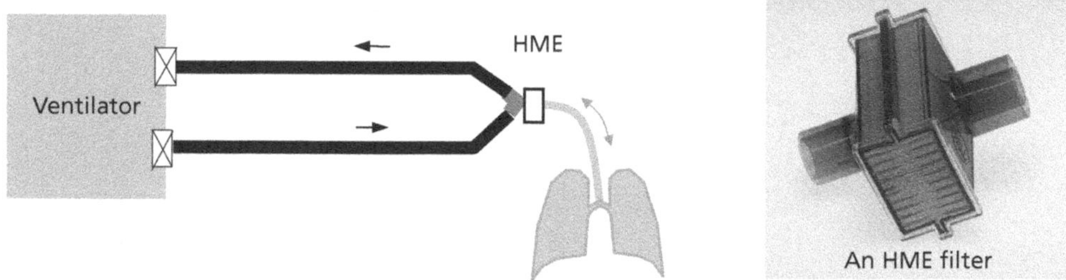

Fig. 5.15 Type D circuit with a heat and moisture exchange (HME) filter.

Table 5.2 Patient populations and corresponding circuit sizes

Patient population	Adult circuit	Paediatric circuit	Infant circuit
Circuit inner diameter	Approximately 22 mm	Approximately 15 mm	Approximately 10 mm

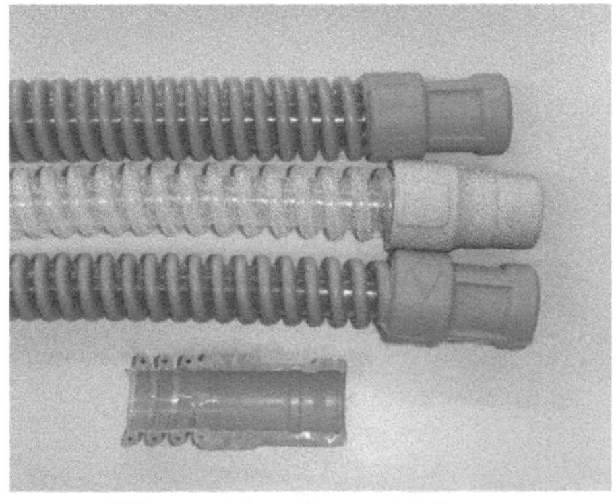

Silicone tubes for multiple use

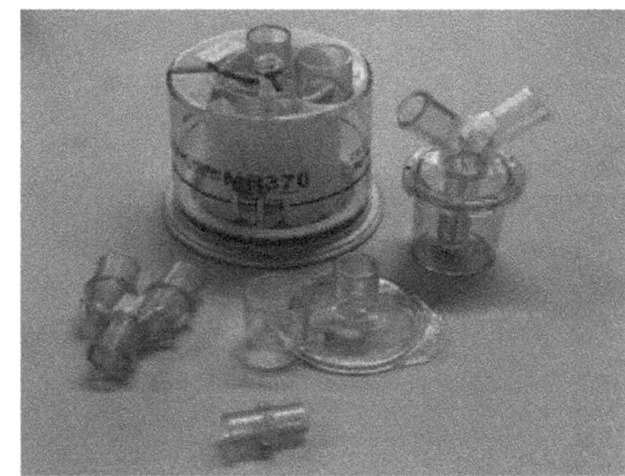

Polysulfone items for multiple use

Fig. 5.16 Circuit components designed for multiple use.

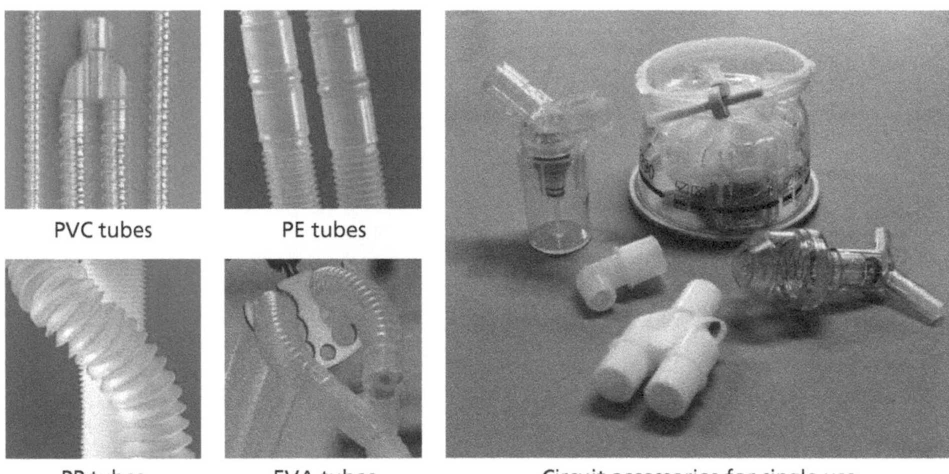

Fig. 5.17 Circuit components designed for single use.
EVA: ethylene vinyl acetate; PE: polyethylene; PP: polypropylene; PVC: polyvinyl chloride.

Generally speaking, reusable breathing circuits are more suitable for mid- and long-term mechanical ventilation, while disposable breathing circuits are for short-term use. Reusable circuits are a bit more complicated to use, because the used components require reprocessing and reassembly. Disposable circuits are simple to use, but they may cost more in the end, and they are environmentally unfriendly.

Single-use circuits are sometimes reused to minimize costs, a practice that especially occurs in the developing world. This is not recommended, because these circuits are not tested for this type of use, and they may not perform as expected. As is true with any misuse of a medical device, any unfortunate consequences become the legal responsibility of the hospital.

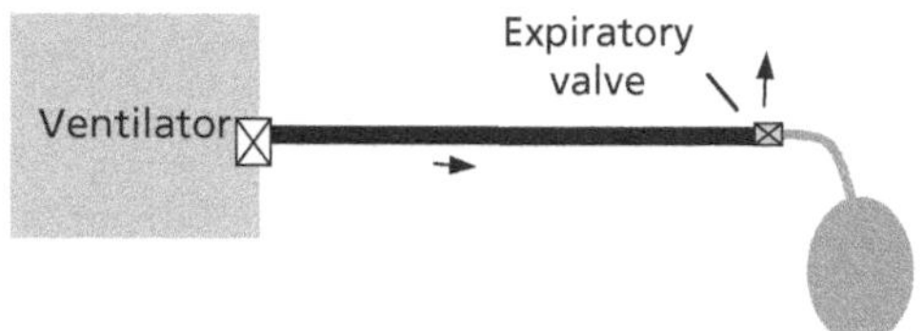

Fig. 5.18 A genuine single-limb circuit.

Single-limb circuit? The *double-limb breathing circuit* structure is the primary one used with most ventilator systems. It is possible, however, to find a special circuit with just one tube connecting the ventilator and the patient. It is called a *single-limb circuit*. A single-limb circuit may be either a genuine single-limb circuit or a pseudo single-limb circuit.

A genuine single-limb circuit has an inspiratory limb only (Fig. 5.18). Expiration occurs through an expiratory valve mounted at the patient end of the limb. Genuine single-limb circuits require a specially designed ventilator, intended for non-invasive ventilation. A typical example is the circuit for the BiPAP (bilevel positive airway pressure) Vision or the Respironics V60 ventilator from Philips Healthcare.

Pseudo single-limb circuits are more common (Fig. 5.19). The circuits have one tube with two separate lumina; one for inspiration and the other for expiration. These circuits retain the basic structure of a classic dual-limb circuit. Pseudo single-limb circuits have two variations: coaxial tube and limb-θ tube, shown in Fig. 5.19.

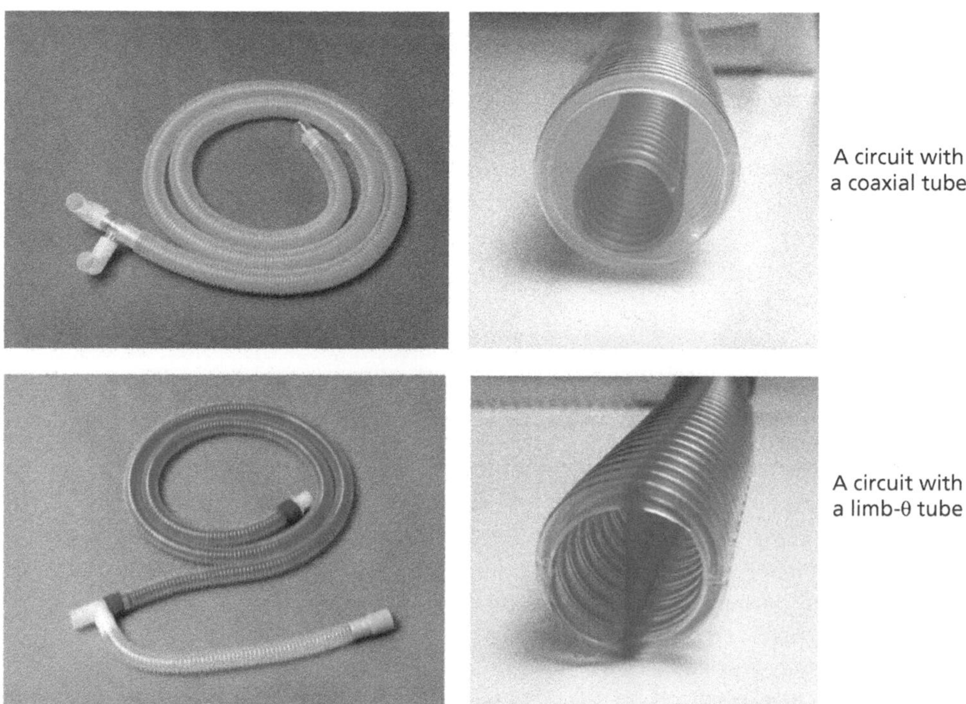

Fig. 5.19 Two pseudo single-limb circuit designs.

We need to be aware that pseudo single-limb circuits have a higher flow resistance due to the decreased effective cross section. In other words, the imposed *work of breathing* is higher, particularly when the ventilated patient has a higher-than-usual flow demand.

Circuit compliance and compliance compensation

All mechanical breaths are either volume or pressure controlled. Here, *controlled* means the way a ventilator controls delivery of inspiratory gas. In Chapter 7 we will discuss this in depth. In a volume breath, a ventilator delivers an exact, predefined volume into the breathing circuit.

Let's assume that we set the tidal volume to 500 ml, and that the ventilator delivers exactly that much gas into the circuit. If we simultaneously measure the volume at the airway, surprisingly the measured tidal volume is only about 450 ml! The patient receives 450 ml instead of the set 500 ml. We check everything and find that the monitoring is accurate. We call this phenomenon *circuit volume loss*.

But where did that extra 50 ml go? During mechanical ventilation, the pressure in a ventilator system fluctuates. In Chapter 2, we learned that gas is compressible. A change in the pressure causes a corresponding change in the gas volume. Further, a positive pressure can slightly expand the elastic tubes of a breathing circuit. The gas compression and tube expansion are responsible for this circuit volume loss.

The lost volume is directly related to the positive pressure applied. We use the term *circuit compliance* to describe this pressure–volume relationship. Every breathing circuit has its own individual circuit compliance.

Like lung compliance, circuit compliance is expressed in ml/cmH_2O. If we assume that the compliance of an adult breathing circuit is 2 ml/cmH_2O, and the inspiratory pressure (the difference between plateau pressure and PEEP) is 25 ml/cmH_2O, then the lost volume would be 50 ml. Generally, the higher the inspiratory pressure, the greater the lost volume.

Note that circuit volume loss is an issue for volume breaths only, not pressure breaths. The lost volume is recognizable only when the tidal volume is measured at the airway.

Lost volume can be compensated automatically if a ventilator has a *circuit compliance compensation* feature. Its principle is simple: the ventilator delivers slightly more gas into the circuit than the set tidal volume so that the patient receives the set tidal volume. Looking at the example discussed, in order for the patient to receive the expected tidal volume of 500 ml, the ventilator actually delivers 550 ml into the circuit.

5.3.5 Artificial airway

Anatomically, the airway (or natural airway) is the *gas passageway* between the atmosphere and alveoli. It may be divided into the upper airway and the lower airway. The upper airway includes the nose, nasal cavity, mouth, pharynx, and larynx. The lower airway includes everything from the trachea, primary bronchi and bronchial tree to the small bronchioles.

Purely from a mechanical viewpoint, the structure of the upper airway may be compared to the letter *X*. The mouth and nose are the two upper legs, while the trachea and oesophagus are the two lower legs. The epiglottis serves as a valve to control which channel intakes of gas, liquid, or food take.

This *X* structure is the anatomic basis of some clinical phenomena closely associated with intubation and mechanical ventilation. Due to this X-like structure, we can place an endotracheal tube (ETT) via either the nose or the mouth. However, the ETT may be misplaced into the oesophagus; positive airway pressure may cause gastric distension; and gastric content may accidentally enter the trachea, causing gastric aspiration.

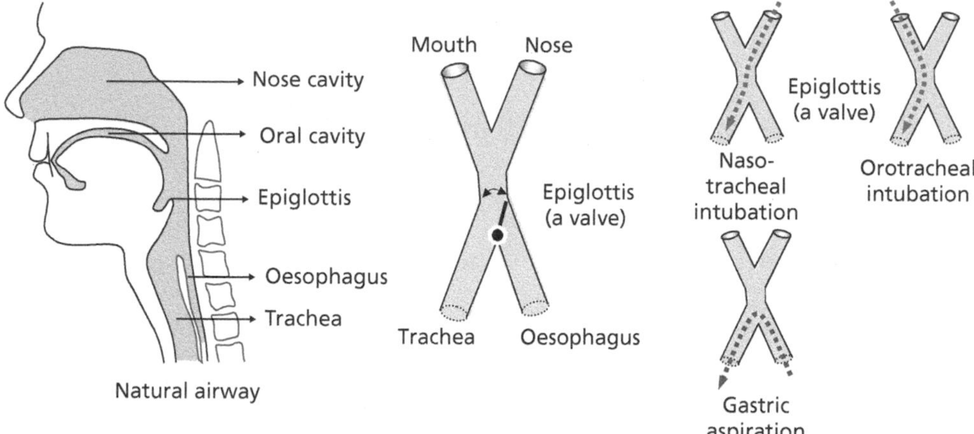

Fig. 5.20 Airway anatomy and the function of the epiglottis.

As Fig. 5.20 shows, orotracheal or nasotracheal intubation bypasses the epiglottis and vocal cords. As a result, the patient cannot speak, and aspiration can occur if the cuff of the ETT or tracheostomy tube (TT) is not inflated properly.

5.3.6 Invasive artificial airway

Mechanical ventilation has two primary forms: invasive and non-invasive. Invasive ventilation requires intubation, while non-invasive ventilation does not.

An *artificial airway* connects the breathing circuit to the natural airway (Fig. 5.21). It includes everything from the Y-piece to the trachea, possibly including an ETT or a TT, a flex tube, a proximal flow sensor, an HME, and a CO_2 adapter.

Endotracheal tube (ETT) and tracheostomy tube (TT) *Intubation* (or *tracheal intubation*) is the placement of a flexible plastic tube into the trachea of a critically ill or anesthetized patient. It keeps the airway open and facilitates invasive mechanical ventilation.

There are two common intubation techniques: inserting an ETT through a nasal or oral route, or introducing a TT into the trachea through a surgically created route. An ETT is typically for emergency or short-term use, while a TT is for mid- or long-term use. These are shown in Fig. 5.22.

Most adult and paediatric ETTs and TTs have a balloon (called a cuff) near the patient end. The cuff should be inflated after tube placement. The inflated cuff seals the airway and prevents aspiration of gastric contents. For the cuff to achieve these goals, an appropriate pressure must

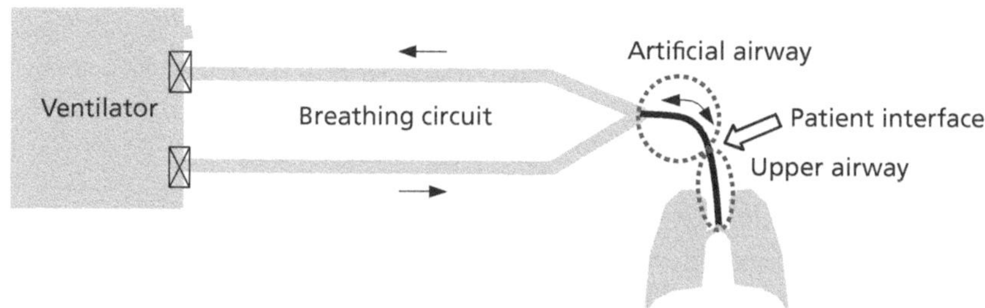

Fig. 5.21 Artificial airway and patient interface.

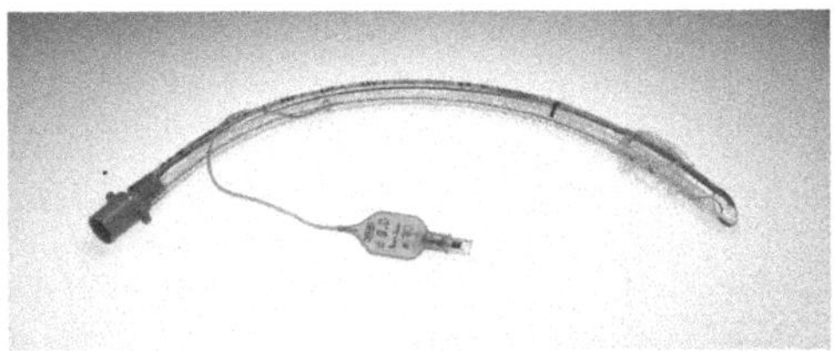

Endotracheal tube (ETT)

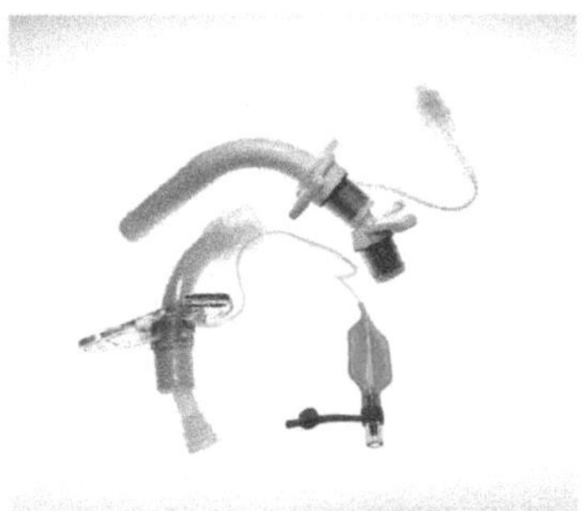

Tracheostomy tube (TT)

Fig. 5.22 An endotracheal tube (ETT) and a tracheostomy tube (TT).

be maintained. Neonatal ETTs are typically uncuffed, as the cricoid cartilage is the narrowest portion of the airway and usually provides an adequate seal for mechanical ventilation.

Although intubation is an effective emergency medical procedure, it may have unwanted complications, including loss of speech; extreme discomfort; loss of air conditioning at the nose; oesophageal or bronchial intubation; broncho- or laryngo-spasm; oesophageal, tracheal, or bronchial perforation; tube obstruction; or aspiration of gastric contents. For this reason intubation should be performed with great care, and the tubes should be kept as short as clinically possible.

Optional components of the artificial airway Besides an ETT or a TT, an artificial airway may also (but does not have to) include a flex tube, a proximal flow sensor, an HME (heat and moisture exchanger), the probe of a mainstream capnograph, and an adapter for a closed tracheal suctioning system. These optional components are shown in Table 5.3.

There are good practical or clinical needs for the optional items. Keep in mind, however, that every component imposes additional dead space, airway resistance, weight, and size to the artificial airway. Finally, a 'fully loaded' artificial airway may be unacceptable. Therefore, use such components only when absolutely necessary.

Intubation and airway resistance Obviously, to be placed into the trachea, an ETT or TT must be thinner than the trachea. Keep in mind that these tubes also have walls. So logically, the inner diameter of the tube must be much smaller than that of the trachea. And a smaller gas airway means a higher resistance to gas flow (Fig. 5.23).

Poiseuille's law states that resistance increases rapidly as diameter decreases, due to the fourth power in the denominator:

$$R = \frac{8nl}{\pi r^4}$$

where: R = resistance, n = viscosity, l = length, and r = radius.

Table 5.3 Optional components of the artificial airway

Item	Graphic	Description and remarks
Flex tube		A flex tube allows the ventilated patient to move their head more easily, and it facilitates tracheal suctioning with the opening at the right angle.
Proximal flow sensor		A proximal flow sensor is a sensor positioned at the artificial airway. This unique position gives it two advantages: (a) monitoring is more sensitive, simply because it occurs close to the signal source, and (b) monitoring (pressure, flow, and volume) is little affected by circuit artefacts such as circuit compliance. To the left you can see proximal flow sensors from Hamilton Medical. They have a variable orifice.
Heat and moisture exchanger (HME)		An HME is a passive gas humidifier that captures and retains the heat and moisture from a patient's expired gas and then releases it into the incoming gas with the next inspired breath. HMEs can provide a humidity of 10 to 31 mg/L at a temperature of 30°C. An HME is a substitute for an active humidifier. An HME has many advantages. It requires no capital investment, is easy to use, requires no cleaning, and eliminates condensed water in the circuit. However, the use of an HME is contraindicated in some cases.
Mainstream CO_2 probe		The probe is a part of the system for continuous CO_2 measurement in respiratory gases. The result may be presented numerically as an $etCO_2$ reading or graphically as a *capnogram*. The probe contains two parts, an infrared sensor and an airway adapter. The monitor may be a standalone device or it may be integrated into another medical device, e.g., an ICU ventilator. In mainstream capnography, the sample cell is installed into an artificial airway.
Closed suctioning system adapter		The adapter shown is part of a closed (tracheal) suctioning system, which is used to remove tracheal secretions from a ventilated patient without airway disconnection. The perceived advantages of closed suctioning include better infection control, continuation of mechanical ventilation, and maintenance of PEEP.

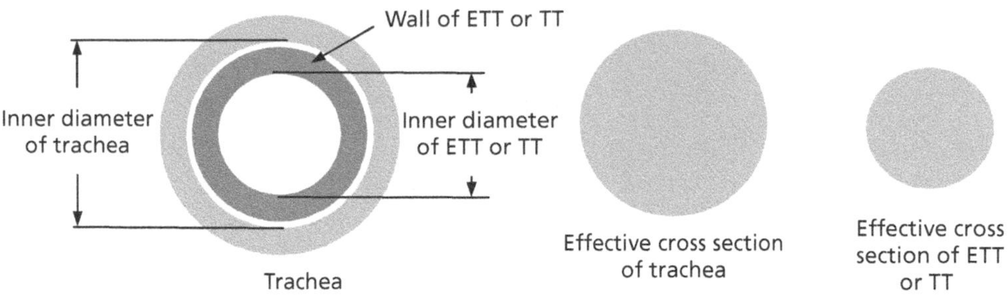

Fig. 5.23 Tracheal intubation significantly decreases the effective cross section, posing higher resistance to air movement.

Overcoming the imposed resistance requires a greater pressure gradient. This means that an intubated patient must breathe harder (i.e. have a greater work of breathing).

Some ICU ventilators have a feature called *ATC* (*automatic tube compensation*) or *TRC* (*tube resistance compensation*) to automatically compensate the resistance imposed by the ETT or TT. Note that tube resistance is not the same as respiratory resistance. In Chapter 10 we will discuss ATC/TRC in depth.

Airway resistance may increase for several other reasons, such as an obstructed or kinked tracheal tube or an HME clogged with secretions or blood clots. These are emergencies, requiring immediate correction.

Instrumental dead space Dead space is defined as the portion of tidal volume that is not involved in gas exchange. In normal human beings, dead space has two parts:

- *Anatomical dead space*: The volume of gas to fill the respiratory tract except for gas exchange areas.
- *Alveolar dead space*: The volume of those alveoli that are ventilated but not perfused, and where, as a result, no gas exchange can occur. Alveolar dead space is negligible in healthy individuals, but can increase dramatically in some lung diseases due to ventilation–perfusion mismatch.

Physiological dead space is the sum of both anatomical and alveolar dead spaces. It is approximately 150 ml in a young adult, and it increases slightly with age.

An intubated patient has yet another type of dead space: *instrumental dead space*. This is the volume of gas that fills the artificial airway, from the Y-piece to the opening of the natural upper airway. Instrumental dead space may noticeably reduce alveolar ventilation per minute, and in turn, CO_2 elimination.

Therefore, alveolar ventilation per minute decreases when total dead space increases, provided that rate and tidal volume remain unchanged:

$$\textit{Total dead space} = \textit{Anatomical dead space} + \textit{Alveolar dead space} + \textit{Instrumental dead space}$$

The following equation is used to calculate alveolar ventilation per minute:

$$\textit{Alveolar ventilation per minute} = \textit{Rate} \times (\textit{Tidal volume} - \textit{Total dead space})$$

As you can see, total dead space increases when instrumental dead space increases, provided that anatomical and alveolar dead spaces remain unchanged.

Table 5.4 Dead space of accessories added to the artificial airway

Accessory	Approximate instrumental dead space
Endotracheal tube	2 ml
Flex tube	16 ml (adult), 7 ml (paediatric)
Proximal flow sensor	10 ml (adult), 1–2 ml (neonate)
Airway CO_2 probe	7 ml (adult), 2 ml (neonate)
Heat moisture exchanger (HME)	2.5–90 ml

Neonates with tiny tidal volumes are very sensitive to any small increase in instrumental dead space.

The amount of instrumental dead space may range from negligible, if the ETT is connected directly to the Y-piece, to considerable, if several accessories (e.g. proximal flow sensor, HME, flex tube, and *capnography* probe) are added to the artificial airway.

Table 5.4 lists the approximate instrumental dead space of some airway components.

5.3.7 Non-invasive interface

Intubation is one way to connect the breathing circuit to the patient's airway, but not the only one. The other way is through a non-invasive patient interface. Normally, the natural airway has two openings, the nose and the mouth. An interface that covers the patient's nose, or mouth, or both with little gas leakage can permit mechanical ventilation without the need for intubation.

Generally speaking, there are four types of *non-invasive interface* (Fig. 5.24):

- *Mouthpieces* and *oral masks*;
- *Nasal masks* and *nasal prongs*, covering the nose only;
- *Full face masks*, also called *oro-nasal masks*, and *total face masks*, which cover both the nose and mouth;
- *Helmet*, enclosing the entire head with a soft seal over the upper chest.

Fig. 5.25 shows typical examples of full and total face masks.

A complete interface includes two main parts: the interface itself and the fixation device. The fixation device should secure the interface properly in the right position even when the patient moves their head. The fixation device is typically *headgear*, which may be of various designs.

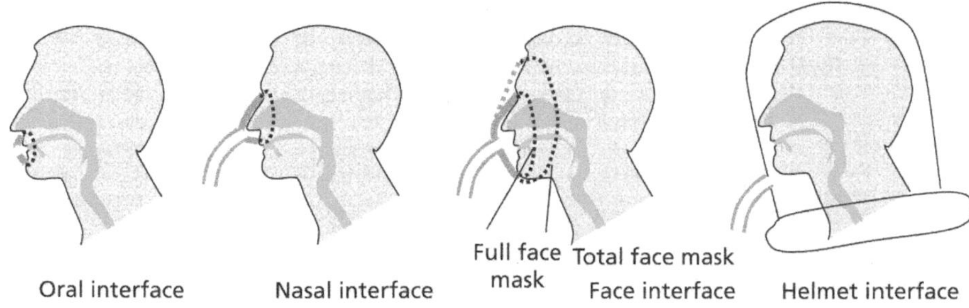

Fig. 5.24 Four basic types of non-invasive airway interface.

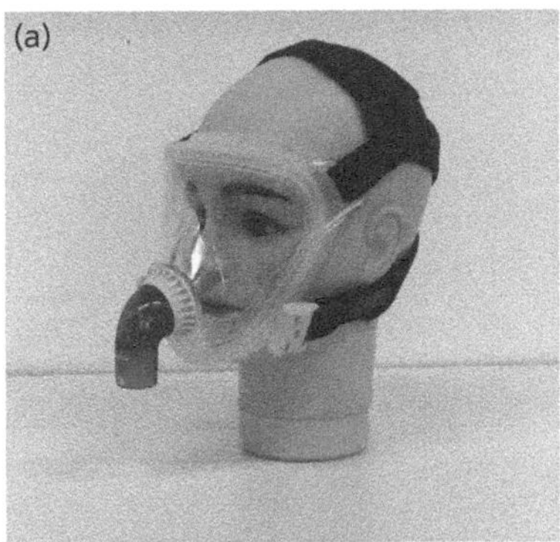

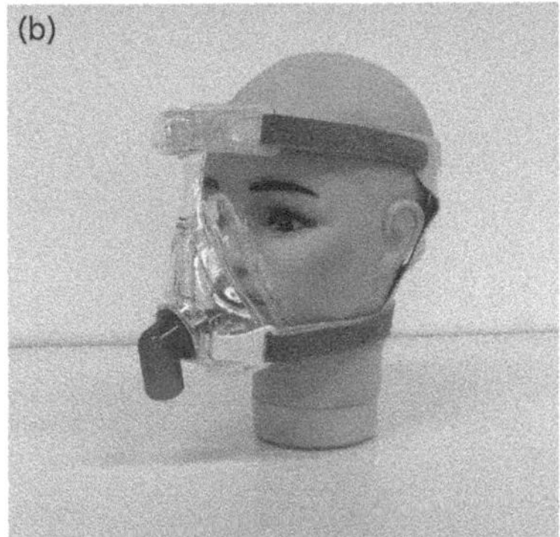

Fig. 5.25 Total face mask (left) and full face mask (right) from Philips Respironics.

In theory it should be possible to use any IPPV ventilator for non-invasive ventilation, assuming the interface is truly gas tight. In reality, however, controlling leakage at the interface is a big challenge, because everybody has a unique face size and profile. It is simply not possible to design one mask that fits all faces; and due to positive internal pressure, even a small face–mask mismatch causes gas leakage at the interface.

Thanks to continuous efforts by mask manufacturers, today's masks and fixation devices are far better than those of one or two decades ago, with technical improvements and innovations certain to continue.

To minimize gas leakage at the interface, three measures may help.

First, have a wide variety of interfaces in different shapes and sizes readily available.

Second, pay attention to the quality of the interface. The quality is often directly related to the cost. You face a tough purchasing decision, deciding between poor but cheap masks and good

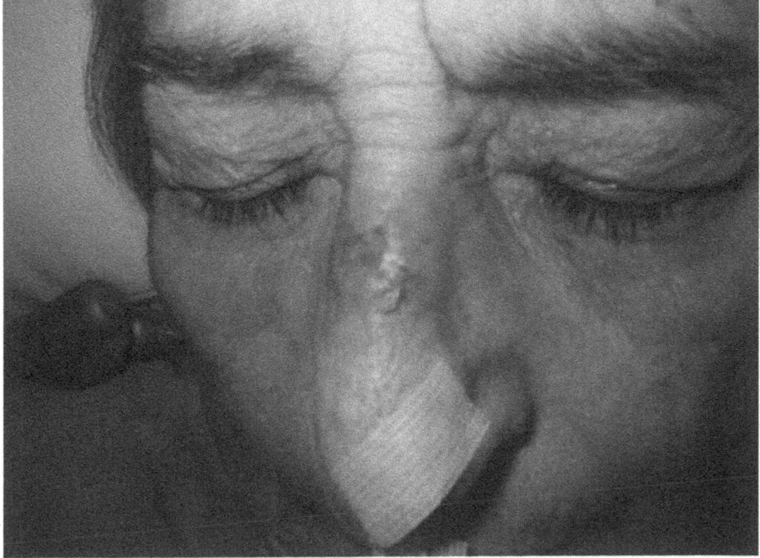

Fig. 5.26 Ischaemic skin lesion during non-invasive mechanical ventilation.

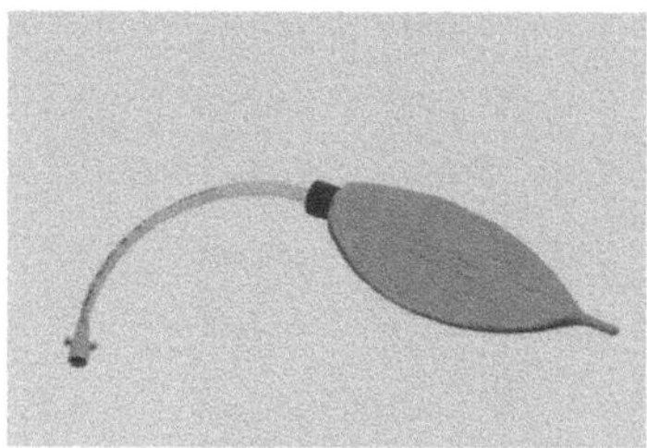

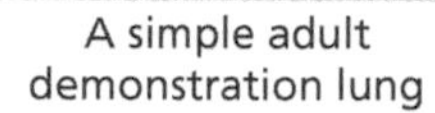

A simple adult demonstration lung

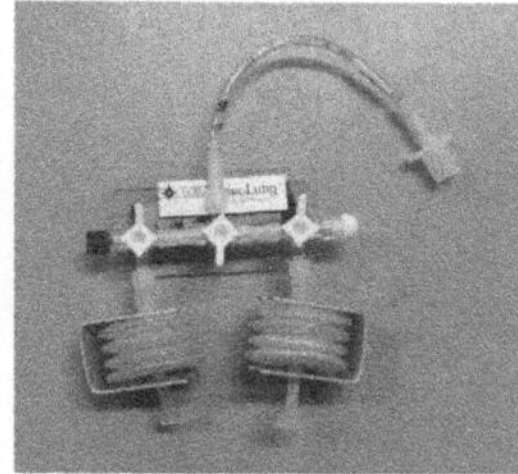

A neonatal demonstration lung

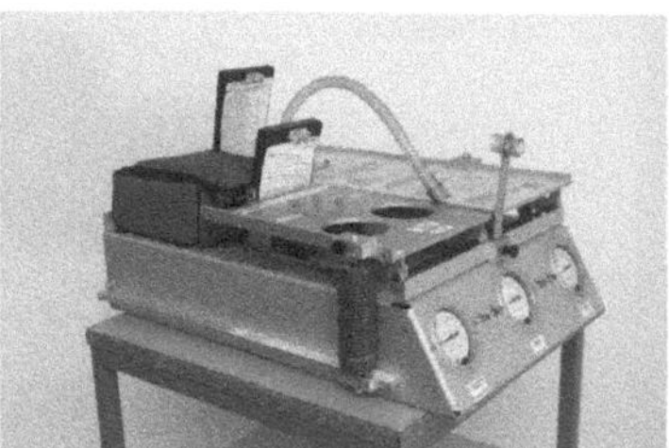

Michigan test lung

Fig. 5.27 Some lung models to mimic a natural airway-lung system.

but expensive ones. This may be the wrong place to save money, because a bad interface can easily cause non-invasive ventilation therapy to fail completely.

Third, refrain from increasing the tension on the headgear in order to control gas leakage. The right solution includes a better fitting mask, better positioning of the mask, and better fixation. Otherwise, ischaemic skin breakdown will be inevitable due to the continuous tension applied (Fig. 5.26).

Non-invasive ventilation requires that the ventilator design be modified so that the ventilator system can work nearly normally even with moderate leakage at the interface. However, beware of some ventilator manufacturers' claims of 'leak compensation'. A ventilator system can tolerate only a certain level of gas leakage. No ventilator system can compensate the maximum possible gas leak, that is, disconnection.

5.3.8 The lungs

The lungs correspond to the balloon in the balloon model we saw earlier. They are also a required part of a ventilator system: the system simply does not work without them. A demonstration lung model or *test lung*, which is typically a rubber bag, may be used to mimic the lungs (Fig. 5.27).

A ventilator system can function normally only if the lungs or a demonstration lung model meet these requirements:

- They have a balloon-like structure.
- They are elastic, so that their volume changes when the internal pressure changes. Pleural effusion or high abdominal tension may significantly limit their inflatability.
- They do not have an abnormal opening to the atmosphere or to another cavity. A pneumothorax and a bronchopleural fistula by a chest drainage tube are two examples of such an abnormality.

Demonstration lungs differ in size for adult, paediatric, and neonatal applications. You need to choose the right one for the intended application.

Chapter 6

Humidification, Nebulization, and Gas Filtering

6.1 Introduction

Humidification, nebulization, and respiratory gas filtering are therapies or techniques that are frequently applied together with mechanical ventilation therapy. Commonly required items for these therapies are listed in Table 6.1.

These techniques are frequently used with mechanical ventilation, but they are not required parts, because a ventilator system can function perfectly or even better without them. They are added to the system for clinical reasons.

The presence of these items, especially those for humidification, noticeably changes the setup of a breathing circuit. And their functional status can greatly affect the performance of a ventilator system.

6.2 Artificial humidification

6.2.1 Air conditioning at nose and intubation

Artificial humidification refers to the technique used to artificially warm and humidify the inspiratory gas.

Why is this necessary? To understand, we need to know that the *nose* has an important but less mentioned physiological function: *air conditioning*. This refers to the warming, humidifying, and filtering of the inhaled air.

Depending on the local climate, the temperature and relative humidity (RH) of the ambient air vary widely. To compensate for such differences, the nose efficiently warms, humidifies, and cleans the inhaled air. By the time air reaches the carina or the end of the trachea, its temperature is approximately 37°C or 98.6°F and its relative humidity is 100%. Warm and humid air is critical for the physiological functioning of the airway and lungs.

Why do we need to pay special attention to inspiratory gas warming and humidifying in intubated and mechanically ventilated patients?

Intubation involves placing a tube in a patient's trachea. Through either an endotracheal tube (ETT) or a tracheostomy tube (TT), the inspiratory gas enters the trachea directly; see Fig. 6.1. In either case, the gas is *not* conditioned.

Now let's measure the temperature and relative humidity of inspiratory gas at the trachea using three different scenarios. In the first scenario, normal breathing, room air is inhaled and conditioned as described above. The second scenario involves a patient who is intubated but not mechanically ventilated, so they inhale unconditioned room air. The third scenario involves a patient who is intubated and mechanically ventilated. The inhaled gas originates from the ventilator's gas source. Typically, such gases are at close to room temperature and are extremely dry (<5% RH). These situations are visualized in Fig. 6.2. Cold and dry gases directly entering the

Table 6.1 Items required for humidification, in-line nebulization, and gas filtering

Therapy or technique	Humidification	Nebulization	Gas filtering
Required items	Active humidifier kit	Pneumatic nebulizer kit	Inspiratory filter
	Heat and moisture exchanger (HME)	Ultrasonic nebulizer kit	Expiratory filter

trachea may cause inspissation of airway secretions, destruction of airway epithelium, atelectasis, and hypothermia. To avoid these complications, inspiratory gas must be sufficiently warmed and humidified before entering the airway, as indicated by the light green arrows.

There are two common techniques to artificially warm and humidify inspiratory gases: an active humidifier set, and a heat and moisture exchanger (HME). For every intubated and mechanically ventilated patient, one of these techniques should be deployed.

The AARC (American Association of Respiratory Care) recommends that: (a) an active humidifier provide a *humidity* level between 33 mg/L and 44 mg/L of water and a gas temperature between 34°C and 41°C at the Y-piece, with RH of 100%; and (b) an HME provide a minimum of 30 mg H_2O/L. This is the goal to achieve for artificial humidification during mechanical ventilation (Restrepo and Walsh, 2012).

6.2.2 Gas humidity and temperature

Now let's learn a few special terms that are frequently used in artificial humidification: condensation, evaporation, absolute humidity, relative humidification, and dew point.

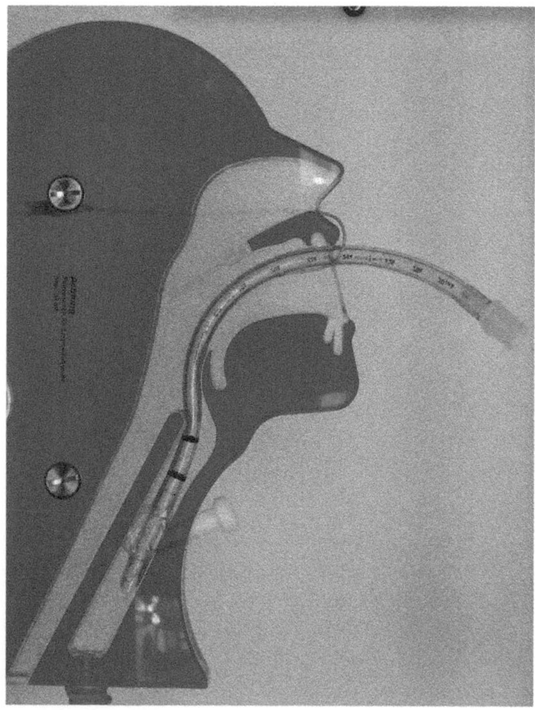

Fig. 6.1 Intubation with an endotracheal tube (ETT).

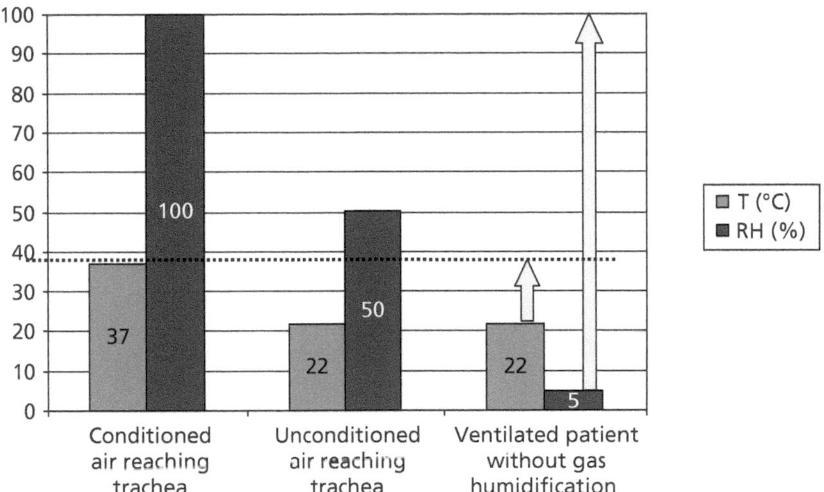

Fig. 6.2 Inspiratory gas temperature (T) and relative humidity (RH) at the trachea in three scenarios. The two light green arrows indicate how much the gas temperature and relative humidity need to be artificially increased during invasive mechanical ventilation.

Condensation is the process by which water is converted from its vapour form to its liquid form (droplets). Essentially, condensation is the consequence of air or gas oversaturation. Condensation typically occurs when warm air comes in contact with a cold surface.

Evaporation is the process by which water is converted from its liquid form to its vapour form. Evaporation increases when (a) gas temperature rises, (b) vapour partial pressure is low, and/or (c) the air moves (wind).

Air can hold a certain amount of water vapour. It is interesting and important to know that the maximum amount of vapour content that a unit volume of air can hold is temperature dependent. Warm air can hold more water vapour than cool air.

Two terms are commonly used to express the gas humidity: absolute humidity and relative humidity.

Absolute humidity (AH) is the water vapour present in a unit volume of air, typically expressed in milligrams per litre (mg/L) or kilograms per cubic metre (kg/m^3). Absolute humidity does not fluctuate with the temperature of the air.

Relative humidity (RH) is the the ratio of the amount of water vapour in air at a given temperature to the maximum amount that the air could hold at that temperature. With a given amount of water vapour, an increase in air temperature leads to a decrease in the RH simply because warm air can hold more water vapour.

$$RH = \frac{\textit{Actual vapor content}\ (\text{mg/L})}{\textit{Maximum vapor content}\ (\text{mg/L})} \times 100\%$$

Relative humidity can be regarded as the level of vapour saturation. A relative humidity of 50% means that the air holds just half of the maximum vapour content it can hold at the current temperature.

Dew point is the temperature at which the air becomes 100% saturated with vapour. For a given vapour content, there is a fixed dew point (temperature).

Fig. 6.3 shows the relationship between temperature, absolute humidity, and relative humidity.

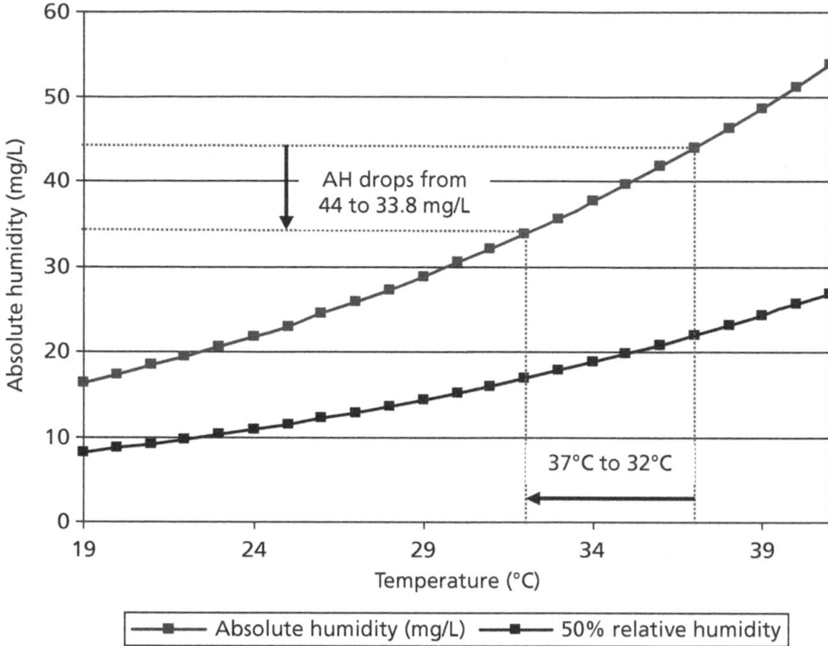

Fig. 6.3 The relationship between temperature, absolute humidity (AH), and relative humidity (RH).

6.2.3 Active humidifier

An *active humidifier*, also known as a *heated humidifier*, is a medical device designed to continuously warm and humidify the gas that a intubated and mechanically ventilated patient inhales. An active humidifier is integrated into the breathing circuit of a ventilator system.

An active humidifier typically includes these items:

- A humidifier base (heater).
- A water reservoir.
- A gas temperature sensor. Initially, this was just an airway gas thermometer positioned at the Y-piece. Modern active humidifiers often have a *dual temperature sensor*, which monitors the gas temperatures at the reservoir outlet and the Y-piece simultaneously. The results are used to regulate heating intensity.
- One or two water traps to remove the condensed water from the circuit tube.
- Heating wire, which is placed in the circuit tube to prevent the air temperature from dropping as the gas travels through the tube.
- (Optional) An expiratory filter and heater to minimize condensation in the expiratory limb.

Which parts are used depends upon the design of active humidifier.

Most active humidifiers work like a kettle, as shown in Fig. 6.4. The relatively cold and dry gas is warmed and humidified when it travels through the water reservoir, which is continuously heated. The passing gas continuously removes heat and water vapour, so that the reservoir must be heated continuously and refilled periodically.

This kettle principle is a common foundation of most active humidifiers, including those from Fisher & Paykel and Hudson RCI (Teleflex). An exception is the Gründler humidifier, where inspiratory gas passes through a sponge through which warm water circulates. The structures of these humidifiers are shown in Fig. 6.5.

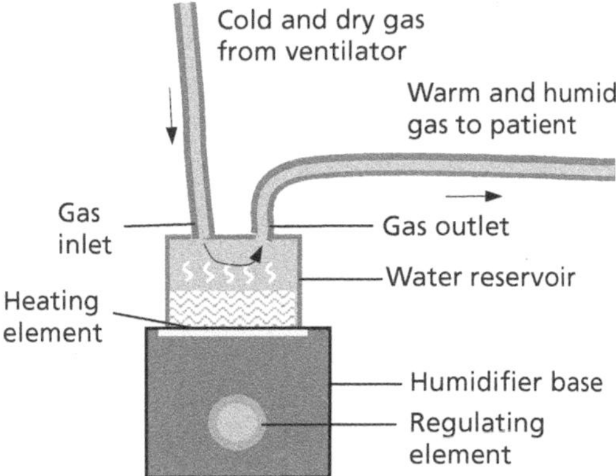

Fig. 6.4 An active humidifier is comparable to a kettle.

A general goal of active humidification is to ensure that the inspiratory gas at the Y-piece is approximately 37°C (or 98.6°F) and 100% in relative humidity (i.e. 44 mg/L in vapour content).

During mechanical ventilation, inspiratory flow is not stable. At a high flow, the passing gas carries away more heat, and vice versa. Therefore, an active humidifier needs to regulate its heating intensity according to the measured gas temperature.

6.2.4 Managing condensation

The water reservoir and the Y-piece are connected with an inspiratory tube, as shown in Fig. 6.6. This tube is relatively cold, so the warm gas cools as it passes through the tube.

In order to offset the cooling effect and ensure that the gas temperature at the Y-piece is 37°C, the gas at the reservoir must be warmer (i.e. up to 45°C). This is technically possible. However, if the gas is fully vapour saturated (100%), we have a new problem—condensation.

As we saw earlier, warmer air can hold more vapour than cooler air. At 45°C one litre of air can hold 66 mg/L, while at 37°C it can only hold a maximum of 44 mg/L. As the gas cools, the surplus vapour of 22 mg/litre condenses into liquid form.

Condensation also occurs in the expiratory limb due to this cooling effect. At the Y-piece, the exhaled gas is approximately 37°C, with vapour content of 44 mg/L. At the expiratory valve, it is approximately 30°C, with vapour content of 30 mg/L. The surplus is 12 mg/L. In both cases condensation is inevitable.

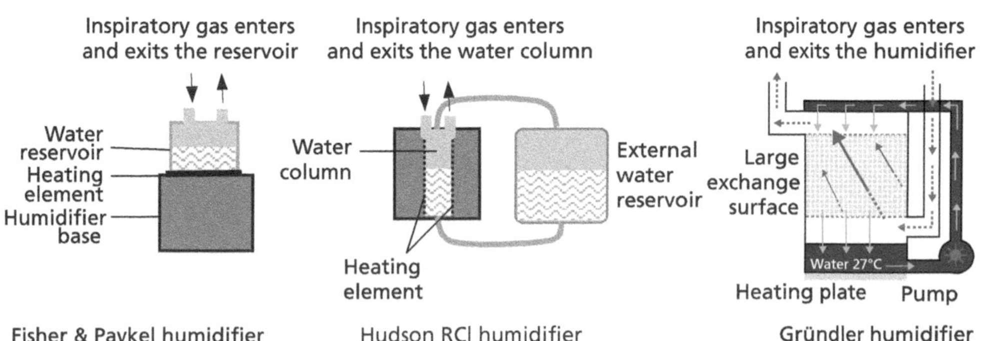

Fig. 6.5 Three active humidifier structures.
Used with permission from Gründler Medical.

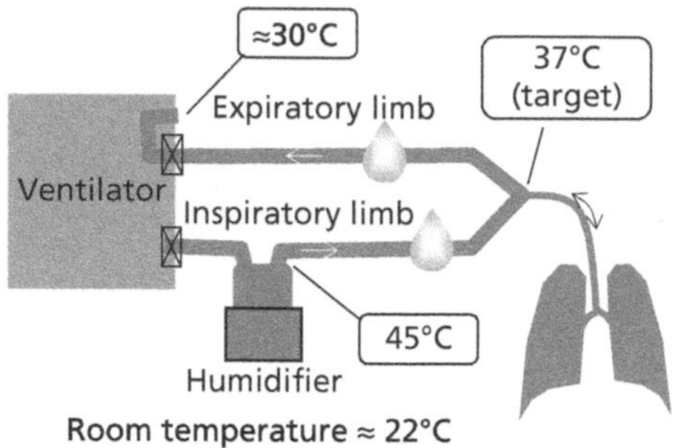

Fig. 6.6 Circuit rainout occurs if saturated, warm gas cools.

Water condensation is a continuous process. Initially, there may be just some drops on the inner surface of the tube. Over time, more and more water accumulates in the circuit tubes. You can easily recognize the water by listening for the sound of water being pushed by the passing gas flow. An accumulation of condensed water in the breathing circuit is called *circuit rainout*.

Does water inside the circuit really matter?

The answer depends entirely on the amount. Condensed water always stays in the lowest parts of the tubes due to gravity (Fig. 6.7). It presents a moving obstacle to the passing gas flow, resulting in local turbulence. If the amount of water is tiny, the influence is negligible. However, a significant amount of water can seriously interfere with gas movement, which is easily visible in a pressure–time waveform (Fig. 6.8). Such interference is an important cause of auto-triggering (i.e. the triggering of the ventilator by pneumatic artefact rather than the patient's inspiratory efforts); we will discuss normal and abnormal triggering in detail in Chapter 7. The clinical consequences of auto-triggering include hyperventilation and high respiratory frequency, along with their corresponding alarms.

If more water accumulates, the tube may become totally occluded. This is an emergency, and requires immediate corrective action.

What can be done to solve the problem of circuit condensation? There are three common solutions: (1) drain off the water, (2) minimize or prevent condensation, and (3) increase evaporation.

1. Use a water trap to drain off the water. A water trap can be used to drain condensed water from the circuit tube in order to minimize the disturbance to gas movement.

A water trap may be designed for single use or multiple uses (see Fig. 6.9). It has a cover and a container. The cover is integrated into the circuit limb. Gas passes through the cover, and the water falls into the container due to gravity. The container can be detached from the cover for emptying. The circuit should remain gas tight when the trap container is detached.

Keep the following in mind when using a water trap:

- Use a water trap whenever circuit condensation may occur.
- Make sure the water trap is always positioned at the lowest part of the circuit, and keep the cover upward, as drainage depends on gravity. This is not as easy as it sounds. Drainage cannot occur if the water trap is in any of the positions shown in Fig. 6.10.

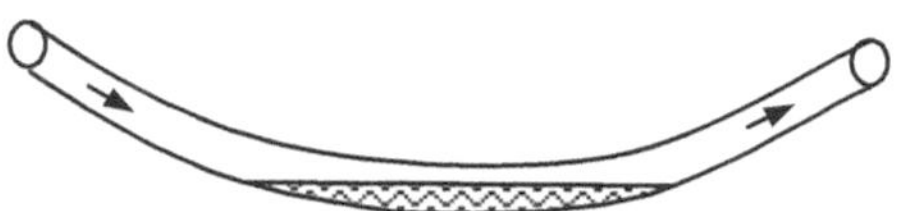

Fig. 6.7 Condensed water accumulates in the lowest part of a tube.

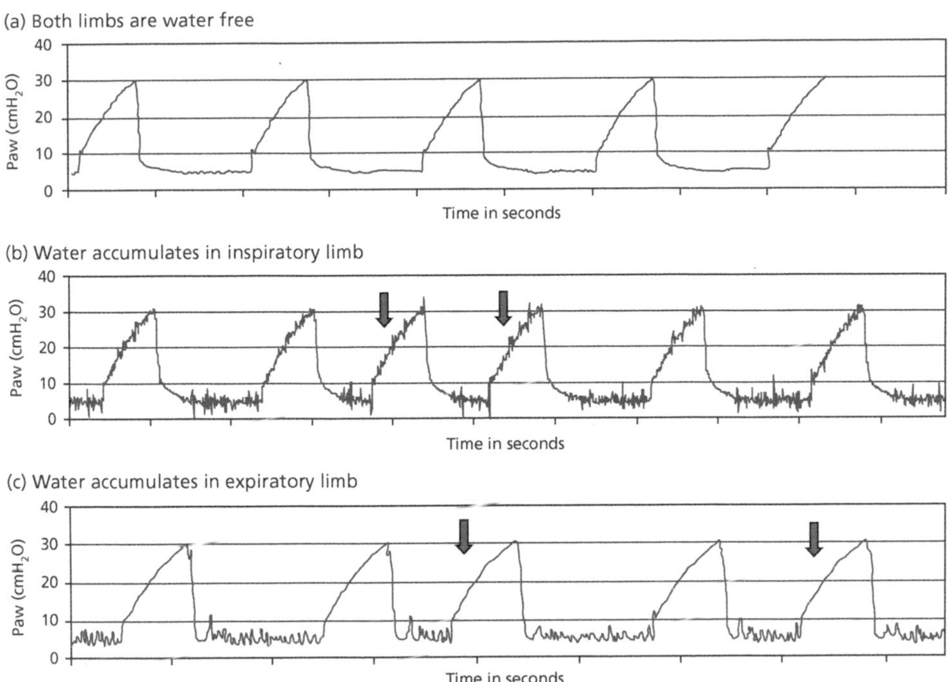

Fig. 6.8 Representative pressure–time waveforms with and without accumulated water in the circuit.

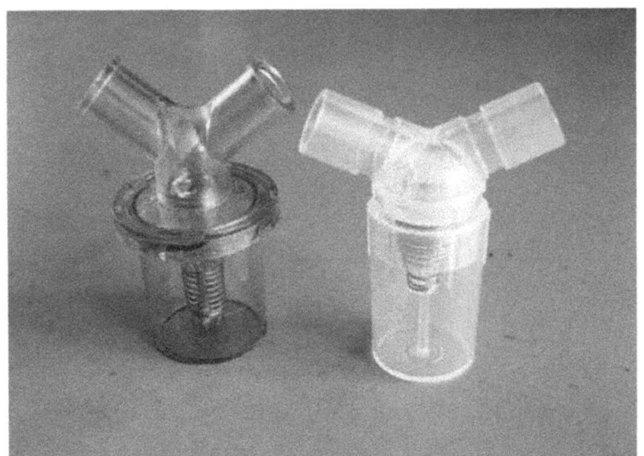

Fig. 6.9 Reusable water trap (left) and single-use water trap (right).

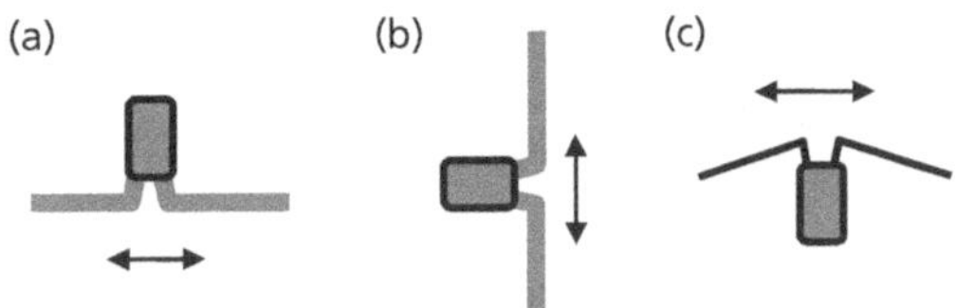

Fig. 6.10 Three incorrect water trap positions (a–c) in which condensed water can hardly enter or stay, resulting in drainage failure.

- Periodically inspect water traps and empty them if necessary.
- After emptying the container, make sure to tightly secure the container to the cover.
- The collected, condensed water is contaminated.
- Discard a water trap if it is cracked or if it leaks.
- Do not reuse water traps that are designed for single use.

2. Use a *heated circuit* to minimize condensation. We know that water condenses when warm and humid gas cools. Logically, if the travelling gas stays as warm as or even warmer than it was when it left the humidifier reservoir, condensation will not occur. This is the basic principle behind the heated circuit.

Fig. 6.11 shows a typical breathing circuit with an active humidifier. Note that the inspiratory limb, between the reservoir and the Y-piece, is heated to approximately 39°C.

Inspiratory limb heating causes two important changes. First, the gas temperature at the reservoir outlet is 37°C rather than 45°C because there is no cooling effect at the tube. Second, the tube heating also slightly warms the gas so that its relative humidity drops from 100% to around 90%. Under these conditions, condensation is unlikely to occur, at least in theory, so a water trap is unnecessary when the inspiratory limb is heated.

Technically, the heated wire solution involves a loop of *heating wire*, which is a special isolated metal wire. The wire becomes hot when an electrical current passes through it. A special cable called an *electrical adapter* connects the heating wire to the humidifier base. The heating wire is powered by the humidifier and the heating intensity is electrically regulated.

Initially, heating wires were designed for multiple use—for use with a reusable circuit with silicone tubes. After use on a patient, such a circuit must be disassembled, reprocessed (i.e. cleaned and disinfected/sterilized), and reassembled.

Today, ready-made, disposable heated circuits dominate the market. They are made of biocompatible polymers and are available in various sizes and designs. The circuits are convenient to use, but not environmentally friendly.

A heating wire that spans a tube's full length imposes additional resistance to flow. In order to eliminate the imposed resistance and to distribute the heat more evenly, some new circuits have the heating wire embedded in the wall of the tube. Fig. 6.12 shows three common heating wires.

3. Increase evaporation with a heated filter. The third solution is effective but less used. It is intended to minimize condensation at the expiratory limb by adding a large filter enclosed in an electrical heater. The filter temperature is maintained between 55°C and 70°C. This can effectively decrease the RH of the passing gas and intensify the evaporation process.

Such a heated filter can be integrated into a ventilator, as in the Puritan Bennett 840 ventilator (Fig. 6.13). Or, it may be added to the expiratory limb, as with the filter heater from VADI Medical (Fig. 6.14).

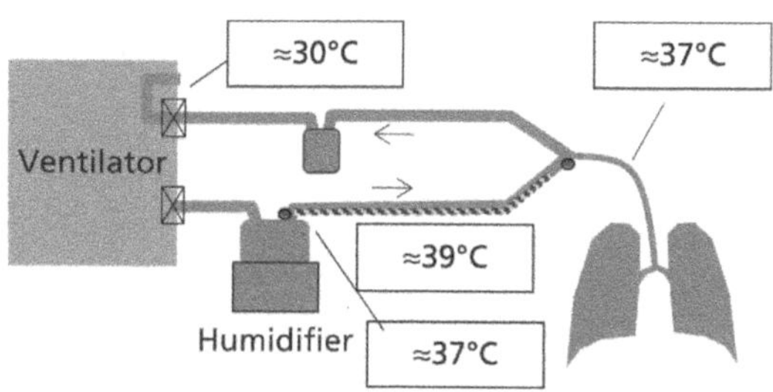

Fig. 6.11 Breathing circuit with inspiratory limb heated.

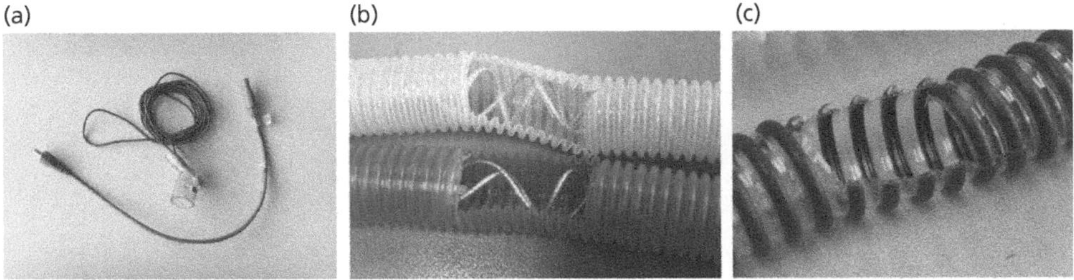

Fig. 6.12 Heating wire in three forms: (a) A reusable heating wire and an electric adapter; (b) A single-use circuit with the heating wire spiral in the lumen; and (c) A single-use circuit with the heating wire embedded in the wall of tube.

The heated filter protects the moisture-sensitive sensors at the expiratory valve and it filters the expiratory gas for staff protection.

Humidification and circuit composition

The composition of the breathing circuit varies based on the active humidifier used. There are three common circuit compositions.

Type A: Neither circuit limb heated In this configuration (Fig. 6.15), the gas temperature at the reservoir outlet must be sufficiently high to offset the tube cooling effect described earlier. Condensation is inevitable in both the inspiratory and expiratory limbs, so we need to install a water trap in both limbs to drain off the water. A typical example of this circuit includes the Fisher & Paykel MR410 humidifier. This circuit may be either reusable or for single use.

Type B: Heated inspiratory limb As shown in Fig 6.16, a large portion of the inspiratory limb, between the reservoir and the Y-piece, is heated by a heating wire.

The inspiratory limb prevents the tube cooling effect and the resultant condensation, so the inspiratory water trap is omitted. The gas temperature at the reservoir outlet is around 37°C.

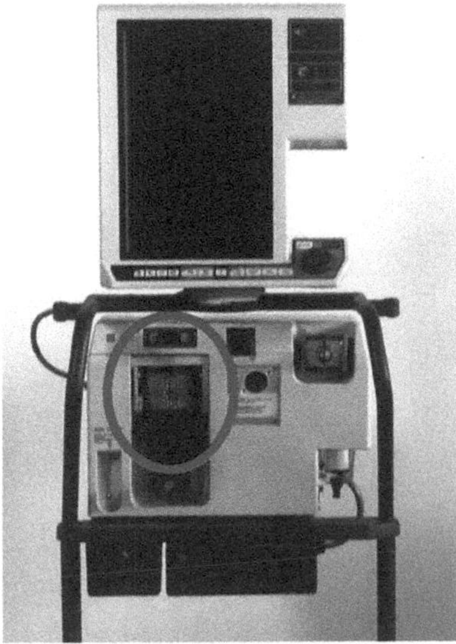

Fig. 6.13 Integrated heated filter in Puritan Bennett 840 ventilator.

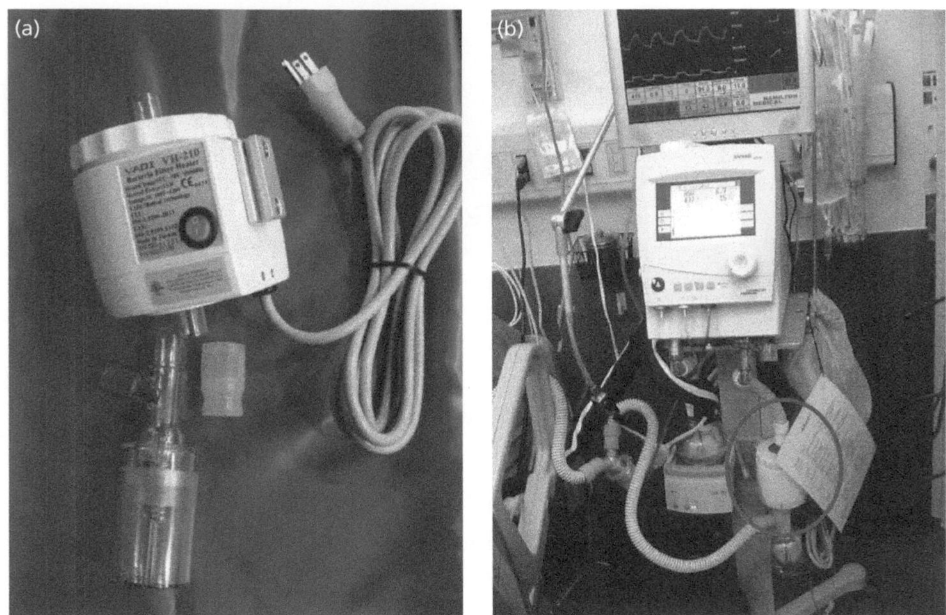

Fig. 6.14 (a) VADI Heated filter installed at expiratory limb (b) to minimize condensed water.
Reproduced with permission from VADI Medical.

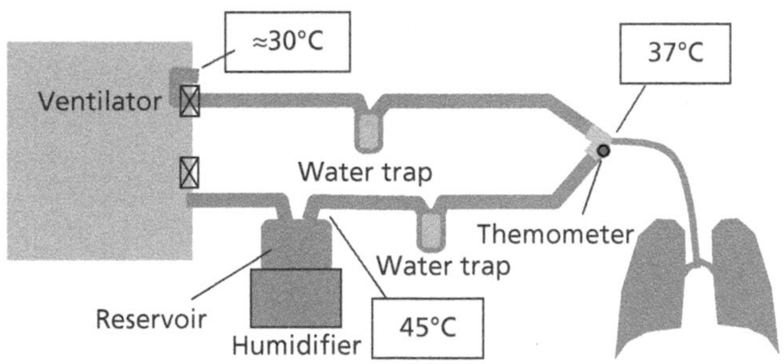

Fig. 6.15 Type A circuit with no heated limb.

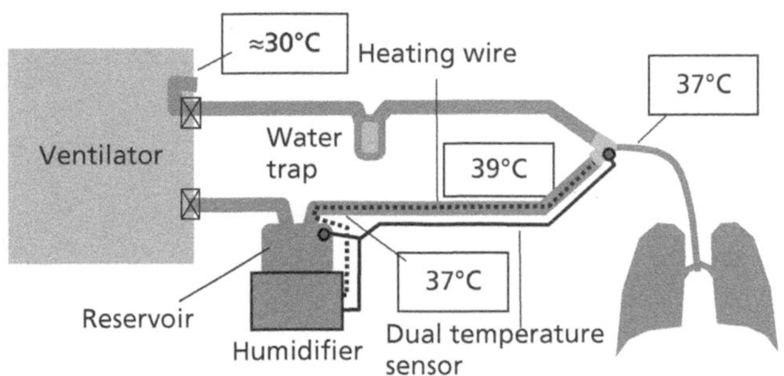

Fig. 6.16 Type B circuit with inspiratory limb heated.

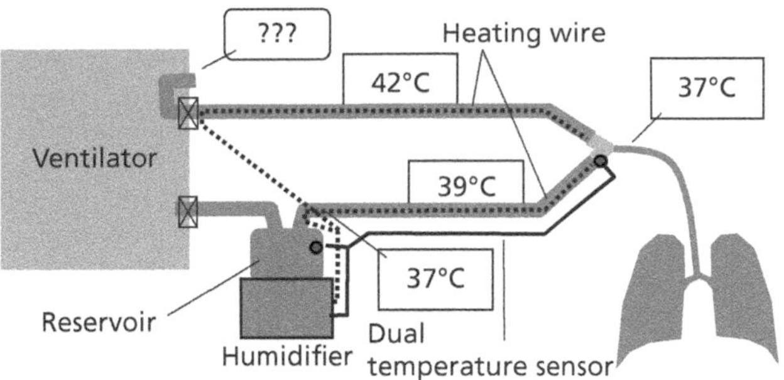

Fig. 6.17 Type C circuit with two heated limbs.

However, the expiratory water trap is still required. A typical example includes the Fisher & Paykel MR730 humidifier. Note that the tube between the ventilator outlet and the reservoir is a part of the inspiratory limb but not heated. This circuit may be either reusable or for single use.

Type C: Both circuit limbs heated As shown in Fig. 6.17, both inspiratory and expiratory limbs are heated so that condensation is not expected. Therefore, this circuit does not have a water trap. A typical example includes the Fisher & Paykel MR850 humidifier. This circuit is typically for single use.

Common problems associated with active humidification

Although the active humidifier serves important clinical needs, it often introduces problems to the ventilator system. The consequences are not only dysfunction of the humidifier, but also disturbance to the functionality of the ventilator system. Table 6.2 lists some common problems.

6.2.5 **Heat and moisture exchangers (HMEs)**

A *heat and moisture exchanger (HME)* is the other common way to warm and humidify the inspiratory gas. It is also known as a *hygroscopic condenser humidifier* or an *artificial nose.*

Technically, an HME is a special filter. Although it may resemble a non-HME airway filter, do not confuse them.

An active humidifier, described above, actively increases the heat and vapour content of inspired gas. An HME, on the other hand, operates passively by storing the heat and moisture from the patient's exhaled gas and releasing them back to the inspired gas in the next breath. An HME should be able to provide a minimum of 30 mg/L. An active humidifier and HME are never used together. An HME is positioned between the Y-piece and the ETT, and it becomes a part of the artificial airway.

When an HME is used, circuit condensation should not occur, so there is no need for a water trap or circuit limb heating. Use of an HME greatly simplifies the breathing circuit (Fig. 6.18).

An HME is most suitable for a patient on short-term mechanical ventilation (i.e. less than 96 hours). Active humidifiers, by contrast, are for both short-term and long-term mechanical ventilation.

An HME is an effective gas conditioning solution for many patients, but it is not recommended for patients with the following:

a. Thick, copious, or bloody secretions;
b. Expired tidal volume less than 70% of the delivered tidal volume (e.g. those with large bronchopleurocutaneous fistulas or incompetent or absent endotracheal tube cuffs);

Table 6.2 Common problems associated with active humidification

Problem	Root cause	Consequences	Corrective actions
No active humidification	The humidifier is not electrically powered due to (a) a plug-socket mismatch at the wall side, (b) accidental unplugging, (c) a nonfunctional socket, (d) poor connection or broken cable, or (d) failure to switch the humidifier on	Cold, dry gas entering the trachea leads to serious lung crusting and infection	Ensure that the humidifier is powered and switched on
	The humidifier is defective		Have the defective humidifier serviced
Inadequate humidification	The humidifier setting is inappropriate		Adjust the humidifier setting
	'Dry heating': the reservoir is empty		Regularly inspect and refill the reservoir
Expiratory humidification	The humidifier is incorrectly installed in the expiratory rather than the inspiratory limb so that the inspiratory gas remains cold and dry		Make sure the humidifier is installed in the inspiratory limb
Excessive condensation	The water trap is full and cannot drain off water	Auto-triggering;Patient-ventilator asynchrony; Occlusion of the gas passageway; Repeated alarms	Regularly inspect and empty the water trap
	The heating wire is defective or inadequately powered		Replace the heating wire (limb) and make sure the wire is properly powered
	The circuit was lengthened, and a part of the tube is not heating as expected		Avoid arbitrary lengthening of the circuit limbs
	The gas temperature is improperly monitored, because (a) the temperature sensor at the Y-piece is too close to the heating wire, or (b) the sensor is in a thermal environment, such as in an incubator or a warming bed in neonatal care. The heating regulation is affected in either case	Auto-triggering; Patient-ventilator asynchrony; Occlusion of the gas passageway; Repeated alarms	Consult the manufacturer of the heated circuit. Avoid placing the sensor directly in a thermal environment
Circuit overheating	Gas flow has stopped (e.g. during ventilator standby), but the humidifier remained active. Gas temperature can rise to a dangerous level, because gas temperature monitored at the Y-piece may be low. When ventilation resumes, the inspiratory gas may be very hot for the first breaths	Circuit melt-down; Airway thermal injury	Start ventilation first, then start humidification. Stop humidification first, then stop ventilation. Always turn off the humidifier when entering standby or switching off the ventilator
Gas leak	Integration of an active humidifier complicates the circuit structure. The additional connections and ports increase the probability of gas leak. The reservoir or water trap is damaged	Auto-triggering;Poor performance of ventilator system	Eliminate the leak. Refer to Chapter 13 for details. Replace the damaged items

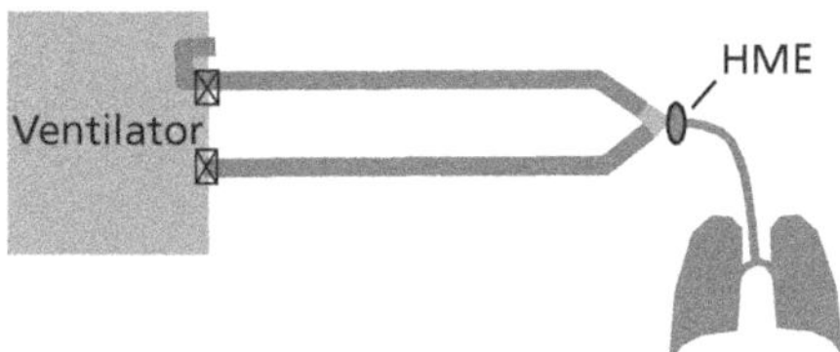

Fig. 6.18 Type D circuit with a heat and moisture exchanger (HME).

c. Body temperature less than 32°C;
d. High spontaneous minute volume (>10 L/min).

An HME must be removed during in-line nebulization.

Use of an HME poses two major risks. First, excessive liquid (secretion or blood clots) from the trachea or medication aerosols can clog an HME partially or even completely, causing dyspnoea or suffocation. Second, an HME contributes to instrumental dead space and decreases alveolar ventilation; see section 5.3.5. This adverse effect is insignificant if the tidal volume is large, but it may be deadly if the tidal volume is tiny, as in neonates.

For further information, refer to the AARC clinical practice guideline, 'Humidification during invasive and noninvasive mechanical ventilation'. (Restrepo and Walsh, 2012).

6.3 In-line nebulization

6.3.1 Aerosol nebulization

Aerosol therapy or *nebulization therapy* is a common therapy to directly administer drugs, or even sterile water, into the upper and lower airway and lungs. Aerosol therapy produces *aerosols*, airborne liquid droplets, or solid particles suspended in a gas. The therapy is widely used to treat pulmonary diseases, especially for outpatients or for home care.

The medical devices required for aerosol generation are called *nebulizers*. They generate medical aerosols with two common techniques.

6.3.2 Pneumatic (jet) nebulizer

A spray or perfume bottle is an everyday example of a *pneumatic nebulizer* or *jet nebulizer*. A pneumatic nebulizer (Fig. 6.19) is typically composed of the following items: a reservoir that contains the liquid to be aerosolized, a thin tube, a very small hole (nozzle), and a compressed

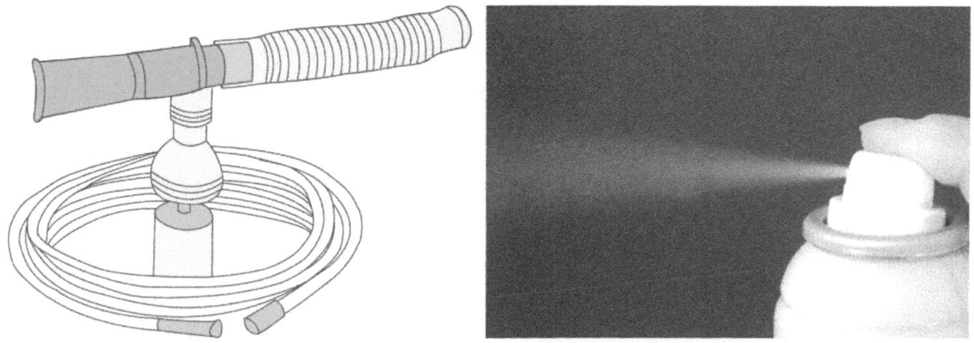

Fig. 6.19 A handheld jet nebulizer set (left) and an aerosol spray can (right).

gas source. Liquid aerosols are generated by passing gas at a high velocity through the small hole. The resulting low pressure at the jet sucks the liquid from the reservoir up through the tube, and the liquid is shattered into liquid particles. The generated aerosols spurt out, carried in an invisible gas stream.

Pneumatic nebulizers for medical use may have more sophisticated designs, but the basic principle remains the same.

Pneumatic nebulizers are simple, effective, compact, and inexpensive.

6.3.3 Ultrasonic nebulizer

Ultrasonic (or *piezoelectric*) *nebulizers* use sound waves at ultrasound frequencies to produce fine medical aerosols. An ultrasonic nebulizer is typically composed of a radio-frequency generator, a shielded cable, a piezoelectric crystal transducer, and a reservoir chamber with an inlet and an outlet. Electric current is converted into sound waves at the crystal transducer. The sound energy is transferred either indirectly through a water-filled reservoir (as shown in Fig. 6.20) or directly to a solution chamber. The gas passing through the chamber carries with it the generated aerosols.

An ultrasonic nebulizer is typically larger, more complicated, and more expensive than a pneumatic nebulizer.

A relatively new type of ultrasonic nebulizer is the *vibrating mesh nebulizer*. This device has a mesh installed at the bottom of a liquid container. When the nebulizer is powered, this mesh, made of a piezoelectric material, vibrates at a high frequency, causing a pumping action. Aerosols are produced when the liquid passes through the mesh. The size and flow of the aerosol particles are determined by the diameter of the exit aperture holes. A typical example is the Aeroneb Solo from Aerogen (Fig. 6.21).

An in-line nebulizer is typically composed of three items, listed in Table 6.3.

6.3.4 Open and in-line nebulization

Aerosol therapy is an effective treatment commonly used for a wide range of respiratory diseases. Integrated into mechanical ventilation, aerosol therapy serves the same purpose and employs

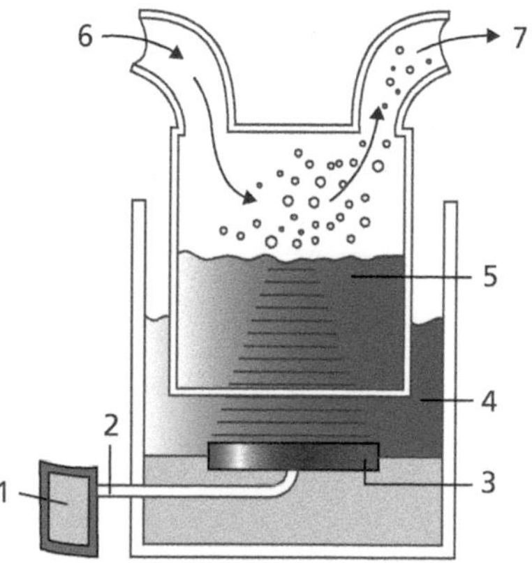

Fig. 6.20 Schematic of ultrasonic nebulizer: 1) radiofrequency generator; 2) shielded cable; 3) piezoelectric crystal transducer; 4) water-filled couplant reservoir; 5) solution chamber; 6) chamber inlet; 7) chamber outlet.

Reprinted with permission from *Egan's Fundamentals of Respiratory Care*, 8th edition, Wilkins R.L., Stroller J.K., and Scanlan C.L., p753. Copyright (2003) with permission from Mosby, Elsevier Inc.

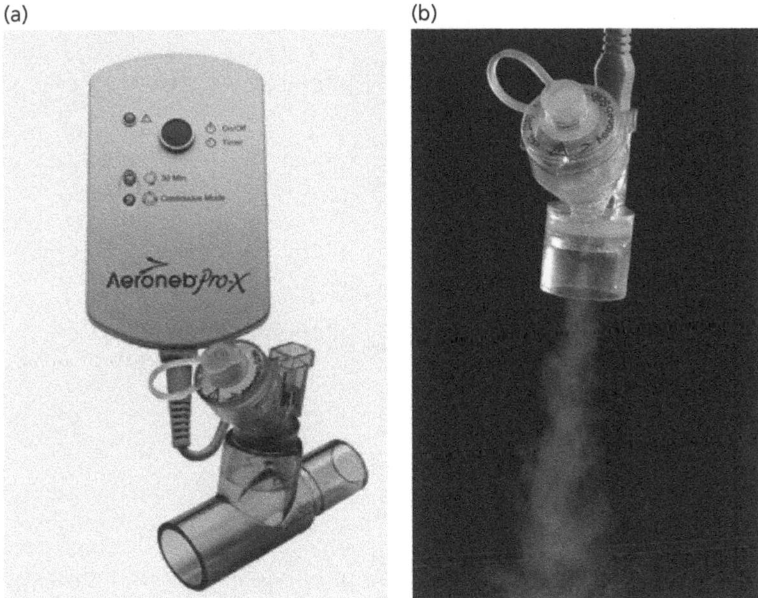

Fig. 6.21 (a) Aeroneb Pro and (b) Aeroneb Solo nebulizers.
Reprinted with permission from Aerogen.

the same techniques. However, there is a fundamental difference between the conventional use of aerosol therapy and that used with mechanically ventilated patients.

During conventional aerosol therapy, a patient's airway is open to the atmosphere, so the patient inhales and exhales the air and the medication aerosols. Conventional aerosol therapy is known as *open nebulization*.

During mechanical ventilation, a patient's airway is connected to a ventilator system, as shown in Fig. 6.22. The patient must inhale and exhale through the connected ventilator system. The nebulizer jar is typically installed in the inspiratory limb. The exhaled gas and aerosols exit the ventilator system exclusively through the expiratory route. Such an arrangement is known as *in-line nebulization*.

It is important to understand the differences between open and in-line nebulization. A failure to understand these differences is the *root cause* of several complications of mechanical ventilation.

Table 6.3 In-line nebulizer components

Pneumatic nebulizer	Ultrasonic nebulizer
A nebulizer jar in which medication aerosols are generated. It is typically installed in the inspiratory path or, infrequently, at the airway	A nebulizer in which medication aerosols are generated. It is typically installed in the inspiratory route or, infrequently, at the airway
A connecting tube	A connecting cable
A source of compressed driving gas, either a standalone compressor or a source integrated into the ventilator	A driving or control device

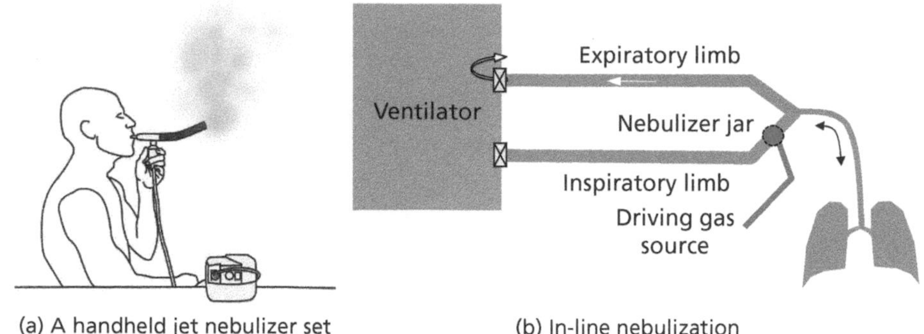

Fig. 6.22 (a) Open and (b) in-line nebulization.

6.3.5 Complications of in-line nebulization

Occlusion of the gas passageway

Occlusion of the gas passageway may occur with both pneumatic and ultrasonic nebulization.

With in-line nebulization using the pneumatic or ultrasonic technique, the nebulizer jar is typically installed in the inspiratory limb of the breathing circuit. The inspiratory gas carries the medication aerosols to the patient's respiratory tract and lungs during inspiration.

Nebulization is intended to deposit therapeutic aerosols at certain locations within the respiratory tract. The depth of penetration of an aerosol particle is inversely proportional to the particle size. The deposition is influenced by a number of factors such as inertial impaction; gravity; the kinetic activity of the particles; the physical nature of the particles; the temperature and humidity of the carrier gas; the patient's ventilatory pattern; and physical characteristics of the patient's airways.

During expiration, the exhaled gas carries out moisture, secretion, *and* residual aerosols: not all aerosols enter the patient's respiratory tract or are deposited. As a result, aerosols are invariably deposited on the inner surface of the expiratory path (Fig. 6.23). Over time, these accumulated aerosols can occlude the expiratory valve, making expiration increasingly difficult. This is an emergency, requiring immediate corrective action.

A typical example of this scenario involves the administration of Mucomyst (acetylcysteine), a medication used to treat various bronchopulmonary disorders. Its solution is very sticky.

Obviously, such an event can potentially occur in any intermittent positive pressure ventilation (IPPV) ventilator, regardless of brand and model, but the following recommendations can minimize that likelihood:

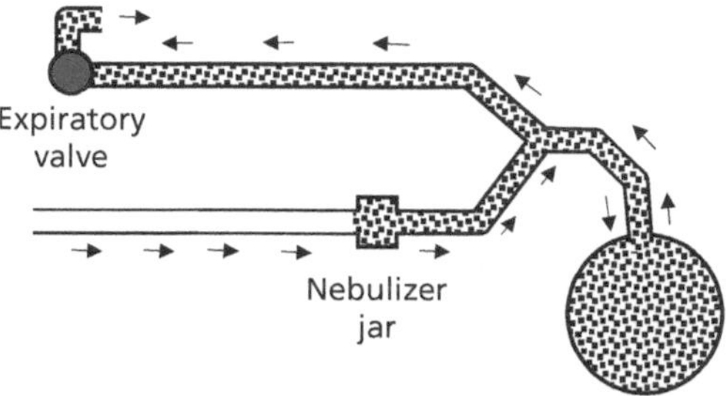

Fig. 6.23 The areas where aerosols are present.

- Make sure your intensive care unit (ICU) staff are well informed about the potential risks of in-line nebulization, how they manifest, and what to do if they occur.
- Make sure any medications intended for in-line nebulization are approved.
- Pay attention to ventilator alarms indicating increased expiratory resistance.
- Check the expiratory valve performance after every episode of in-line nebulization.
- Replace the expiratory valve (block) if the expiratory resistance exceeds the threshold permitted.

Installation of a filter just before the expiratory valve may be an effective measure, but it also has its drawbacks. The filter can prevent medication aerosols from being deposited at the expiratory valve, but the aerosols can gradually block the filter instead. An expiratory filter should be used if it is difficult to inspect and replace the expiratory valve. If you do use an expiratory filter, be sure to periodically check the performance of the filter and replace it if resistance increases noticeably.

Nebulization volume

The use of a pneumatic nebulizer in a volume mode may increase the tidal volume delivered to the patient beyond the set level.

You may recall that during open nebulization, the carrier gas dissipates into the atmosphere, while in-line nebulization occurs in a closed system. In order to generate the aerosols, a pneumatic nebulizer needs driving gas flow, which enters the circuit too. This means that the gas delivered into the breathing circuit comes from two sources. The primary source is the ventilator, and the secondary one is the nebulizer. The total delivered gas volume is the sum of the two.

This additional nebulization volume is determined by:

- The flow rate of the driving gas. It is usually constant at 4–8 L/min, or 67–134 ml/second.
- The time pattern of in-line nebulization: nebulization is activated continuously or intermittently during inspiration only.

This additional nebulization volume has an effect during inspiration, but not expiration, because it is vented when the expiratory valve opens.

Let's assume that a ventilator is set to a volume mode, with a T_i of 1 second. The nebulizer flow is 6 L/min or 100 ml/second. The pneumatic nebulization adds 100 ml gas to the current tidal volume.

Does the *nebulization volume* really matter? The impact of the nebulization volume depends on the set tidal volume. The smaller the tidal volume, the greater the impact is. Let's say you ventilate a baby in a volume mode (unusual) with a tidal volume of 20 ml, a rate of 30 b/min, and a T_i of 0.5 second. The nebulizer flow is constant at 6 L/min or 100 ml/second. The nebulization volume becomes 50 ml per breath, which is much larger than the tidal volume. For this reason, it is not recommended to use pneumatic nebulization in neonates and small children. Ultrasonic nebulization is the recommended alternative, as it introduces no additional volume.

Pneumatic nebulization and F_iO_2

Pneumatic nebulization can impact the F_iO_2 of the delivered gas. As we have seen, a pneumatic nebulizer requires driving gas. Depending on the design of ventilator, the driving gas can be either pure oxygen, pure air, or a mixture.

With either pure oxygen or air, pneumatic nebulization can cause the F_iO_2 to deviate from its initial setting. This deviation depends on the set tidal volume, the difference between the set F_iO_2 and the O_2 concentration of the driving gas, and the nebulization gas flow. F_iO_2 monitoring cannot detect this deviation.

This deviation can be entirely eliminated if the gas from the nebulizer and the gas from the ventilator have the same F_iO_2. This is the case with the GALILEO ventilator.

Moving from open nebulization to in-line nebulization is a natural process. However, we need to understand the difference between these applications and the possible consequences. The clinical efficacy of in-line nebulization depends on such factors as humidification, nebulizer type, position of the nebulizer jar, ventilator settings, continuous versus synchronized nebulization, and the properties of the medications to be administered. To answer these questions, extensive studies are necessary.

6.4 **Respiratory gas filtering**

In mechanical ventilation, one or more gas filters, also known as breathing system filters, may be installed in the breathing circuit or artificial airway. We need to understand some basics about use of these filters.

- Why do we want to filter the gas?
- When should we use a filter?
- Where should we install a filter?
- What are the expected benefits from using a filter?
- What are the potential risks?
- How can we minimize the potential risks?

Let's take a look at some answers.

6.4.1 **Introduction**

A *filter* is a device that removes something from whatever passes through it. In our context, a gas filter is used to remove particles, including droplets, secretions, microgerms, or medication aerosols, from respiratory gas.

A filter is composed of three essential components: the housing, the filtering medium, and adapting ports (Fig. 6.24). The housing may be enlarged in the middle to increase the filtering surface.

Breathing system filters may be classified into two types (electrostatic and mechanical), based on the filtering medium used.

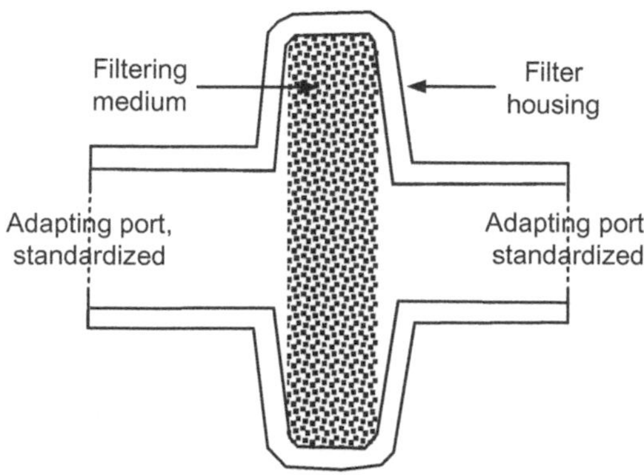

Fig. 6.24 Structure of a gas filter.

Electrostatic filters have a loosely woven medium whose fibres are permanently bipolar charged. The static electric charge causes this type of filter to retain the particles in the passing gas.

Mechanical (pleated paper) filters, whose medium is constructed of tightly packed layers of mixed strands of glass fibre filter paper. The medium acts as a sieve, retaining unwanted particles while allowing gases and humidified air to travel through with minimal obstruction.

Regardless of the type, all breathing system filters have four key characteristics to consider:

- Filtration efficiency: how efficiently the filter captures intended particles under normal conditions of use;
- Pressure drop (resistance): the resistance to gas flow imposed by the filter;
- Internal volume: the dead space that the filter adds when installed at the artificial airway;
- Filter size and weight.

Filter manufacturers should provide this information. Fig. 6.25 is an example of such specifications.

A filter may be mounted in one of three positions in a breathing circuit for different purposes (Fig. 6.26).

The first position is the artificial airway. This is the position of an HME filter for short-term airway humidification. Refer to section 6.2.4.

The second position is the beginning of the inspiratory limb. The inspiratory filter is intended to separate the ventilator and the ventilated patient. On one hand, use of an inspiratory filter can prevent the ventilator from being contaminated. Bear in mind that disinfection or sterilization of the gas passageway inside the ventilator is almost impossible. In addition, it can prevent particles from the source gases or ventilator from reaching the patient.

Code	1944000	1944003
Box Qty.	70	70
Luer lock port		✔
Bacterial and viral filtration efficiency	>99.999%	>99.999%
Resistance to flow at 30 L/min	1.1 cmH_2O	1.1 cmH_2O
Resistance to flow at 60 L/min	2.1 cmH_2O	2.1 cmH_2O
Compressible volume	67 ml	68 ml
Weight	40 g	41 g
Connectors	22F-22M/15F	22F-22M/15F
Minimum tidal volume	200 ml	200 ml

Fig. 6.25 Specifications of filters from Intersurgical.
Reprinted with permission from InterSurgical.

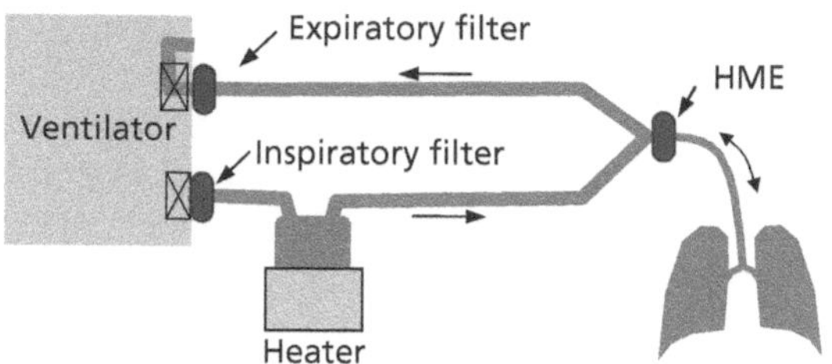

Fig. 6.26 Three possible positions for a gas filter.

The third position is the end of the expiratory limb. An expiratory filter can safeguard the medical staff by filtering the expired gas. This is particularly valuable if the patient has infectious diseases, especially airborne transmitted diseases such as SARS (severe acute respiratory syndrome) or H1N1 flu. It also protects delicate sensors. On many ventilators, the primary flow sensor is located at the expiratory valve. This flow sensor may be very sensitive to droplets, secretions, microgerms, or medication aerosols. In this case, an expiratory filter is required.

6.4.2 Safety concerns when using a filter

For all their benefits, breathing circuit filters also introduce risks. An occluded filter may be the most common root cause of circuit occlusion (Williams and Stacey, 2002; Peady, 2002; Walton et al., 1999). As we mentioned earlier, an invasively ventilated patient has no choice but to breathe through the ventilator system, so an occlusion can become a life-threatening emergency to the patient. A ventilated patient cannot inhale with a completely occluded inspiratory limb. The patient cannot exhale with a completely occluded expiratory limb. And they can neither inhale nor exhale with a completed occluded airway.

The purpose for placing a filter in a gas passageway is to remove particles from the gas that passes through it. Where do the particles go? Clearly, the particles accumulate at the surface of the filter material.

A vacuum cleaner is a perfect example. To assure the normal functioning of a vacuum cleaner, we must periodically replace or empty its dust bag, which is comparable to a filter. When the bag is new, empty, and clean, the resistance is negligible. Over time, the resistance increases progressively when the dust bag fills up.

In a ventilator system, the gas at the airway and the expiratory limb contains particles, including moisture, secretion, microgerms, blood clots, and medication aerosols. Filters installed at these two locations will gradually occlude. So, the question is not *whether* the occlusion will occur, but *when* or *how fast* the occlusion will become clinically relevant. An inspiratory filter, by contrast, is seldom blocked because inspiratory gas is typically clean and dry.

Be aware too that an HME at the artificial airway is also a filter, although its purpose is to warm and humidify the inspiratory gas. Note that the use of an HME is contraindicated under some conditions. One of the conditions is that the ventilated patient has bloody, thick, or copious sections.

In-line nebulization dramatically increases the probability of the filter occlusion, evidenced by the case report in Box 6.1.

Box 6.1 A case report of an obstructed breathing circuit filter

A 56-year old man required postoperative mechanical ventilation. He had been treated with antibiotics, chest physiotherapy, nebulised acetylcysteine (Parvolex), and salbutamol. During weaning from mechanical ventilation, he became progressively agitated, tachypnoeic, and hypertensive. Auscultation of the lungs showed a widespread wheeze and poor air entry to both lungs.

There was no apparent obstruction of either the tracheal tube or breathing tubes. Salbutamol, aminophylline, hydrocortisone, and magnesium were given, but none was effective. Therefore, the patient was sedated and paralysed but airway pressures increased further. Hypercapnia with normal oxygenation was noted. Manual ventilation was difficult. By close inspection, we noticed a small bubble in a breathing system filter (Pall BB 100 filter), which had been placed between the catheter mount and the Y-piece. Normal breathing was promptly obtained by replacing the filter.

Pall Biomedical hypothesised, after extensive investigation of this device, that nebulised acetylcysteine might have broken down viscous mucus, which was present on the patient side of the hydrophobic filter element, and produced a fluid of low surface tension. This product then might have entered the pores of the filter membrane[1] and increased the filter resistance. Acetylcysteine is not licensed for nebulisation by the manufacturer (Evans Medical Ltd) and therefore Pall had not tested this factor before this incident.

We inform readers that obstruction could occur when a breathing system filter is used during nebulisation of acetylcysteine, and we recommend that acetylcysteine is delivered only during inspirations.

[1]DHSS. Pall Ultipor breathing system filter (BB50/BB50T/BB22-15): warning on the use of ipratropium bromide (Atrovent). HN(HAZARD)(85)7 1985.

Reproduced from *Canadian Journal of Anesthesia*, 43, 12, Stacey M.R.W, 'Obstruction of a breathing system filter', p. 1276. Copyright (1996) with permission from Springer and Canadian Anesthesiologists.

6.4.3 How to recognize filter occlusion

The risk of occlusion exists any time a filter is used at the airway or in the expiratory limb. Therefore, whenever the ventilated patient shows signs of *respiratory distress syndrome (RDS)*, we should check or replace the filter or HME in order to eliminate that possibility.

6.4.4 Preventive recommendations

Follow these recommendations to prevent possible filter occlusion:

- Do not use an HME on patients with thick, copious, or bloody secretions.
- Use a filter only when the potential benefits outweigh the potential risks.
- Ensure that all clinicians involved are sufficiently informed about the potential risks of using filters at the airway or in expiratory limb.
- Inspect the filter periodically, and document the inspection. Remove or replace the filter immediately if you suspect occlusion.
- Remove any HME and expiratory filter from the circuit during in-line nebulization.
- Immediately disconnect the ventilated patient at the airway opening whenever severe respiratory distress syndrome appears, and continue ventilation manually.

References

Peady CJ. Another report of obstruction of a heat and moisture exchange filter. *Can J Anesth* 2002: **49**; 1001.

Restrepo RD, Walsh BK. AARC Clinical practice guidelines: Humidification during invasive and noninvasive mechanical ventilation. *Respir Care* 2012: **57**; 782–8.

Walton JS, Fears R, Burt N, Dorman BH. Intraoperative breathing circuit obstruction caused by albuterol nebulization. *Anesth Analg* 1999: **89**; 650–1.

Williams DJ, Stacey MRW. Rapid and complete occlusion of a heat and moisture exchange filter by pulmonary edema (Clinical report). *Can J Anesth* 2002; **49**; 126–31.

Chapter 7

Essential Variables and Breath Types

7.1 Introduction

We have learned that mechanical ventilation can be realized with one of three operating principles: intermittent positive pressure ventilation (IPPV), intermittent negative pressure ventilation (INPV), and high-frequency ventilation (HFV). Most ventilators today are IPPV based.

Lung ventilation refers to the gas movement in and out of the lungs. During IPPV, lung *inflation* and *deflation* occur due to the interaction of two processes.

The first process is the fluctuation of airway opening pressure (P_{ao}), which is generated by the ventilator system (Fig. 7.1). Gas moves into the lungs when P_{ao} increases, and moves out when P_{ao} decreases.

The second process is the fluctuation of alveolar pressure (P_{alv}), which is generated by the respiratory muscles and the elastic recoil force. Gas moves into the lungs when P_{alv} decreases, and moves out when P_{alv} increases.

The basic unit of mechanical ventilation is the *mechanical breath,* which is defined as a breath realized through a ventilator system. Mechanical ventilation can be viewed as a series of mechanical breaths.

There are several mechanical breath types. The type of mechanical breath is determined by five essential *variables*:

1. *Triggering*: defines when inspiration begins;
2. *Cycling*: defines when inspiration ends;
3. *Controlling*: defines how delivery of inspiratory gas is controlled;
4. *Targeting*: defines the size of a mechanical breath;
5. *Baseline*: defines the baseline pressure at which mechanical breaths occur.

This chapter will focus on these essential variables and mechanical breath types.

Why do you, a clinician, need to know them?

These essential variables are the foundation of mechanical breaths. In turn, mechanical breaths are the foundation of ventilation modes. To help us understand the relationship between essential variables, mechanical breaths, and ventilation modes, let's look at a two-storey house. The variables serve as the basement, mechanical breaths are the first floor, and ventilation modes are the top floor (Fig. 7.2). Further, the essential parameters are the very basis of control parameters.

7.2 Essential variables

Let's start our discussion by looking at those five essential variables that form the 'basement' of our house and that are the building blocks of mechanical breath types. As Table 7.1 shows, various mechanisms are associated with these variables.

Every type of mechanical breath represents a unique combination of these variables.

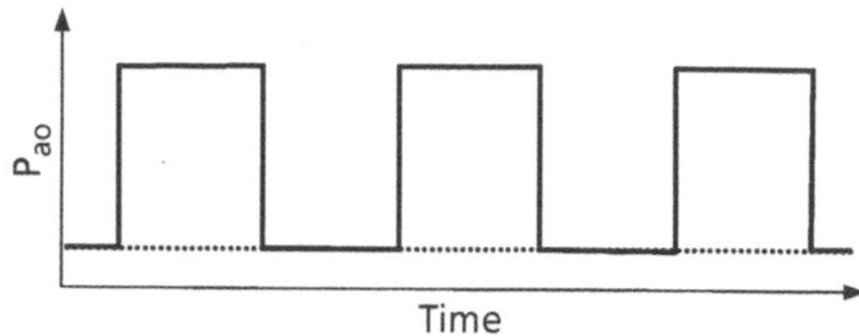

Fig. 7.1 Intermittent positive pressure applied to airway opening.

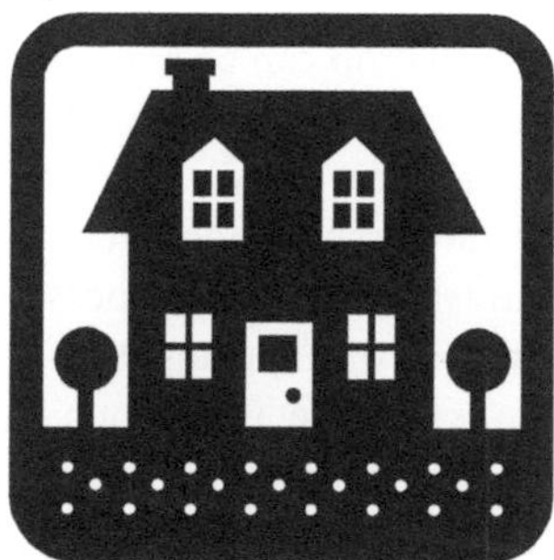

Fig. 7.2 A two-floor house shows the relationship among the essential variables, breath types, and ventilation modes.

Table 7.1 Essential variables and their common mechanisms

Variable	Triggering	Cycling	Controlling	Targeting	Baseline
Common mechanisms	◆ Time triggering ◆ Pressure triggering ◆ Flow triggering ◆ Manual triggering	◆ Time cycling ◆ Flow cycling	◆ Volume controlling ◆ Pressure controlling ◆ Adaptive controlling ◆ Hybrid controlling	◆ Tidal volume ◆ Inspiratory pressure ◆ Target tidal volume	Positive end-expiratory pressure (PEEP)

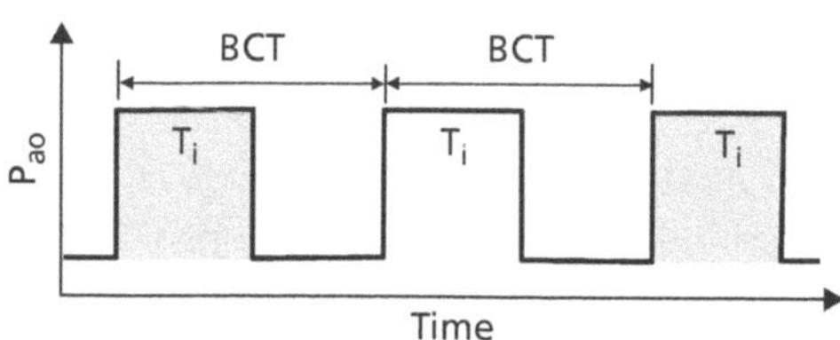

Fig. 7.3 The relationship between breath cycle time (BCT), inspiratory time (T_i), and expiratory time (T_e).

7.2.1 Triggering

Every mechanical breath takes a certain time to complete. We call the duration of a mechanical breath the *breath cycle time* or BCT. Do not confuse breath cycle time with *cycling*, which is an essential variable.

A breath cycle time contains two *phases* (Fig. 7.3):

Inspiratory time (T_i), when a ventilator delivers gas into the breathing circuit so that P_{ao} increases and the lungs are inflated; and

Expiratory time (T_e), when the ventilator allows the gas to exit from the system, and P_{ao} drops to the baseline pressure. The lungs are deflated.

The relationship between BCT, T_i, and T_e is simple: BCT = $T_i + T_e$. There are two general conventions in this regard. First, T_i comes before T_e. Second, there is no time gap between two consecutive mechanical breaths. Therefore, if T_i is fixed, an increase in BCT results in the same increase in T_e.

Triggering is defined as the time point when inspiration begins. It has four common mechanisms: time triggering, pressure triggering, flow triggering, and manual triggering.

A less common triggering mechanism is NAVA (neurally adjusted ventilatory assist) from Maquet. NAVA detects the patient's phrenic nerve signal with a special oesophageal catheter sensor and uses this signal for triggering. NAVA is an innovation with great potential, but it is still in its infancy.

Time triggering

Time triggering is also known as *ventilator triggering.*

With time triggering, the ventilator initiates inspiration at a preset, fixed interval.

As Fig. 7.4 shows, the BCT equals the interval between two consecutive triggers. Therefore, once the BCT is defined, the triggering interval is defined as well.

The BCT can be defined in several ways. The most common one is by setting a rate in breaths per minute. When you set the rate, you define the BCT and the triggering interval.

You can easily convert this set rate to BCT or a triggering interval with a simple equation:

$$BCT\ (s) = 60/Set\ rate\ (b/min)$$

Table 7.2 lists commonly used rates and corresponding BCTs.

In order to improve patient comfort and safety, all ventilation modes allow *patient triggering*, although you may be able to deactivate it. The set rate serves as a backup. Consequently, even under normal conditions, the actual or monitored respiratory rate is often higher than the set rate in active patients. The monitored rate and the set rate are equal only in passive patients.

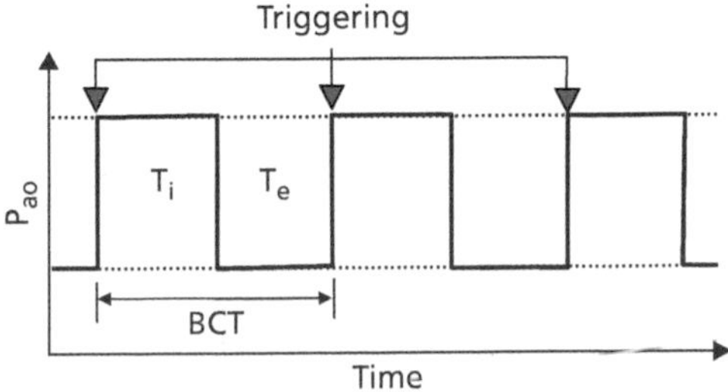

Fig. 7.4 Triggering refers to beginning an inspiration and also beginning a mechanical breath.
BCT: breath cycle time; P_{ao}: airway opening pressure; T_i: inspiratory time; T_e: expiratory time.

Table 7.2 Commonly used rates and corresponding breath cycle times (BCT)

Commonly used rate (breaths/minute)	6	10	12	15	20	30	60
Corresponding BCT (seconds)	10	6	5	4	3	2	1

Pressure triggering

Pressure triggering is a form of patient triggering (Fig. 7.5). It relies on the monitoring of circuit or airway pressure.

To understand pressure triggering, think about sucking on an empty wine bottle. Your effort generates a negative internal pressure but little gas flow. The stronger you suck, the more negative the pressure. If pressure triggering is activated, the breathing circuit serves as the bottle. The patient's inspiratory efforts cause the airway pressure to drop from the current baseline pressure.

To use pressure triggering, you need to activate it and set the pressure *trigger sensitivity*. The sensitivity is a negative value in cmH_2O, such as −0.5, −1.0, or −2.0 cmH_2O. The value represents a virtual pressure threshold below the current *PEEP (positive end-expiratory pressure)*. For instance, if the set PEEP is 5 cmH_2O, and the triggering sensitivity is set to −2.0 cmH_2O, the ventilator starts delivering inspiratory gas if the airway pressure drops to or below 3 cmH_2O. The smaller the absolute value of the sensitivity, the more sensitive the triggering, and vice versa. So, a pressure trigger of −0.5 cmH_2O is more sensitive than −2.0 cmH_2O.

With a high sensitivity, the patient can trigger the ventilator very easily. The price to pay, however, is the increased probability of an adverse event known as *auto-triggering*. Auto-triggering typically manifests as a series of quick, rhythmic mechanical breaths. It occurs if the ventilator is not triggered as expected by the patient's inspiratory efforts, but by pneumatic artefacts due to a gas leak, accumulated condensed water in the circuit, or even cardiac oscillation. The best solution for auto-triggering is to remove the root cause. If this is not feasible, lower the sensitivity until auto-triggering disappears.

Flow triggering

Flow triggering is another form of patient triggering (Fig. 7.6). It relies on circuit or airway flow monitoring. To help us understand flow triggering, let us first specify three types of flow:

- Flow A: The gas flow measured at the inspiratory limb of the circuit;
- Flow B: The gas flow measured at the expiratory limb of the circuit;
- Airway flow: The gas flow measured at the airway. It can be either inspiratory or expiratory.

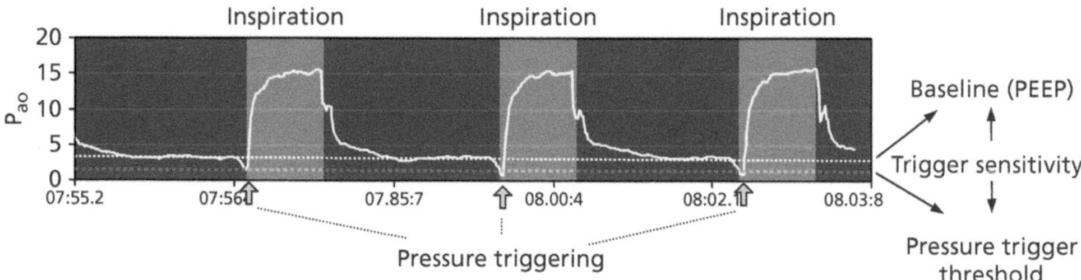

Fig. 7.5 The principle of pressure triggering.

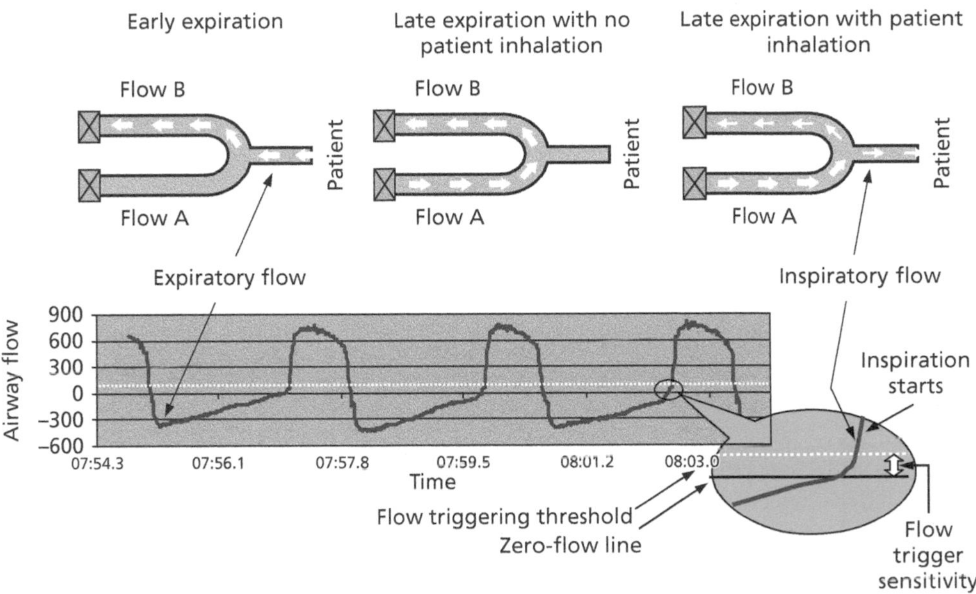

Fig. 7.6 The principle of flow triggering with base flow.

Now, let's further divide T_e into early expiration and late expiration.

At early expiration, the ventilator closes its inspiratory valve and fully opens the expiratory valve for maximum expiratory flow. The high circuit pressure drives the gas out of the system, and the airway pressure drops sharply. Both flow B and expiratory airway flow rise quickly to their maximum or *peak expiratory flow*, and then decrease gradually as the circuit pressure drops.

At late expiration, the ventilator tries to rebuild and maintain the set baseline pressure by (a) reducing the expiratory valve opening for a high resistance against the expiratory flow, and (b) slightly opening the inspiratory valve for a constant base flow, which is crucial for flow triggering.

If the patient does not inhale, both flow A and flow B are equal to the base flow, and the airway flow is zero.

If the patient inhales, a part of base flow goes to the patient, resulting in an inspiratory airway flow and a decreased flow B.

If the detected inspiratory airway flow or the difference between flow A and B reaches a defined threshold, the ventilator is triggered.

To use flow triggering, you need to activate it and then set the flow trigger sensitivity. The sensitivity is expressed in litres per minute, such as 0.5, 1.0, 2.0, or 5.0 litres per minute. The smaller the set value, the more sensitive the flow trigger, and vice versa.

If flow triggering is set to an extremely sensitive setting, auto-triggering can also occur due to gas leakage, water in the circuit, or cardiac oscillation. The best solution for auto-triggering is to remove the root cause. If this is not feasible, lower the sensitivity until auto-triggering disappears.

Is flow triggering superior to pressure triggering, or the other way around? The answer is controversial. To arrive at an answer, we have to ask two more questions:

- Which mechanism requires less effort for the patient to trigger the ventilator?
- Which mechanism is prone to auto-triggering?

With pressure triggering, a patient sucks an empty bottle to generate a negative pressure, while with flow triggering, the patient sucks the bottle with a hole (i.e. the *base flow*) to generate an inspiratory flow. Clearly, flow triggering requires less sucking effort. Controversy over which mechanism is the easiest for the patient may stem from differences in the technical performance of individual ventilators and the sensitivity settings used in these studies. You can easily verify the difference yourself by putting yourself on a ventilator in the pressure support ventilation (PSV) mode and trying both triggering mechanisms at various sensitivity levels. Most likely you will conclude that flow triggering is easier.

Auto-triggering can occur with both pressure and flow triggering. It is the author's personal experience that auto-triggering occurs more readily with pressure triggering under the same conditions.

Do not confuse the sensitivity values of triggering mechanisms. For instance, a pressure trigger of -0.5 cmH_2O is not interchangeable with a flow trigger of 0.5 L/min. They are fundamentally different.

Note: A ventilator system cannot differentiate patient triggering from auto-triggering. You need to verify whether the ventilator is triggered by the patient's genuine inspiratory efforts or pneumatic artefacts.

Manual triggering

Some ventilators provide a *manual triggering* function that allows an operator to directly trigger the ventilator. Such ventilators usually have a special 'Manual' button or key on their user interface.

When this button or key is pressed, the ventilator delivers an additional mechanical breath, either immediately or at the next opportunity.

Triggering abnormalities

Generally speaking, time triggering and manual triggering are highly reliable. Abnormal triggering is almost always associated with flow or pressure triggering, and it takes one of two forms (see Table 7.3):

Auto-triggering: The ventilator triggers without patient inspiratory effort, as mentioned above.

Unresponsive or missed triggering: The ventilator does not trigger when the patient inhales. A variation is that the ventilator does respond to the patient's effort but with a significant delay—delayed triggering.

7.2.2 Cycling

Cycling refers to the end of inspiration and determines the length of T_i (Fig. 7.7). *Time cycling* and *flow cycling* are commonly used cycling mechanisms. Because BCT is the sum of T_i and T_e, if BCT is given, an increase in T_i causes a corresponding decrease in T_e, and vice versa.

Table 7.3 Common root causes of abnormal triggering

Auto-triggering	Unresponsive or delayed triggering
◆ Overly sensitive trigger setting ◆ Unstable PEEP ◆ Noticeable gas leak at the circuit or airway ◆ Circuit rainout ◆ Abnormal ventilator monitoring	◆ Insensitive trigger setting ◆ Hyperdistention of the lungs ◆ Weak patient inspiratory effort ◆ Blocked signal transmission route (e.g. kinked endotracheal tube in neonates) ◆ Abnormal ventilator monitoring

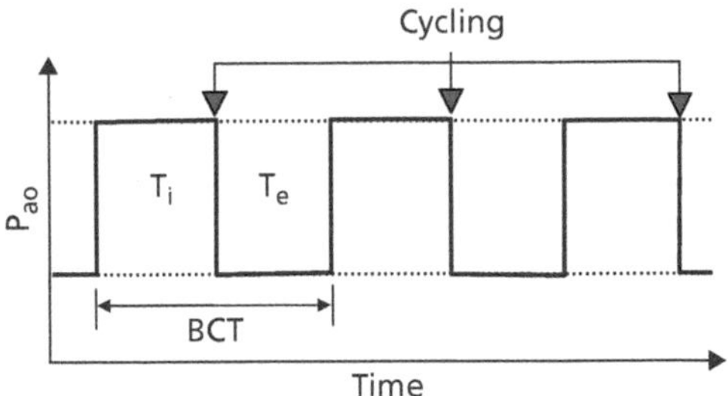

Fig. 7.7 Cycling refers to the end of inspiration.
BCT: breath cycle time; P_{ao}: airway opening pressure; T_i: inspiratory time; T_e: expiratory time.

Time cycling

Time cycling is the simplest form of cycling: a ventilator switches from inspiration to expiration when the set T_i is over. Time cycling applies to all control breaths and all assisted breaths. Time cycling can be realized with four methods: (a) the T_i method, (b) the I:E (inspiratory/expiratory) ratio method, (c) the $\%T_i$ method, and (d) the peak flow method. The I:E ratio and T_i methods are more popular.

The T_i method With this method an operator directly sets T_i in seconds. The ventilator ends inspiration and starts expiration once the set T_i ends.

The T_i method applies to volume breaths, pressure breaths, and adaptive breaths.

The I:E ratio method BCT is the sum of T_i and T_e. With any BCT, there is always a ratio between the T_i and T_e portions. This is the I:E ratio. The number to the left of colon represents the T_i portion, and the number to the right represents the T_e portion. Assume that we set the rate to 10 breaths per minute and the I:E ratio to 1:2. The resultant BCT is 6 seconds, the T_i is 2 seconds, and the T_e is 4 seconds. Table 7.4 shows the I:E ratios, T_i, and T_e for a rate of 10 breaths per minute.

The I:E ratio method has two major advantages: (a) a change in the I:E ratio and/or BCT causes corresponding changes in both T_i and T_e; and (b) the relationship between T_i and T_e is clearly shown. Its disadvantage is that you do not see T_i and T_e in seconds without mental calculation. Note: if the patient is active, the actual BCT, T_i, and T_e may differ from the settings.

The I:E ratio method applies to volume breaths, pressure breaths, and adaptive breaths.

The $\%T_i$ method This method expresses BCT, T_i, and T_e as percentages, regardless of their actual length in seconds. The BCT, regardless of its length in seconds, is always considered to be 100%. Therefore, if $\%T_i$ is set to 50%, T_e becomes 50%. If $\%T_i$ is set to 33%, T_e becomes 67%.

You can also calculate T_i and T_e in seconds with a given BCT:

$$T_i(s) = Set\ \%T_i \times BCT$$
$$T_e(s) = Remaining\ \%Te \times BCT$$

Table 7.4 Relationship between inspiratory time (T_i), expiratory time (T_e), and I:E ratio for rate of 10 breaths per minute

Set I:E ratio	**1:3**	**1:2**	**1:1**	**2:1**	**3:1**
T_i (seconds)	1.5	2.0	3.0	4.0	4.5
T_e (seconds)	4.5	4.0	3.0	2.0	1.5
BCT (seconds)	6.0	6.0	6.0	6.0	6.0

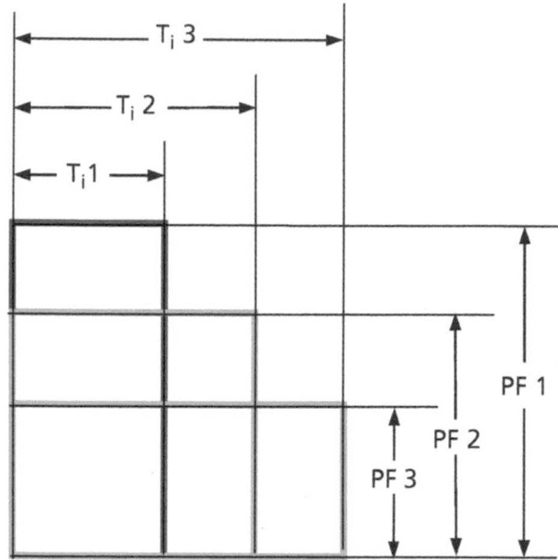

Fig. 7.8 Relationship between peak flow (height), T_i (width), and tidal volume (total area).

Much like the I:E ratio method, the %T_i method gives you a sense of both T_i and T_e. Determining the durations of T_i and T_e in seconds, however, requires a mental calculation.

Use of the %T_i method is limited, although it can apply to volume breaths, pressure breaths, and adaptive breaths.

The peak flow method This method is a bit confusing at first glance. You may wonder how T_i can be defined by setting peak flow.

Peak flow refers to peak inspiratory flow. This method applies to volume breaths with constant inspiratory flow. With these breaths, the delivered tidal volume is the product of the set T_i and the set peak flow rate.

$$V_T = T_i \times Set\ peak\ flow$$
$$or$$
$$T_i = V_T \,/\, Set\ peak\ flow$$

This means that T_i increases when peak flow decreases and/or V_T (tidal volume) increases. T_i decreases when peak flow increases and/or V_T decreases (Fig. 7.8).

Let's look at an example. We set V_T to 600 ml and peak flow to 36 L/min (600 ml/s). The resultant T_i is 1.0 second. At the set inspiratory flow, it takes 1.0 second to complete delivery of the set V_T (600 ml).

Now, if we reduce V_T to 300 ml but keep the same peak flow (36 L/min), the resultant T_i drops to 0.5 s. Or, if we keep the V_T of 600 ml unchanged but raise the peak flow to 72 L/min (1200 ml/s), the resultant T_i is 0.5 s as well.

Flow cycling

Flow cycling is designed for active patients and is a key feature of support breaths, which we will discuss later.

In a pressure breath, the inspiratory flow is uncontrolled. Typically, inspiratory flow rises quickly to the peak at the beginning of inspiration, and then drops gradually back to zero. Flow cycling works with the descending part of inspiratory flow (Fig. 7.9). The peak inspiratory flow, regardless of its absolute height, is taken as 100%. A ventilator cycles from inspiration to expiration when the inspiratory flow falls to a preset percentage.

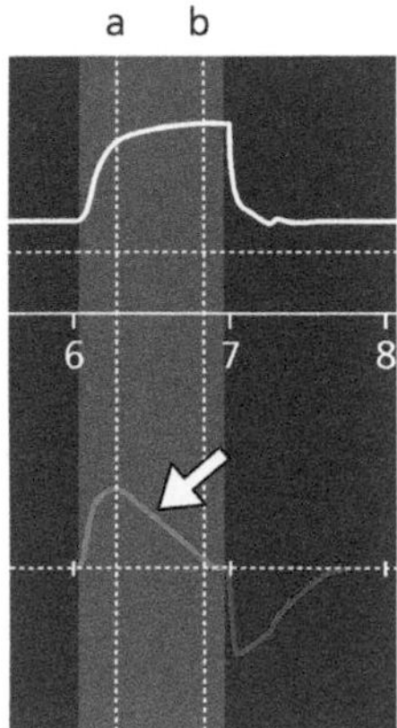

Fig. 7.9 Flow cycling works with the descending part of inspiratory flow (between a and b).

Flow cycling is adjustable in some ventilators and fixed in others. If flow cycling is adjustable in your ventilator, it will have a control setting in any mode that offers support breaths. The flow cycling control has different names on different ventilators, as we will see in Chapter 9. If flow cycling is not adjustable, the level is fixed, typically at 25%.

A flow cycling control lets you influence T_i in support breaths to a certain extent; the higher the set percentage, the shorter the actual T_i, and vice versa (refer to Fig. 7.10). This technical feature helps optimize patient-ventilator synchrony in spontaneously breathing patients.

If the set percentage is very low (e.g. 10%) and there is a massive leak at the circuit or airway, flow cycling can fail because the inspiratory flow does not fall to the set level. The consequence is endless inspiration, which is clinically unacceptable.

An operator should do two things to prevent this potential complication: (a) set flow cycling to a minimum of 40%, and (b) try everything possible to minimize the gas leak.

Because flow cycling can fail, backup time cycling should be part of the ventilator design. In some ventilators the operator can set this time with a control that may be called *maximum inspiratory time* (T_i max); if flow cycling fails, the ventilator can still cycle based on this setting. In other ventilators, this parameter may not be operator adjustable.

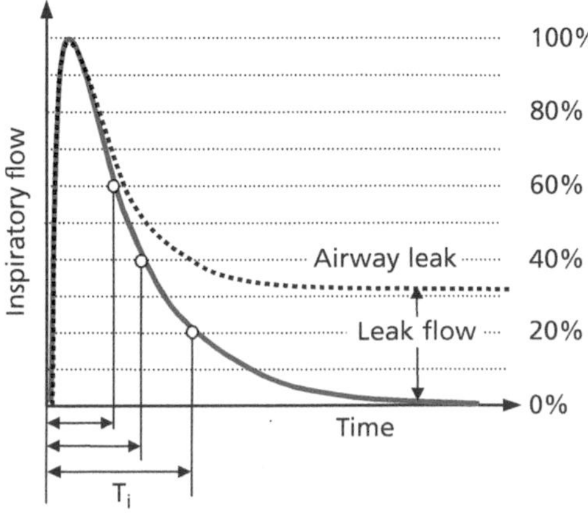

Fig. 7.10 Various flow cycling settings for different inspiratory times (T_i).

Pressure cycling

Typically *pressure cycling* is used as a protective measure in a volume breath.

In a volume mode, the ventilator precisely controls the inspiratory gas flow. The resultant peak pressure varies, depending on the set peak inspiratory flow and the patient's respiratory resistance and compliance. As we know, a persistent high peak pressure can cause barotrauma to the lungs.

To prevent this possible complication, the set upper limit of peak airway pressure serves not only as the alarm threshold but also the threshold for pressure cycling. This means that when the peak pressure reaches the threshold, the ventilator immediately cycles from inspiration to expiration, resulting in a (much) shorter T_i and a (much) smaller V_T than the settings. In this case, three alarms may be active: high airway pressure, low tidal volume, and low minute volume.

Caution: Unless you can immediately identify and remove the cause of the excessive peak pressure, hypoventilation is inevitable and the annoying alarms will persist.

7.2.3 Controlling

Unlike triggering and cycling, which dictate the timing of ventilation, the third variable, *controlling*, refers to the mechanism with which a ventilator controls delivery of inspiratory gas.

Fundamentally there are only two types of controlling: *volume controlling* and *pressure controlling*. At any given time, a ventilator can control only volume or pressure, but not both. Pressure controlling has a variant called *adaptive controlling*. Finally, a few ventilators use *hybrid controlling*. We will explain them individually.

Volume controlling

A better name for volume controlling is *flow controlling*, because during inspiration a ventilator controls the flow of inspiratory gas that is delivered into the circuit. At the end of inspiration, delivery of the set tidal volume is completed.

Volume controlling uses three primary parameters: V_T, T_i, and peak flow. Typically we set either V_T and T_i, or V_T and peak flow. The ventilator calculates the third automatically.

Volume controlling has a secondary parameter: (inspiratory) *flow pattern*, which is the inspiratory flow profile of the flow-time waveform. The most common flow pattern is square flow (i.e. constant inspiratory flow). The square flow pattern is the only one available for volume breaths in some ventilators. However, some modern ventilators may also provide other flow patterns. Some common flow patterns are shown in Fig. 7.11.

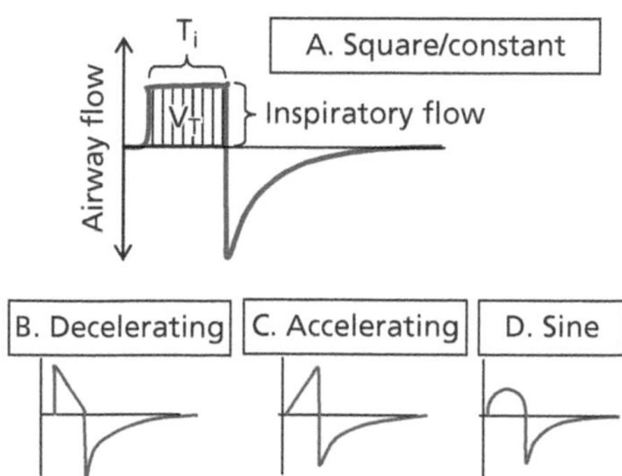

Fig. 7.11 Volume breaths have four common patterns of inspiratory flow.

The major perceived advantage of volume controlling is stable tidal and minute volumes, which makes clinicians more comfortable. However, volume controlling has four inherent disadvantages:

- With volume controlling, a ventilator dictates all important aspects of inspiratory gas delivery. This is hardly acceptable if the patient is active. This explains why patient-ventilator asynchrony often occurs in volume modes.
- Even under normal conditions, the delivered tidal volume is always higher than the tidal volume that the patient actually receives, due to gas compression in the elastic breathing circuit. If the patient is to get the intended V_T, the ventilator must deliver more gas volume into the circuit than the set V_T.
- Leak compensation is impossible with volume controlling. The ventilator delivers exactly the set gas volume into the circuit. A gas leak can sharply decrease the tidal volume that the patient receives—hypoventilation.
- The peak pressure varies with volume controlling. If the peak pressure stays high, the lungs may be damaged.

Pressure controlling

Because of the disadvantages, the volume controlling mechanism has slowly but steadily given way to pressure controlling.

With pressure controlling, a ventilator first draws a target airway pressure profile according to the settings. When inspiration begins, the ventilator dynamically adjusts the inspiratory gas flow, aiming to close the gap between the actual airway pressure and the target pressure profile (Fig. 7.12). The ventilator increases the inspiratory flow if the monitored pressure is much below the target pressure. It decreases the flow if the monitored pressure is a bit below the target pressure. It stops the flow if both pressures are equal.

Pressure controlling is shaped by two primary parameters: T_i and *inspiratory pressure*. Inspiratory pressure is defined as the applied positive pressure above baseline pressure (PEEP). Inspiratory pressure drives gas into the lungs. Inspiratory pressure is expressed in cmH_2O, and its abbreviation is P_{insp}. In Hamilton Medical ventilators, P_{insp} has two names: pressure support (or $P_{support}$) for support breaths and pressure control (or $P_{control}$) for control breaths and assist breaths.

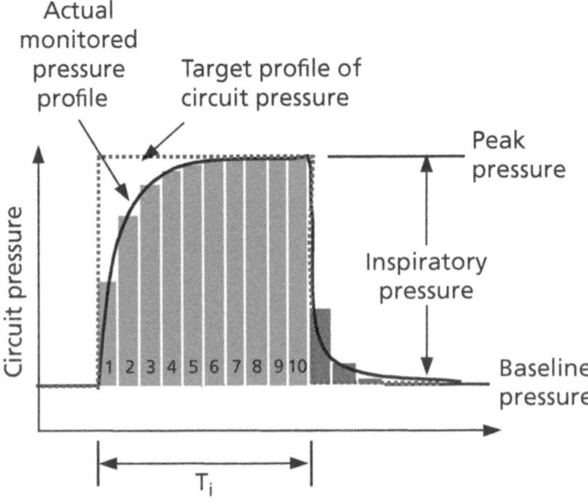

Fig. 7.12 The mechanism to generate inspiratory pressure in a pressure breath.

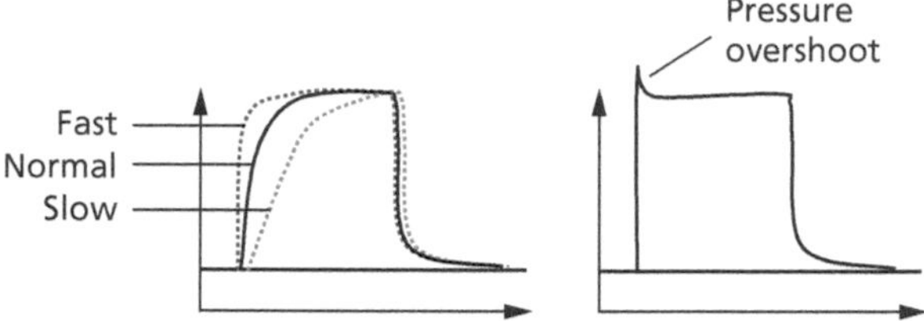

Fig. 7.13 The meaning of rise time and pressure overshoot.

The pressure control mechanism has a secondary parameter: *pressure ramp* (P_{ramp}) or *rise time* (Fig. 7.13). It is defined as the time required for airway pressure to rise to a target pressure at the beginning of inspiration. A short P_{ramp} means a fast pressurization, and vice versa. The P_{ramp} control is used to change the speed of pressurization.

If we compare volume controlling to a dictator, we would call pressure controlling somewhat of a liberal, because V_T and inspiratory flow are variable as per the patient's demand. This means that actively breathing patients may influence the inspiratory flow and tidal volume they receive, resulting in better patient-ventilator synchrony.

When the system has a leak, causing circuit pressure to drop, the ventilator responds with an increased inspiratory flow. This is how 'leak compensation' works. With pressure controlling, a ventilator can effectively compensate a moderate leak.

With pressure controlling, the price to pay for patient comfort is variable tidal volume. The critical factors that can influence the tidal volume include: (a) the applied inspiratory pressure, (b) the patient's respiratory mechanics, and (c) the patient's breathing efforts. Under unfavourable conditions, the resultant tidal volume may be much smaller or greater than desired. To safeguard the patient, you need to appropriately set the upper and lower limits of the tidal volume alarm and minute volume alarm.

Adaptive controlling

Adaptive controlling resulted from efforts to exploit the advantages and to minimize the disadvantages of both volume controlling and pressure controlling. By nature, adaptive controlling is a variant of pressure controlling.

With classic pressure controlling, the inspiratory pressure is set, the peak pressure stays stable, and the resultant V_T may vary. With adaptive controlling, by contrast, the operator sets a target V_T instead of inspiratory pressure. After every breath, the ventilator compares the monitored V_T to the target V_T and regulates the inspiratory pressure with the aim to minimize the gap between the monitored and target V_T. The ventilator increases inspiratory pressure if the monitored V_T is below the target V_T. It decreases the inspiratory pressure if the monitored V_T is above the target V_T. It keeps the inspiratory pressure unchanged if both tidal volumes are equal. The regulation of inspiratory pressure is fully automated, breath by breath.

Adaptive controlling may be misperceived as volume controlling, because both require setting of tidal volume. Other than that, however, the two mechanisms have nothing in common. Typical flow and pressure waveforms for volume, pressure, and adaptive controlling are shown in Fig. 7.14.

The major advantages of adaptive controlling include: (a) the actual V_T can be stabilized at the desired level, especially in passive patients; and (b) adaptive controlling retains most advantages of pressure controlling.

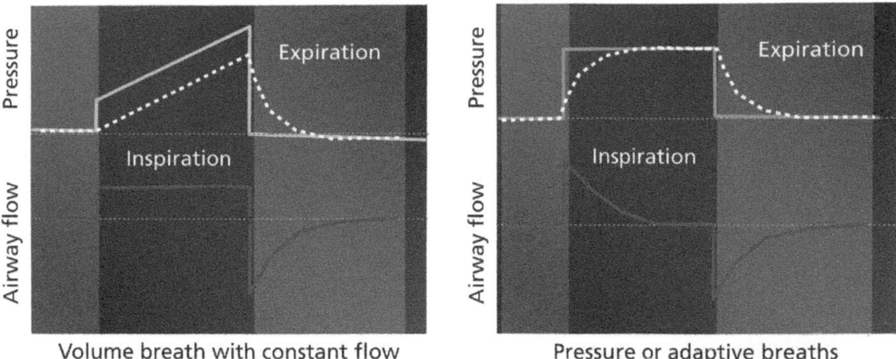

Fig. 7.14 Pressure and flow waveforms of a volume breath with constant flow (left) and a pressure/adaptive breath (right) in a passive model. The white dotted curves indicate alveolar pressure.

For optimal performance, adaptive controlling imposes a hard but little mentioned requirement on the operator: they must adapt the target volume to the patient's current ventilatory demand, which may change over time.

A suboptimal scenario is where the target volume is set lower than the current demand. The patient has to breathe harder to satisfy the demand. Because the monitored V_T exceeds the set target, the ventilator reduces the inspiratory pressure. In the end, the patient does all work of breathing, and the ventilator does little.

Hybrid controlling

Hybrid controlling is a mechanism where the ventilator switches between volume controlling and pressure controlling within a single breath. Examples of hybrid controlling include the volume-assured pressure support (VAPS) mode on the Bird 8400 ST_i ventilator, the volume control mode on Maquet ventilators, and pressure-limited ventilation (PLV) on Dräger ventilators. Fig. 7.15 shows VAPS waveforms. Hybrid controlling can be difficult to understand and has not yet become popular.

Robert Chatburn's taxonomy of mechanical ventilation calls hybrid controlling *dual control* (Chatburn, 2007).

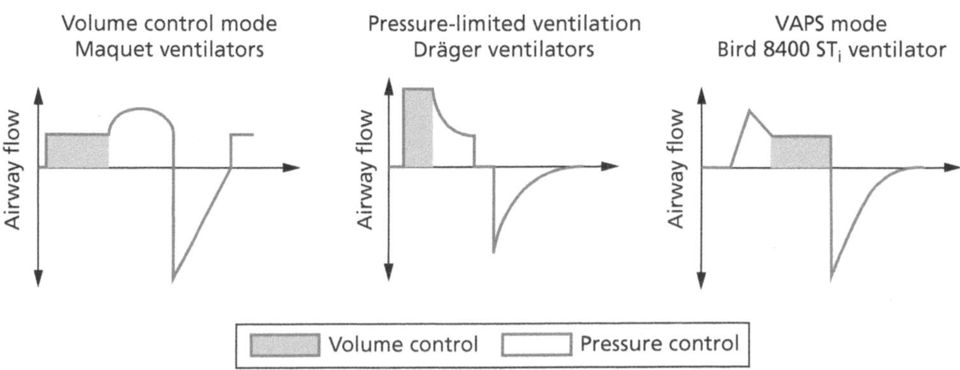

Fig. 7.15 Flow waveforms of three mechanical breaths with hybrid controlling.

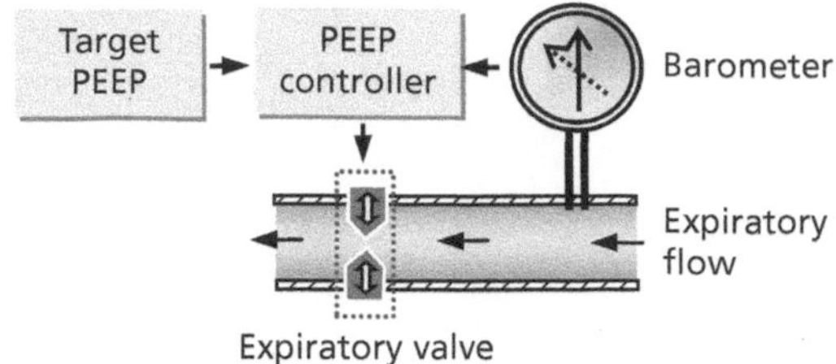

Fig. 7.16 Dynamic regulation of expiratory valve to maintain a stable baseline at the desired level.

7.2.4 Targeting

Targeting is sometimes also called *limiting*.

The controlling mechanisms define *how* a ventilator controls delivery of inspiratory gas. With any controlling mechanism, a ventilator can deliver a large or small breath. The targeting parameter defines *how much* or the size of the mechanical breath.

The targeting parameter depends entirely on the controlling mechanism used. With volume controlling, the targeting parameter is tidal volume. With pressure controlling, it is inspiratory pressure. With adaptive controlling, it is *target tidal volume.*

When the set targeting parameter is reached, the ventilator typically stops further gas delivery into the circuit. Expiration may or may not start immediately, depending on the set T_i.

7.2.5 Baseline pressure (PEEP)

Positive end-expiratory pressure (PEEP) is the baseline pressure above which positive pressure is applied intermittently. Positive end-expiratory pressure is adjustable in all ventilators, and it is relative to atmospheric pressure. It is generated by interaction between the expiratory gas flow and the resistance imposed by the ventilator's expiratory valve (Fig. 7.16).

PEEP alone is therapeutic, as it can increase functional residual capacity (FRC), improve alveolar gas exchange, keep the lung units open, and even improve lung compliance.

A moderate level of PEEP, 3–5 cmH_2O, is preferred for all ventilated patients without apparent lung disease. A high PEEP may be clinically necessary for patients with restrictive lung disease, such as acute respiratory distress syndrome (ARDS). It is possible to set PEEP to zero, but zero PEEP is not recommended for intubated and ventilated patients.

7.3 From variables to mechanical breaths

So far we have looked at all five essential variables. With this knowledge, we are ready to proceed to the next storey of our house: mechanical breath types. Actually, we need just three variables for this discussion, triggering, cycling, and controlling, because PEEP applies to all breath types and targeting is controlling dependent. Table 7.5 classifies mechanical breath types.

Table 7.5 The eight types of mechanical breath

Breath types	Control breaths	Assist breaths	Support breaths
Volume breath	Volume control breath	Volume assist breath	—
Pressure breath	Pressure control breath	Pressure assist breath	Pressure support breath
Adaptive breath	Adaptive control breath	Adaptive assist breath	Adaptive support breath

Table 7.6 Characteristics of mechanical breath types

Breath type	Triggering	Cycling	Controlling/limiting
1. Volume control	Time	Time	Volume
2. Volume assist	Pressure or flow	Time	Volume
3. Pressure control	Time	Time	Pressure
4. Pressure assist	Pressure or flow	Time	Pressure
5. Pressure support	Pressure or flow	Flow	Pressure
6. Adaptive control	Time	Time	Adaptive
7. Adaptive assist	Pressure or flow	Time	Adaptive
8. Adaptive support	Pressure or flow	Flow	Adaptive

Depending on the triggering and cycling mechanisms applied, a mechanical breath can be a control breath, an assist breath, or a support breath, as follows:

- A *control breath* is a mechanical breath that is time triggered and time cycled.
- An *assist breath* is a mechanical breath that is patient (pressure or flow) triggered and time cycled.
- A *support breath* is a mechanical breath that is patient (pressure or flow) triggered and flow cycled.

Depending on the controlling mechanism applied, a mechanical breath can be a volume breath, a pressure breath, or an adaptive breath, as follows:

- A *volume breath* is a mechanical breath with volume controlling.
- A *pressure breath* is a mechanical breath with pressure controlling.
- An *adaptive breath* is a mechanical breath with adaptive controlling.

Combining the two dimensions, we get eight breath types, as shown in Table 7.6.

There is no volume support breath, because inspiratory flow is strictly controlled in volume breaths, so that flow cycling is impossible.

Do not confuse mechanical breath types with ventilation modes that have similar or identical terms. For instance, adaptive support *breath* is similar to adaptive support *ventilation* (ASV), which is a *mode* on Hamilton Medical ventilators. We just stated that a volume support *breath* does not exist. However, Maquet ventilators have a *mode* called 'volume support'.

These mechanical breath types are of paramount importance, because they are the foundation of almost all ventilation modes, which will be described in Chapter 8.

When facing an unknown ventilation mode, if you can correctly identify its essential variables and breath types, you know pretty much what it does and where it should be used, regardless of its given name.

References

Chatburn RL. Classification of ventilator modes: update and proposal for implementation. *Respir Care* 2007: 5; 301–23.

Chapter 8

Mechanical Ventilation Modes

8.1 Ventilation modes in general

In Chapter 7, we learned that:

- Mechanical breaths are characterized by five essential variables. Each variable uses one or more mechanisms.
- Eight mechanical breath types are defined by various combinations of these variables.
- A ventilator mode is characterized by its mechanical breath type or types.

This chapter is devoted to ventilation modes, a hotly debated topic in mechanical ventilation today.

8.1.1 Ventilation modes: just one of many important issues

Ventilation modes, also called *modes of ventilation* or *ventilator modes*, are a hot topic, and 'new modes of mechanical ventilation' is the subject for many talks at professional congresses of intensive care medicine and respiratory care.

Ventilation modes, however, are just one of many important issues in mechanical ventilation. To achieve the best possible outcomes from a mechanical ventilator you must pay attention to all important issues, not just ventilation modes. These issues are shown in Fig. 8.1.

In this chapter, we will unveil ventilation modes, focusing on their definitions, classifications, and applications.

8.1.2 Definition of ventilation modes

Let's start by defining ventilation modes.

First, we need to exclude what are *not* considered to be ventilation modes.

- Basic pneumatic principles of mechanical ventilation are *not* ventilation modes. Such basic principles include IPPV (intermittent positive pressure ventilation), INPV (intermittent negative pressure ventilation), and HFV (high-frequency ventilation).

Note that Evita ventilators (Dräger) have a mode called 'IPPV', which is very similar to the volume assist/control mode described in this book.

- Invasive mechanical ventilation and non-invasive mechanical ventilation are *not* ventilation modes. They represent two different ways to connect an artificial airway to a natural airway, and both can work with multiple ventilation modes.
- Ventilation functions such as tube (resistance) compensation, in-line nebulization, and apnoea backup are *not* ventilation modes. They may be activated in multiple modes.

It is a bit surprising that in the literature you cannot find a globally standardized definition of ventilation mode. So we do not have a clearly defined and widely agreed answer to the question of 'what is a ventilation mode?' Here is how some respected authors have answered this question:

- During mechanical ventilation, the mode is one of the principal ventilator settings (Hess and Kacmarek, 2002).

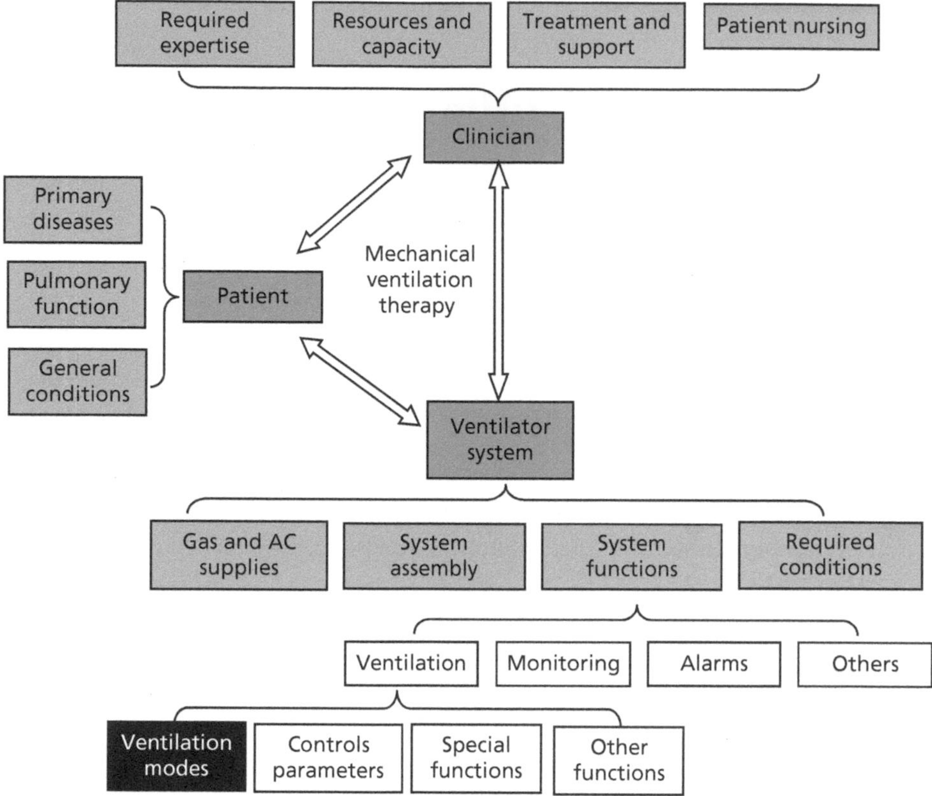

Fig. 8.1 The true position of ventilation modes in the big picture.

- A ventilator mode can be defined as a set of operating characteristics that control how the ventilator functions. An operation mode can be described by the way a ventilator is triggered into inspiration and cycled into exhalation, what variables are limited during inspiration, and whether or not the mode allows only mandatory breaths, spontaneous breaths, or both (Chang, 2006).
- Modes of ventilation describe the pattern of breath delivery to a patient. The use of the terms associated with ventilator modes indicates the type of breath being delivered and how the breaths are triggered, controlled, and cycled (Pilbeam, 2004).
- Modes of ventilation are shorthand terms or acronyms used to describe how a ventilator is behaving in a certain situation . . . A mode is a particular set of control and phase variables (Pilbeam, 1998).
- A ventilation mode represents a specific operation logic for the mechanical ventilator, based on one or more kinds of respiratory cycle management (Iotti, 2003).
- A specific combination of breathing pattern, control, and operational algorithms (Chatburn, 2007).
- The relationship between various possible breath types and inspiratory-phase variables are referred to as modes of ventilation (Kacmarek and Chapman, 2006).

This author's definition is:

> A ventilation mode is a set of ventilator operations with one or more predefined mechanical breath types.

You can come to your own conclusion after reading this chapter.

8.1.3 Mode classification and categorization

Mode classification

It is almost impossible to know the exact number of ventilation modes that have ever existed—old modes disappear and new ones emerge—but that number may be well over 100.

The terminology of ventilation modes is not globally standardized. Ventilator manufacturers and researchers enjoy the freedom to name new modes of ventilation even for trivial changes or innovations. The consequence is that some modes with similar names behave very differently, while other modes with dissimilar names can behave similarly. This chaotic situation of mode terminology confuses clinical ventilator users and is potentially dangerous. Considerable efforts to standardize the terminology of ventilation modes have been made in the last decades. Robert Chatburn, in particular, has done some valuable work in this area. Unfortunately, for practical reasons and reasons of commercial interest, the chaotic situation may not end anytime soon.

This book uses a simple method to classify ventilation modes. It is based on analysis of mechanical breath types in individual ventilation modes. We focus on what the modes are and what they do, but not on what they are named.

Mode categorization

All common ventilation modes can be divided roughly into three categories: (a) conventional ventilation modes, (b) adaptive ventilation modes, and (c) biphasic ventilation modes (Fig. 8.2).

Conventional ventilation modes refer to the most mature and widely used ventilation modes. In a conventional mode, the ventilator works exactly according to the operator's setting, that is, none of the ventilator settings is automatically regulated. Conventional modes are the foundation of the modes in the other categories.

Adaptive ventilation modes are basically conventional modes in which one or more control settings are automatically regulated. For example, inspiratory pressure is automatically regulated in the adaptive assist/control mode. Another example is CareFusion's $CLiO_2$. With this optional function, the ventilator automatically regulates F_iO_2 in neonates. In more advanced adaptive ventilation modes, the ventilator can automatically adjust several control settings at the same time. For instance, tidal volume, respiratory rate, and inspiratory time are automated in the ASV (adaptive support ventilation) mode of Hamilton Medical.

Biphasic ventilation modes may be thought of as a special form of *continuous positive airway pressure* (CPAP) where the *baseline pressure* alternates intermittently between two positive pressure levels according to the operator's settings. The ventilated patient can breathe spontaneously

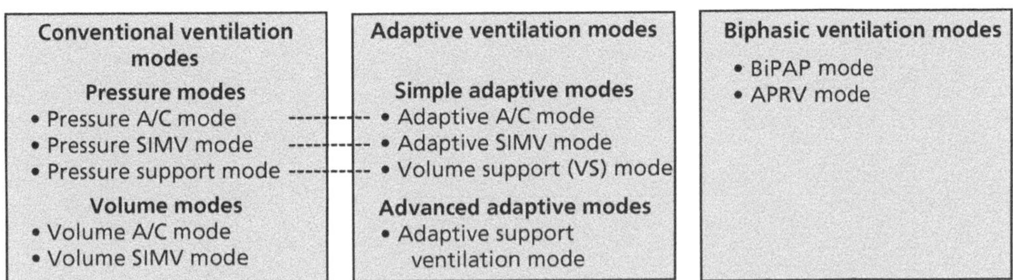

Fig. 8.2 Categories of ventilation mode. The dotted lines indicate the inherent relationships between pressure modes and adaptive modes.

APRV: airway pressure release ventilation; BiPAP: bilevel positive airway pressure; SIMV: synchronized intermittent mandatory ventilation.

at either level. This category includes *bilevel positive airway pressure* (BiPAP) and *airway pressure release ventilation* (APRV).

8.1.4 Ventilation mode terminology

As we mentioned earlier, the terminology of ventilation modes is not globally standardized. Our solution is to focus on the essence rather than the names of ventilation modes. Table 8.1 shows the names of the ventilation modes as they are implemented in popular ventilators.

8.1.5 Graphic symbols for mechanical breaths

To help us understand the building blocks of modes, let's assign a specific symbol to each mechanical breath type (Fig. 8.3).

Table 8.1 Terminology of common ventilation modes

Vendor	Hamilton Medical	Dräger	CareFusion	Covidien	Maquet	GE
Ventilation model	GALILEO/ HAMILTON-G5	Evita XL	AVEA	Puritan Bennett 840	SERVO-i	Care-station
Volume A/C	(S)CMV or A/C	IPPV*	Volume/A/C	AC/VC	Volume control**	VCV
Pressure A/C	P-CMV or P-A/C	BiPAP (mimicking)	Pressure A/C	AC-PC	Pressure control	PCV
Pressure support	SPONT	CPAP, CPAP/P.Supp.	CPAP PSV	SPONT PSV	Pressure support CPAP	CPAP/PSV
Volume SIMV	SIMV	SIMV, SIMV/PS	Volume SIMV	SIMV-VC	SIMV (Volume control)	SIMV-VC
Pressure SIMV	P-SIMV	Not specified	Pressure SIMV	SIMV-PC	SIMV (pressure control)	SIMV-PC
Adaptive A/C	APVcmv	IPPV/AutoFlow***	PRVC A/C	AC-VC+	PRVC	PCV-VG
Adaptive SIMV	APVsimv	SIMV/AutoFlow***	PRVC SIMV	SIMV-VC+	SIMV (PRVC)	SIMV-PCVG
Adaptive support	—	—	—	—	Volume support	—
Biphasic	DuoPAP	BiPAP	APRV/BiPhasic	BiLevel	Bi-vent	BiLevel
	APRV	APRV				

* IPPV in Dräger ventilators is volume assist/control with one distinction: if the Pmax pressure limit is activated, the peak pressure is not allowed to exceed the set Pmax level;

** Volume control in the Maquet SERVO-i ventilator is volume assist/control with one distinction: the ventilated patient, if active, can modify the inspiratory flow and timing;

*** AutoFlow is a mode addition. By adding it, a pressure mode is converted to an adaptive mode.

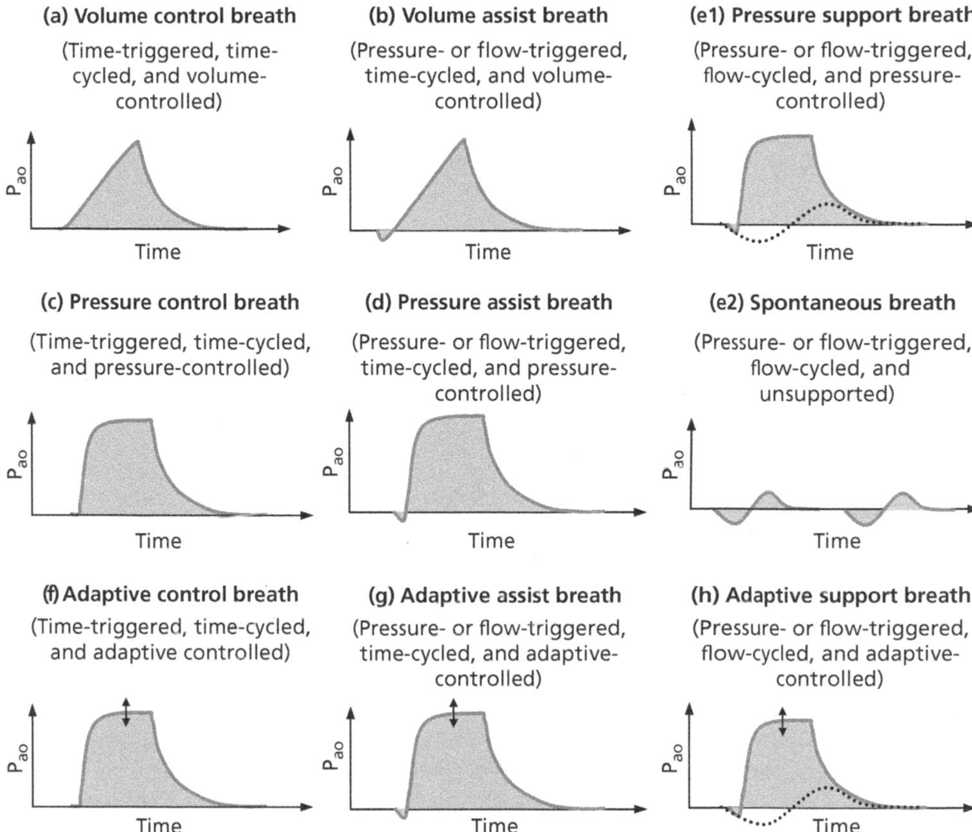

Fig. 8.3 Graphic symbols for breath types.

You may wonder why we have nine symbols for eight breath types. This is because a *pressure support breath* may be either a supported spontaneous breath (e1) or an unsupported spontaneous breath (e2). In the latter case, the ventilated patient must generate tidal volume by their own inspiratory muscle activities.

8.2 Conventional ventilation modes

Conventional ventilation modes are mature and the most popularized. In conventional modes, the baseline stays at a set level, and none of the variables is adjusted automatically. There are five conventional modes: volume assist/control; pressure assist/control; pressure support ventilation; volume synchronized intermittent mandatory ventilation (SIMV); and pressure SIMV.

8.2.1 Volume assist/control (A/C) mode

The *volume A/C mode* has different names (see Table 8.2).

The volume *A/C* mode allows two breath types: *volume control breaths* and *volume assist breaths*. Their characteristics are given in Table 8.3.

In this mode, the operator sets:

a. Tidal volume
b. Rate
c. T_i (or I:E ratio or peak flow)

Table 8.2 Volume A/C mode has different names

Ventilator model	GALILEO/HAMILTON-G5	Evita XL	AVEA	Puritan Bennett 840	SERVO-i	Care-station
Volume assist/control	(S)CMV or A/C	IPPV*	Volume A/C	AC-VC	Volume control**	VCV

* IPPV in Evita ventilators is volume assist/control mode with one distinction: if the Pmax pressure limit is activated, the peak pressure is not allowed to exceed the set Pmax; ** Volume control in the Maquet SERVO-i ventilator is volume assist/control with one distinction: the ventilated patient, if active, can modify the inspiratory flow and timing.

d. Patient trigger type and sensitivity
e. PEEP (positive end-expiratory pressure)
f. F_iO_2
g. Flow pattern (possibly).

Mechanical ventilation may be regarded as a series of mechanical breaths. In Chapter 7, we learned how pressure and flow triggering works in a single mechanical breath. If two or more consecutive mechanical breaths are involved, we need to learn about another important concept of patient triggering, that is, the *triggering window* or *trigger window*.

The triggering window is a defined time slot at late expiration, when the ventilator responds to patient triggering—either by pressure or flow. If the ventilator detects a valid pneumatic signal within the triggering window, it delivers a volume assist breath. If not, it delivers a volume control (time-triggered) breath according to the preset rate. The triggering window is an important technical feature in terms of patient-ventilator synchrony. In a passive patient, all breaths are volume control breaths, and the monitored rate and the set rate are equal. In an active patient, some or all breaths are volume assist breaths, and the monitored rate is higher than the set rate.

Fig. 8.4 shows a typical waveform in volume A/C mode.

In the volume A/C mode, the baseline pressure (PEEP) is constant.

The volume A/C mode is intended for ventilated patients who are passive or partially active. It is not a good choice for active patients, especially those with a strong drive, because the patient may not tolerate the inflexible manner of inspiratory gas delivery. *Patient-ventilator asynchrony* is highly probable.

It is critical to set tidal volume and rate so that the resultant alveolar ventilation matches the patient's current demand. Note that the demand may vary during mechanical ventilation. If so, you need to adjust the ventilator settings.

Table 8.3 Volume A/C mode allows two breath types

Variable	Volume control breath	Volume assist breath
Triggering	Time	Pressure/flow
Cycling	Time	Time
Controlling	Volume	Volume

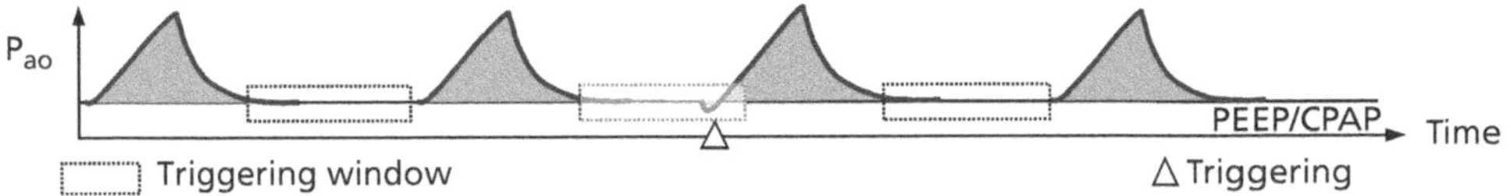

Fig. 8.4 Typical pressure-time waveform in volume A/C mode.

The volume assist/control mode allows the operator to directly control tidal volume, rate, and T_i for a desired minute volume. It was a primary mode in the past. Over time, its disadvantages have become apparent:

- There is a high incidence of patient-ventilator asynchrony in active patients with a strong drive.
- The resultant peak airway pressure can be uncomfortably high. Therefore, it is important to set the upper limit of the airway pressure alarm to avoid resultant *barotrauma*.
  Caution: In some ventilators, the set alarm limit is used for pressure cycling (i.e. the ventilator cycles immediately to expiration whenever the monitored airway pressure reaches this limit, even if the desired tidal volume is not completely delivered).
- In this mode, leakage compensation is impossible.

8.2.2 Pressure assist/control (A/C) mode

The *pressure A/C mode* has different names (see Table 8.4).

The pressure A/C mode also allows two breath types: *pressure control breaths* and *pressure assist breaths*. Their characteristics are given in Table 8.5.

In this mode, the operator sets:

a. Inspiratory pressure (often called *pressure control*)
b. Rate
c. T_i (or I:E)
d. Patient trigger type and sensitivity
e. PEEP
f. F_iO_2
g. Rise time (possibly).

Like the volume A/C mode, the pressure A/C mode has a triggering window, which opens at late expiration. If the ventilator detects a valid pneumatic signal during the triggering window, it delivers a pressure assist breath. If not, it delivers a pressure control (time-triggered) breath according to the set rate. The set $P_{control}$ applies to both breath types.

Table 8.4 Pressure A/C mode has different names

Ventilator model	GALILEO/HAMILTON-G5	Evita XL	AVEA	Puritan Bennett 840	SERVO-i	Care-station
Pressure assist/ control	P-CMV or P-A/C	BiPAP (mimicking)	Pressure A/C	AC-PC	Pressure control	PCV

Table 8.5 Pressure A/C mode allows two breath types

Variable	Pressure control breath	Pressure assist breath
Triggering	Time	Pressure/flow
Cycling	Time	Time
Limiting/control	Pressure	Pressure

In the pressure A/C mode, all breaths are pressure controlled if the ventilated patient is passive, and the monitored rate and the set rate are roughly equal. If the patient is active, some or all breaths are pressure assist breaths, and the monitored rate is typically higher than the set rate.

In the pressure A/C mode, the baseline pressure (PEEP) is constant.

Fig. 8.5 shows a typical waveform in the pressure A/C mode.

The pressure A/C mode is suitable for passive or partially active patients. It can also be used in active patients with weak respiratory drive, because this mode allows the patient to influence rate, inspiratory flow, and tidal volume. Compared to the volume assist/control mode, pressure assist/control has a considerably lower incidence of patient-ventilator asynchrony. Another advantage of pressure assist/control is that this mode enables the ventilator to compensate for moderate levels of gas leakage.

The perceived disadvantage of this mode is that an operator cannot directly control tidal volume. The resultant tidal volume may be unstable when the patient's breathing effort and/or respiratory mechanics change. Therefore, you should carefully set the upper and lower limits of the tidal volume alarm.

8.2.3 Pressure support ventilation (PSV) mode

The *PSV* mode has different names (see Table 8.6)

The pressure support ventilation mode allows just one breath type: pressure support breaths. Its characteristics are given in Table 8.7.

In this mode, an operator sets:

a. Inspiratory pressure (also known as *pressure support*)
b. Patient trigger type and sensitivity
c. PEEP
d. F_iO_2
e. Flow cycling criteria
f. Rise time (possibly).

The pressure support ventilation mode is indicated for active patients only. It is the most comfortable mode for this patient population, because they can influence the actual rate, inspiratory time, inspiratory flow, and tidal volume. Obviously, it is contraindicated for the passive patients.

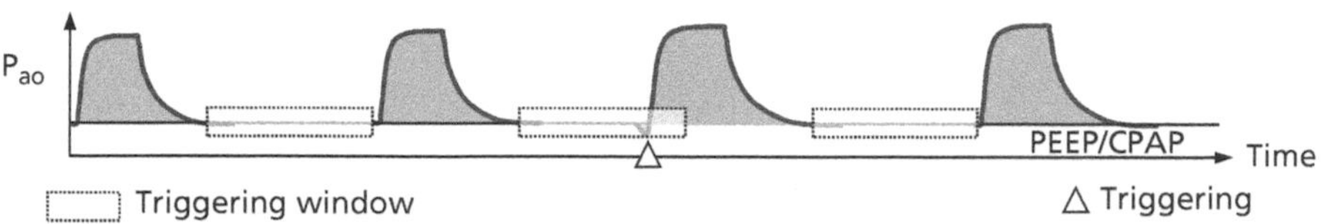

Fig. 8.5 Typical pressure-time waveform in pressure A/C mode.

Table 8.6 SV mode has different names

Ventilator model	GALILEO/HAMILTON-G5	Evita XL	AVEA	Puritan Bennett 840	SERVO-i	Carestation
Pressure support	SPONT	CPAP, CPAP/P.Sup.	CPAP PSV	SPONT PSV	Pressure support CPAP	CPAP/PSV

Apnoea (backup) ventilation should be activated in this mode. This mode enables the ventilator to adequately compensate for moderate levels of gas leakage.

In pressure support ventilation, the baseline pressure (PEEP) is constant.

You may notice that in some ventilators this mode is called CPAP + PSV. CPAP stands for continuous positive airway pressure. The patient breathes unsupported at an elevated baseline pressure. PSV stands for pressure support ventilation. The patient's spontaneous breaths are mechanically supported. In this mode, both CPAP and PSV can be realized by changing the pressure support setting.

Spontaneous breaths

If pressure support is set to zero or close to zero, the patient has to do all the required work of breathing to satisfy the ventilatory demand. Unsupported mechanical breaths are *spontaneous breaths*, often abbreviated as *Spont*. Spontaneous breaths in ventilated patients are a great challenge, and should be used only in patients who are stable and in good clinical condition. Their typical application is for weaning trials, also known as spontaneous breathing trials.

Typically the patient breathes spontaneously at a moderate positive baseline pressure (PEEP).

Fig. 8.6 shows a typical waveform for pressure-supported breaths in the pressure support mode.

For invasive mechanical ventilation, an endotracheal tube imposes an additional airway resistance to the gas flow in both directions. Refer to section 10.6 for details. Even when your intention is to let the patient breathe unsupported, setting a pressure support of 3 or 5 cmH_2O may be advised to offset the resistance imposed by the ETT.

Technologically, spontaneous breathing is a performance challenge to a ventilator system. Good PEEP performance requires excellent sensitivity and system responsiveness. Ideally, the baseline pressure should remain stable even when the patient inhales and exhales intensively.

Pressure-supported breaths

If you set pressure support to 10 cmH_2O or higher, the patient's spontaneous breaths are pressure *supported*. In this case, the ventilator takes over a significant part of the required work of breathing.

Table 8.7 PSV mode allows one breath type

Variable	Pressure support breath
Triggering	Pressure/flow
Cycling	Flow
Limiting/control	Pressure

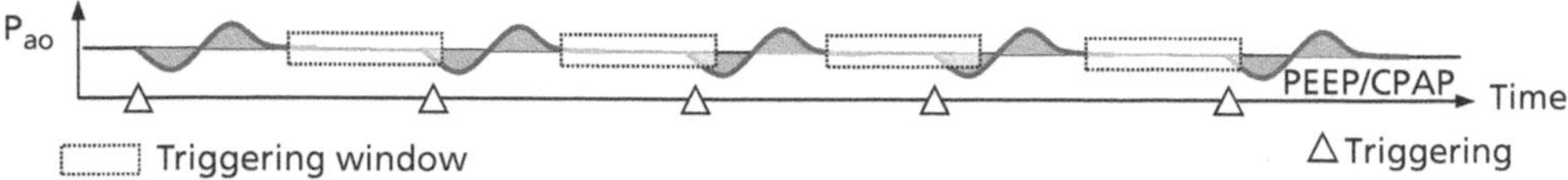

Fig. 8.6 Typical pressure-time waveform for spontaneous breaths in the PSV mode.

Pressure-supported breathing is indicated when the ventilated patient is active, but their own efforts are inadequate to meet their required ventilatory demand.

Fig. 8.7 shows a typical waveform for pressure-supported breaths in the pressure support mode.

By design, a ventilator in the PSV mode delivers a mechanical breath only when it is pressure or flow triggered. Obviously, this is clinically dangerous because an active patient can stop breathing activity (apnoea) at any time for various clinical reasons. To prevent this potential risk, it is strongly recommended that you activate a protective mechanism called *apnoea backup* or *apnoea ventilation* when ventilating in pressure support mode. We will discuss apnoea backup in section 10.5.

In this mode, the set pressure support level represents the amount of mechanical support. How high should pressure support be? To answer that question, we must consider three factors:

- The patient's ventilatory demand: The demand can vary considerably during mechanical ventilation (e.g. it increases with fever and agitation).
- The current status of the pulmonary system: The functionality of the pulmonary system can be seriously diminished in ventilated patients.
- The current objective of mechanical ventilation therapy: Mechanical ventilation therapy has different objectives at different phases. We set the pressure support high when we intend to relax an exhausted patient in an acute phase. We may reduce the pressure support in steps in the weaning phase.

Finally, pressure support ventilation is a common foundation of several newer ventilation modes, including SmartCare, neurally adjusted ventilatory assist (NAVA), and proportional assist ventilation (PAV).

8.2.4 **Volume SIMV mode**

The *volume SIMV mode* has different names (see Table 8.8).

SIMV stands for *synchronized intermittent mandatory ventilation*. It is derived from IMV (*intermittent mandatory ventilation*). In modern ventilators, SIMV is replacing IMV entirely.

The SIMV mode has three forms: volume SIMV, pressure SIMV, and adaptive SIMV. They are discussed in sections 8.2.4, 8.2.5, and 8.3.4, respectively.

The volume SIMV mode allows three breath types: volume control breaths, volume assist breaths, and pressure support breaths. Their characteristics are given in Table 8.9.

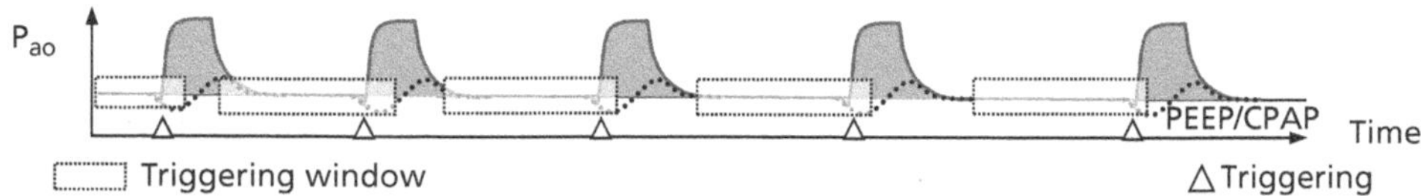

Fig. 8.7 Typical pressure-time waveform for pressure-supported breaths in the PSV (pressure support ventilation) mode.

Table 8.8 Volume SIMV mode has different names

Ventilator model	GALILEO/ HAMILTON-G5	Evita XL	AVEA	Puritan Bennett 840	SERVO-i	Care-station
Volume SIMV	SIMV	SIMV, SIMV/ PS	Volume SIMV	SIMV-VC	SIMV (Volume control)	SIMV-VCV

In this mode, an operator sets:

a. Tidal volume
b. Rate (also known as SIMV rate)
c. T_i (or I:E)
d. $P_{support}$
e. Patient trigger type and sensitivity
f. Flow cycling
g. Rise time (possibly)
h. PEEP
i. F_iO_2.

Volume control breaths are defined by control settings (a), (b), and (c). Volume assist breaths are defined by control settings (a), (c), and (e). Pressure support breaths are defined by control settings (d), (e), (f), and (g).

In the volume SIMV mode, the ventilator delivers volume control breaths at the set SIMV rate. However, if the ventilator detects a valid pressure or flow trigger signal within the triggering window, it delivers a volume assist breath instead. The patient is allowed to breathe spontaneously, with or without pressure support, between two consecutive volume control or assist breaths.

The behaviour of the volume SIMV mode can vary considerably depending on the set rate, known as the SIMV rate.

If the set rate is high, the interval between two consecutive control or assist breaths is so short that no pressure support breath can be inserted (Fig. 8.8). The mode behaves like the volume assist/control mode.

If the set rate is very low, the interval between two consecutive control or assist breaths is long enough that several pressure support breaths can be inserted (Fig. 8.9 and Fig. 8.10). The mode behaves like the pressure support mode.

The volume SIMV mode has two major advantages. First, the volume SIMV mode is versatile: it behaves like the volume assist control mode or the pressure support mode, depending on the set SIMV rate. This single mode can be used from intubation through to extubation; for this reason it has been called the 'universal mode'. Clinicians embrace the volume SIMV mode,

Table 8.9 Volume SIMV mode allows three breath types

Variable	Volume control breath	Volume assist breath	Pressure support breath
Triggering	Time	Pressure/flow	Pressure/flow
Cycling	Time	Time	Flow
Limiting/control	Volume	Volume	Pressure

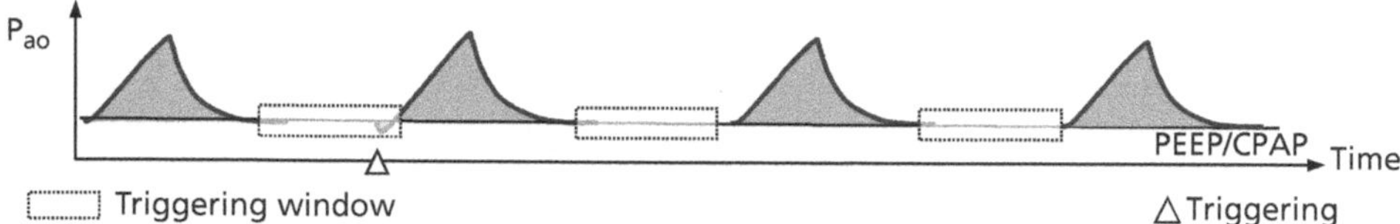

Fig. 8.8 Typical pressure-time waveform for volume SIMV (synchronized intermittent mandatory ventilation) mode with a high set rate.

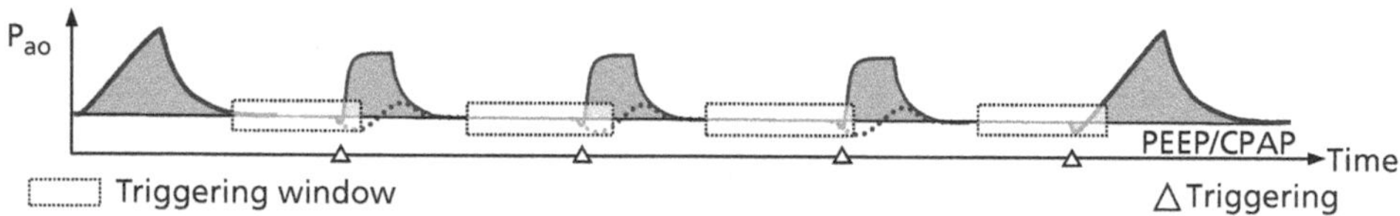

Fig. 8.9 Typical pressure-time waveform for volume SIMV with a low set rate. The inserted breaths are pressure support breaths.

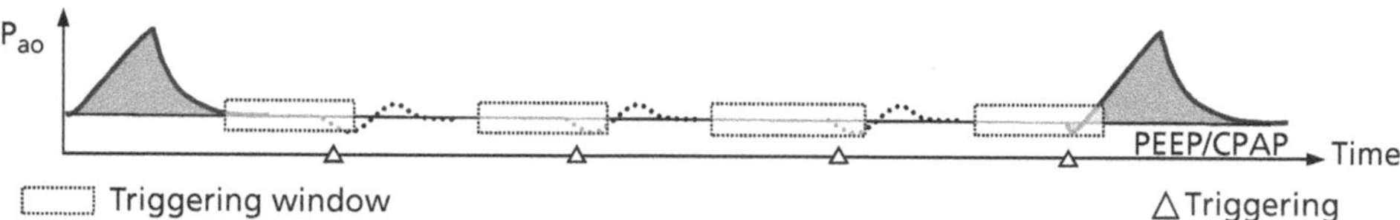

Fig. 8.10 Typical pressure-time waveform for volume SIMV mode with a low set rate. The inserted breaths are spontaneous breaths.

Table 8.10 Pressure SIMV mode has different names

Ventilator model	GALILEO/HAMILTON-G5	Evita XL	AVEA	Puritan Bennett 840	SERVO-i	Care-station
Pressure SIMV	P-SIMV	PCV +/P.Supp.	Pressure SIMV	SIMV-PC	SIMV (pressure control)	SIMV-PC

Table 8.11 Pressure SIMV mode allows three breath types

Variable	Pressure control breath	Pressure assist breath	Pressure support breath
Triggering	Time	Pressure/flow	Pressure/flow
Cycling	Time	Time	Flow
Limiting/control	Pressure	Pressure	Pressure

because it removes the need for mode change, which is sometimes a difficult decision. Therefore, the actual minute volume could be much greater than the minimum.

The major disadvantage of volume SIMV mode is that its mixture of volume and pressure breaths may be uncomfortable for the patient.

Further, the volume SIMV mode has a number of control parameters. Setting and adjusting these appropriately requires a thorough understanding of the controls.

8.2.5 Pressure SIMV mode

The *pressure SIMV mode* has different names (see Table 8.10).

The pressure SIMV mode allows three breath types: pressure control breaths, pressure assist breaths, and pressure support breaths. Their characteristics are given in Table 8.11.

In this mode, an operator sets:

a. $P_{control}$
b. Rate (also known as SIMV rate)
c. T_i (or I:E)
d. Pressure support
e. Patient trigger type and sensitivity
f. Flow cycling
g. Rise time (possibly)
h. PEEP
i. F_iO_2.

Pressure control breaths are defined by control settings (a), (b), (c), and (g). Pressure assist breaths are defined by control settings (a), (c), (e), and (g). Pressure support breaths are defined by control settings (d), (e), (f), and (g).

In the pressure SIMV mode, the ventilator delivers pressure control breaths at the set SIMV rate. However, if the ventilator detects a valid pressure or flow trigger signal within the triggering window, it delivers a pressure assist breath instead. The patient is allowed to breathe spontaneously, with or without pressure support, between two consecutive pressure control or assist breaths.

The behaviour of the pressure SIMV mode can vary considerably, depending on the set rate, known as the SIMV rate.

If the set SIMV rate is high, the interval between two consecutive control or assist breaths is so short that no pressure support breaths can be inserted (Fig. 8.11). The mode behaves like the pressure assist/control mode.

If the set SIMV rate is very low, the interval between two consecutive control or assist breaths is long enough for several additional pressure support breaths (Fig. 8.12 and Fig. 8.13). The mode behaves like the pressure support mode.

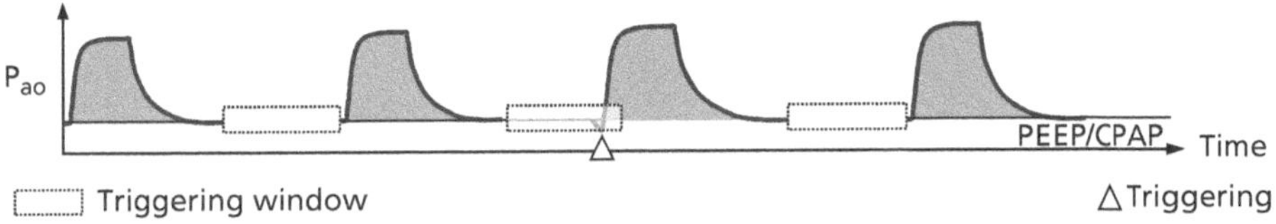

Fig. 8.11 Typical pressure-time waveform for pressure SIMV (synchronized intermittent mandatory ventilation) mode with a high set SIMV rate.

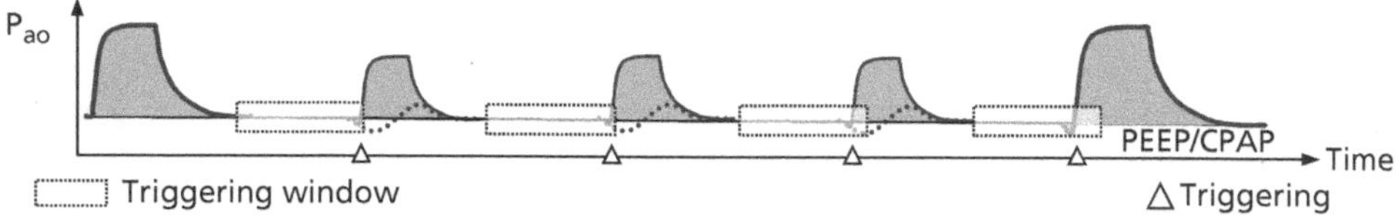

Fig. 8.12 Typical pressure-time waveform for pressure SIMV mode with a low set rate. The inserted breaths are pressure support breaths.

Like the volume SIMV mode, the pressure SIMV mode can also be used from intubation through to extubation, avoiding the need for a mode change.

The obvious difference between these two modes is that in pressure SIMV mode all types of mechanical breath are pressure controlled. This means it is not possible to guarantee a minimum minute volume. On the plus side, this mode prevents the patient discomfort from repeated switching between volume and pressure breaths.

The pressure SIMV mode also requires the operator to set many control parameters. Thus, setting and adjusting these parameters appropriately requires a thorough understanding of the mode.

8.3 Adaptive ventilation modes

8.3.1 Adaptive ventilation modes in general

The definition

An *adaptive ventilation mode* is an advanced ventilation mode where, at a minimum, one primary control parameter is automatically adjusted based on the monitoring inputs and special algorithms. All adaptive ventilation modes are derived from pressure-controlled modes.

Adaptive ventilation mode can be defined in two ways. In its narrowest sense, an adaptive ventilation mode is a mode where inspiratory pressure is automatically regulated based on monitoring input, to assure the target tidal volume. We will use this definition in this book. In its general sense, however, adaptive ventilation modes include all modes in which one or more major controls are automatically regulated, based on monitoring inputs.

What problem do they solve?

During the course of mechanical ventilation, patient conditions can change, either alone or jointly (Fig. 8.14):

- The patient's ventilatory demand;
- The respiratory mechanics (airway resistance and respiratory compliance);
- The functional status of the patient's pulmonary system;
- The patient's breathing activities;
- The functional status of the ventilator system.

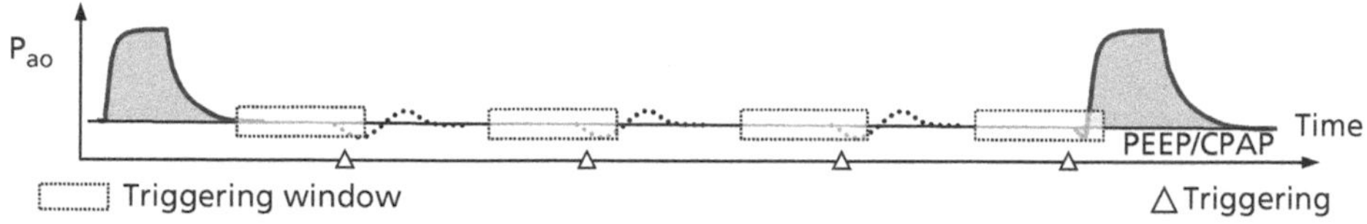

Fig. 8.13 Typical pressure-time waveform for pressure SIMV mode with a low set rate. The inserted breaths are spontaneous breaths.

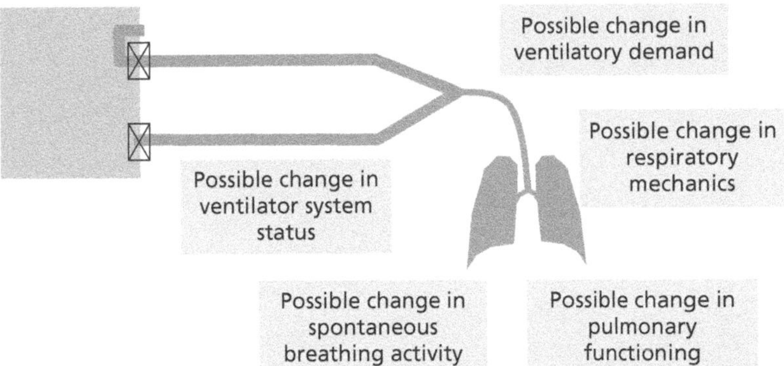

Fig. 8.14 In practice, a ventilator system is often dynamic.

By traditional design concept, a ventilator system is a 'rigid' tool for mechanical ventilation. The ventilator system is 'rigid', because it must carry out its task precisely according to the operator's settings, whether or not they are appropriate. This means that only an operator can change or influence the behaviour of a ventilator system.

Assume that an operator sets a ventilator system optimally. A few hours later, however, the settings may become suboptimal or even unacceptable due to changes in patient status. Now the operator must readjust the settings. This work is labour intensive, especially in acute and unstable patients.

Furthermore, ventilator setting readjustment requires highly specialized knowledge. Optimal ventilator setting is possible only by very knowledgeable operators. Inappropriate readjustment of ventilator settings may worsen the situation.

Is it possible for a smart or intelligent ventilator to automatically readjust the settings without an operator's intervention? This question has shaken that traditional concept of ventilator design and ushered in a new era of intelligent or automatic mechanical ventilation.

The operating principle

The common basis for all adaptive ventilation modes is *closed-loop control* theory. This is also the foundation of industrial automation.

Fig. 8.15 illustrates the basic principles of closed-loop control, which has six components:

1. The operator's command to define the target (e.g. target tidal volume).
2. The controller: A software algorithm that takes in the monitoring input, compares it to the set target, determines how to respond, and sends instructions to the executer.

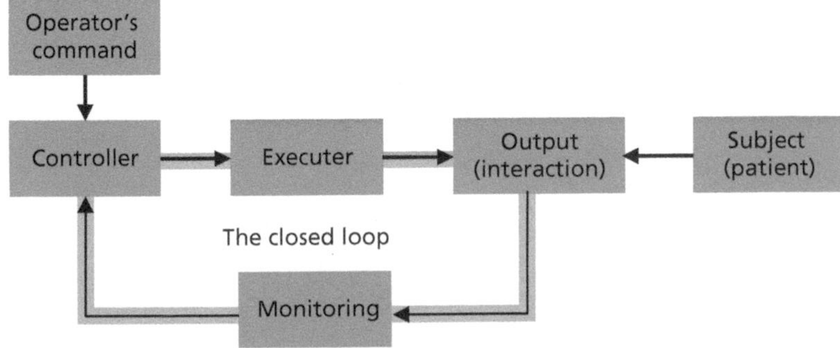

Fig. 8.15 Diagram of closed-loop ventilation control.

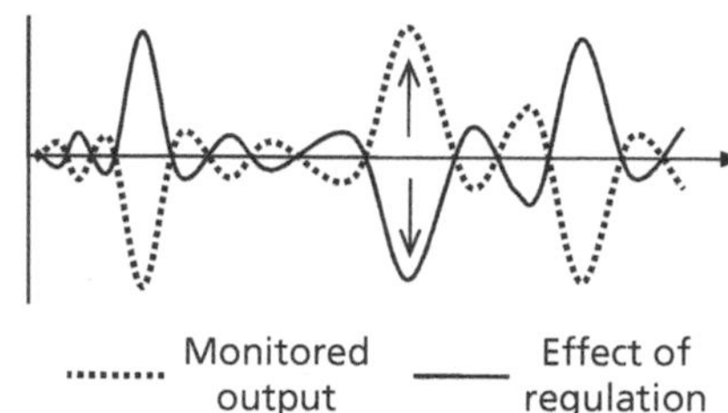

Fig. 8.16 Negative feedback regulation for *stabilization* purposes.

3. The executer: The ventilator system, which carries out the mechanical ventilation according to operator settings and auto-regulation.
4. The subject: The patient's pulmonary system.
5. The output: The result of interaction between the executer and the subject. It changes if either or both sides change.
6. Monitoring: The component that closes the loop. With it, the output can directly influence or change the behaviour of the ventilator system without the operator's involvement.

Closed-loop regulation has two basic forms of regulation: a *negative feedback loop* and a *positive feedback loop*.

Negative feedback loop With negative feedback loop regulation, if the output is less than the target, the executer intensifies its performance. If the output is greater than the target, the executer weakens its performance. Thus, the monitored output and the effect of regulation are in opposite directions (Fig. 8.16). The system tends to stabilize at the target.

Human physiology applies extensive regulation by negative feedback loops in the regulation of blood pressure, blood sugar, $PaCO_2$, and body temperature, among others. Adaptive ventilation modes apply negative feedback loop regulation in a limited sense. A familiar, non-medical example is the cruise control in a car.

Positive feedback loop With positive feedback loop regulation, the executer's performance is proportional to the intensity of the monitored signal, with a gain factor set by an operator. The stronger the signal, the greater the effect of regulation. Both are in the same direction (Fig. 8.17).

Human physiology also, although rarely, applies regulation by positive feedback loop. Blood clotting and childbirth are two examples. Proportional assist ventilation (PAV) and tube resistance compensation (TRC) are based on a positive feedback loop. A non-medical example is power steering in a car.

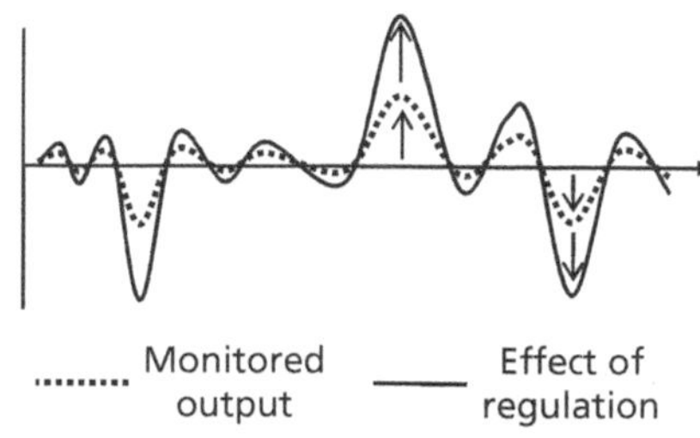

Fig. 8.17 Positive feedback regulation for *amplification* purposes.

Advantages of adaptive ventilation modes

Proper use of adaptive modes can considerably reduce the staff's workload, improve the therapy quality, and decrease the incidence of ventilator alarms. Note that these advantages relate exclusively to ventilator setting. Adaptive modes are not superior in terms of non-setting issues.

Adaptive mode or pressure mode plus a mode addition

In most ventilators, adaptive ventilation modes are independent modes, for simplicity. In some other ventilators, you may have to activate a mode addition feature to convert a pressure mode to an adaptive mode. In Dräger ventilators, this feature is called 'AutoFlow'.

The relationship between adaptive modes and pressure modes plus the feature is simple:

$$\textit{Pressure mode} + \textit{Mode addition} \Leftrightarrow \textit{Adaptive mode}$$

The pressure regulation ceiling

In adaptive ventilation modes, the ventilator automatically regulates the inspiratory pressure so that the monitored tidal volume matches the target tidal volume. However, this automation must be restricted to a defined range for patient safety. In this case, we need to define a pressure ceiling (i.e. the peak pressure is not allowed to exceed this ceiling).

Typically, the pressure ceiling for adult patients is set at 35–40 cmH_2O. Below the ceiling, the controller can freely regulate the inspiratory pressure. However, the peak pressure is not allowed to exceed the ceiling, even if this is necessary to generate the target tidal volume. Should this happen, the ventilator typically informs the operator of this situation. For example, Hamilton Medical ventilators display the message '*APV*: unable to achieve target'. The operator has three choices: (a) identify and remove the cause of the high airway pressure (e.g. low compliance or high resistance); (b) reduce the target tidal volume; and (c) increase the ceiling with caution.

The ceiling may be either set directly or defined by the upper limit of the airway pressure alarm. In the latter case, the ceiling is typically 10 cmH_2O below the alarm limit.

The ceiling may be shown on the ventilator display. HAMILTON-G5 and GALILEO ventilators display a blue bar in the pressure-time graph to visualize both the pressure regulation ceiling and the alarm limit (Fig. 8.18).

8.3.2 Adaptive assist/control (A/C) mode

The *adaptive assist/control mode* (also called the *adaptive pressure ventilation mode* (APV)) is derived from the pressure A/C mode. It is based on closed-loop control with negative feedback (Table 8.12).

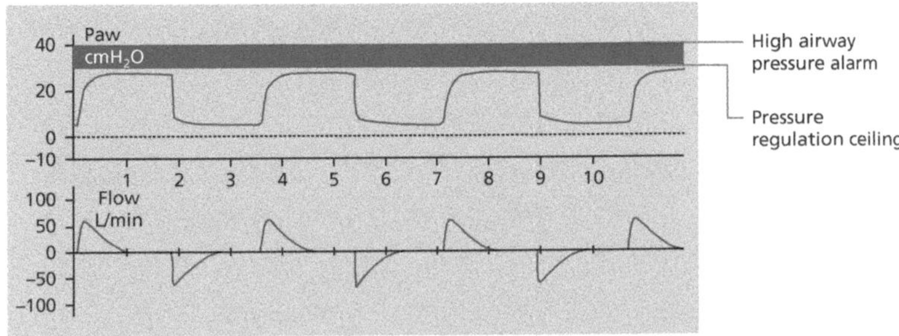

Fig. 8.18 The set high pressure alarm limit and pressure regulation ceiling in an adaptive mode.

Table 8.12 Adaptive A/C mode has different names

Ventilator model	GALILEO/HAMILTON-G5	Evita XL	AVEA	Puritan Bennett 840	SERVO-i	Care-station
Adaptive A/C mode	APVcmv	AutoFlow*	PRVC A/C	AC-VC+	PRVC	PCV-VG

* AutoFlow is a mode addition. It can be added to a pressure mode to convert it to an adaptive mode.

The adaptive A/C mode allows two breath types: *adaptive control breaths* and adaptive assist breaths. Their characteristics are given in Table 8.13.

In this mode, an operator sets:

a. (Target) tidal volume
b. Rate
c. T_i (or I:E)
d. Patient trigger type and sensitivity
e. Rise time
f. PEEP
g. F_iO_2.

In the adaptive A/C mode, a triggering window opens at late expiration with every breath. If a valid patient trigger is detected within the window, the ventilator delivers an adaptive assist breath. Otherwise, it delivers an adaptive control breath. In a passive patient, every breath is an adaptive control breath. The actual respiratory rate is roughly equal to the set rate. In an active patient, however, every breath may be an adaptive assist breath. The actual respiratory rate may be higher than the set rate.

The ventilator automatically regulates the inspiratory pressure breath by breath to minimize the gap between the monitored tidal volume (output) and the target tidal volume. With this mechanism, the actual tidal volume is stabilized at the target level even when the patient's lung mechanics change.

In this mode, the baseline pressure is constant.

Fig. 8.19 shows a typical pressure waveform in adaptive A/C mode.

Like the pressure A/C mode, the adaptive A/C mode is indicated for passive and partially active patients. It may not be a good choice for active patients with a strong drive.

Target tidal volume is a particularly important control in adaptive A/C mode. As we know, alveolar minute volume is determined by tidal volume, respiratory rate, and total dead space. There are three possible scenarios:

1. Alveolar minute ventilation is lower than the current ventilatory demand (i.e. hypoventilation). An important cause is that the set target tidal volume and/or rate are inadequate.

Table 8.13 Adaptive A/C mode allows two breath types

Variable	Adaptive control breath	Adaptive assist breath
Triggering	Time	Pressure/flow
Cycling	Time	Time
Limiting/control	Adaptive	Adaptive

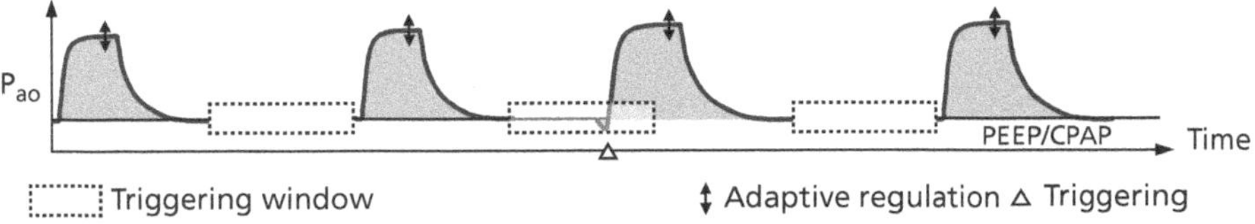

Fig. 8.19 Typical pressure-time waveform in adaptive A/C mode.

2. Alveolar minute ventilation matches the current ventilatory demand.
3. Alveolar minute ventilation is higher than the current ventilatory demand (i.e. hyperventilation). An important cause is that the set target tidal volume is too high.

How does adaptive A/C mode respond to hypoventilation?

Assume that we use the adaptive A/C mode to ventilate an active patient, and the set target tidal volume is inadequate. The patient has to breathe harder to get sufficient minute ventilation. According to the closed-loop control principle, however, the ventilator reduces the inspiratory pressure because the actual tidal volume is greater than the target tidal volume. The harder the patient works, the less mechanical support they receive from the ventilator. Finally, the patient does more or less all the work of breathing, while the ventilator does little. Some clinicians may suspect that this undesirable behaviour is caused by a ventilator design flaw. In fact, the adaptive A/C mode is behaving exactly as specified. The problem disappears if you increase the target tidal volume.

What if hyperventilation is present? The ventilator regulates the inspiratory pressure so that the monitored tidal volume is stabilized at the target level, which is higher than the demand. $PaCO_2$ will decrease, suppressing the patient's spontaneous breaths.

For these reasons, the adaptive A/C mode may not be the best choice for an active patient with a strong drive.

8.3.3 Adaptive SIMV mode

This mode is derived from the pressure SIMV mode and has different names (see Table 8.14)

The adaptive SIMV mode allows three breath types: adaptive control breaths, adaptive assist breaths, and pressure support breaths. Their characteristics are given in Table 8.15.

In this mode, an operator sets:

a. Target tidal volume
b. Rate (also known as SIMV rate)
c. T_i (or I:E)
d. Pressure support

Table 8.14 Adaptive SIMV mode has different names

Ventilator model	GALILEO/HAMILTON-G5	Evita XL	AVEA	Puritan Bennett 840	SERVO-i	Care-station
Adaptive SIMV mode	APVsimv	SIMV/AutoFlow	PRVC SIMV	SIMV-VC+	SIMV (PRVC)	SIMV-PCVG

Table 8.15 Adaptive SIMV mode allows three breath types

Variable	Adaptive control breath	Adaptive assist breath	Pressure support breath
Triggering	Time	Pressure/flow	Pressure/flow
Cycling	Time	Time	Flow
Limiting/ control	Adaptive	Adaptive	Pressure

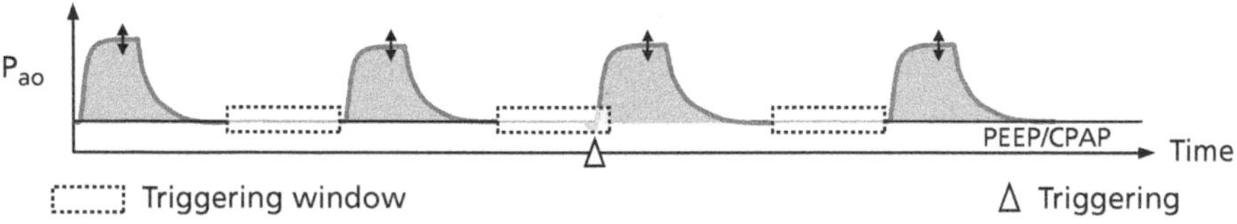

Fig. 8.20 Typical pressure-time waveform in adaptive SIMV with a high rate setting.

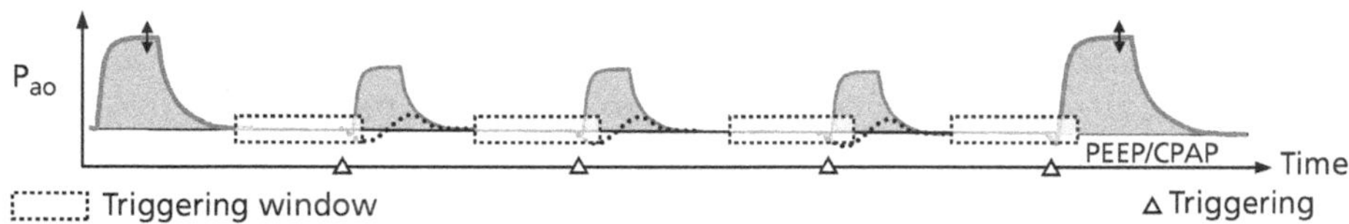

Fig. 8.21 Typical pressure-time waveform in adaptive SIMV mode with a low rate setting and additional pressure-supported breaths.

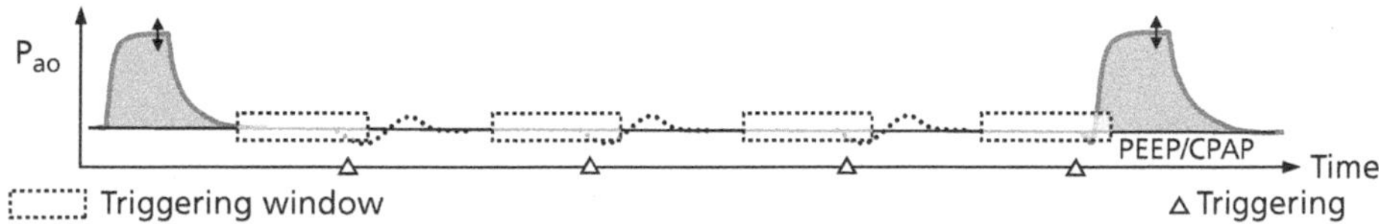

Fig. 8.22 Typical pressure-time waveform in adaptive SIMV mode with a low rate setting and additional unsupported breaths.

Table 8.16 Volume support mode allows one breath type

Variable	Adaptive support breath
Triggering	Pressure/flow
Cycling	Flow
Limiting/control	Adaptive

e. Patient trigger type and sensitivity
f. Flow cycling criterion
g. Rise time
h. PEEP
i. F_iO_2.

The adaptive control breath is defined by (a), (b), (c), and (g). The adaptive assist breath is defined by (a), (c), (e), and (g). The adaptive support breath is defined by (d), (e), (f), and (g).

In the adaptive SIMV mode, the ventilator delivers adaptive control breaths at the set SIMV rate. However, if it detects a valid patient trigger while the triggering window is open, it delivers an adaptive assist breath instead. The patient is allowed to breathe spontaneously, with or without pressure support, between any two consecutive adaptive control or assist breaths.

The behaviour of the adaptive SIMV mode can vary considerably, depending on the set SIMV rate. If the SIMV rate is set high, the interval between two consecutive adaptive control or assist breaths is so short that there is practically no time for additional pressure support breaths (Fig. 8.20). The adaptive SIMV mode resembles the adaptive A/C mode. If the SIMV rate is set very low, the interval between two consecutive control or assist *mandatory breaths* is long enough to accommodate several additional pressure support breaths (Fig. 8.21 and Fig. 8.22). In this case, the adaptive SIMV mode resembles the pressure support mode.

Like other forms of SIMV, the adaptive SIMV mode can be used from intubation through to extubation, avoiding the need for a mode change.

Adaptive SIMV behaves very similarly to pressure SIMV, except for the automatic regulation of inspiratory pressure in all adaptive control and adaptive assist breaths. If the set SIMV rate is very low, this regulation may be fairly slow.

8.3.4 Volume support mode

Following our naming rules, this mode should be called the 'adaptive support mode'. We'll keep the name 'volume support' for two reasons. For one, Maquet ventilators have had a volume support mode for decades. In addition, Hamilton Medical has an advanced adaptive ventilation mode called adaptive support ventilation (ASV).

The *volume support mode* allows just one breath type: an adaptive support breath. Its characteristics are given in Table 8.16.

In this mode, an operator sets:

a. Target tidal volume
b. Patient trigger type and sensitivity
c. Flow cycling criteria
d. Rise time
e. PEEP
f. F_iO_2.

The volume support mode is derived from the pressure support mode, so the two modes behave similarly. The only difference is the automatic regulation of inspiratory pressure in volume support mode.

Fig. 8.23 shows a typical pressure waveform for the volume support mode.

The volume support mode is indicated for active patients only. As in pressure support ventilation, in volume support you should also activate apnoea backup. Be particularly cautious when setting the target tidal volume. An inappropriate target tidal volume may cause hypo- or hyperventilation, as mentioned earlier. This is not the case in the pressure support ventilation mode.

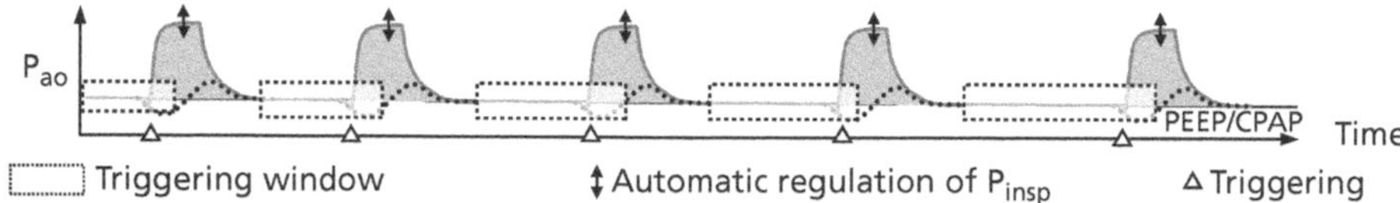

Fig. 8.23 Typical pressure-time waveform for volume support mode.

8.4 Biphasic ventilation modes

8.4.1 Biphasic modes in general

Conventional pressure alteration

All three categories of mode—conventional, adaptive, and biphasic—are IPPV based. That is, the lungs are intermittently inflated and deflated by alternation of airway pressure between a defined baseline pressure and a defined peak pressure. This alternation of airway pressure can be achieved either in a conventional way or a biphasic way.

The conventional method is applied in conventional and adaptive modes (Fig. 8.24). In short, during inspiration, the ventilator closes the expiratory valve and opens the inspiratory valve. The ventilator delivers inspiratory gas according to the operator's settings. During expiration, the ventilator closes the inspiratory valve and opens the expiratory valve. The high internal pressure drives the gas to exit. At late expiration, the ventilator dynamically regulates the opening of the expiratory valve for the desired baseline pressure (PEEP). Refer to section 7.2.2.

The conventional method works well in passive patients. However, if the ventilated patient is active, the closed expiratory valve during inspiration may cause patient-ventilator asynchrony. Below are two examples.

- An active patient coughs during inspiration. The muscular force does not generate the desired expiratory flow, but pressure spikes, because the expiratory valve is closed.
- An active patient starts to exhale before the defined cycling point. The muscular force does not generate the desired expiratory flow, but pressure spikes because the expiratory valve is closed. This phenomenon is known as 'delayed cycling'. See Fig. 8.25.

Both phenomena are very uncomfortable for the ventilated patient.

Biphasic pressure alternation

The biphasic method of airway pressure alternation is applied exclusively in biphasic modes. It is critical that we understand two things in order to truly understand biphasic modes.

First, an active patient can breathe (inhale and exhale) freely at PEEP (positive end-expiratory pressure)—just recall the spontaneous breaths in the PSV mode. During expiration, the

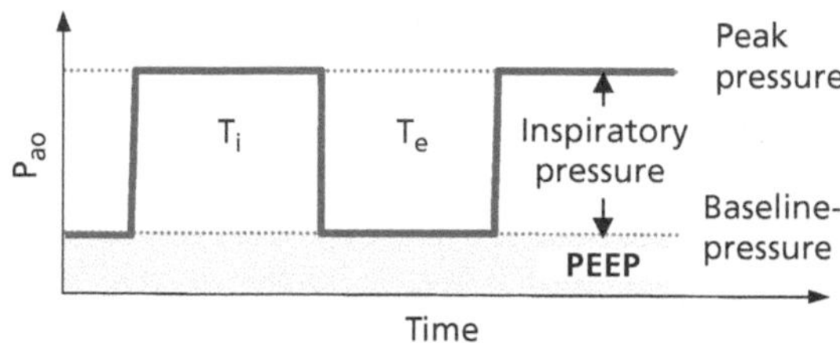

Fig. 8.24 Inspiratory pressure and baseline pressure in non-biphasic modes.

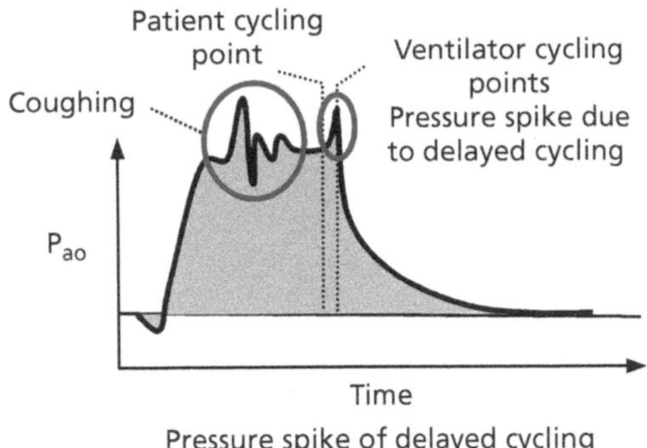

Fig. 8.25 Pressure spike due to delayed time cycling.

ventilator dynamically regulates the expiratory opening to create and maintain the desired PEEP. It seldom, or never, actually closes the valve completely.

Second, during mechanical ventilation, an operator can set and freely modify PEEP in all modes. One option is to manually adjust PEEP up and down after every 3 seconds, producing the pressure waveform shown in Fig. 8.26. Note that the pressure alternation strictly involves PEEP changes with no applied inspiratory pressure.

In a functioning ventilator system, an airway pressure change generates a corresponding lung volume change. So PEEP alternation can also generate the wanted lung volume change.

Biphasic modes

In biphasic modes, the ventilator itself performs this PEEP alternation according to the operator's settings. This spares the operator the work of repeated PEEP adjustment.

Biphasic modes have four unique controls to define how PEEP should alternate (Fig. 8.27):

- *PEEP-high*: the high level of PEEP;
- *PEEP-low*: the low level of PEEP;
- T-high: the duration of PEEP at the high level;
- T-low: the duration of PEEP at the low level.

In non-invasive ventilation, PEEP-high and PEEP-low are also called *inspiratory positive airway pressure (IPAP)* and *expiratory positive airway pressure (EPAP)*. Keep in mind that both pressures are PEEP, so you set these pressures relative to atmospheric pressure. By contrast, you set inspiratory pressure relative to PEEP.

In biphasic modes, an active patient can inhale and exhale spontaneously at low PEEP as well as high PEEP. So, if the patient coughs at high PEEP during the inspiratory phase, delayed cycling is less of a problem. Technically, this mechanism has another name: *active exhalation valve*. An active exhalation valve can open to release gas as the patient requires, even during the inspiratory phase. In theory biphasic modes are more comfortable than other modes for active patients.

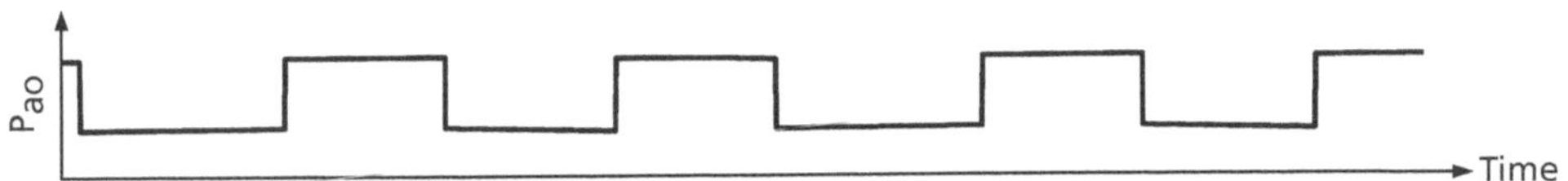

Fig. 8.26 The result of manual positive end-expiratory pressure (PEEP) adjustment.

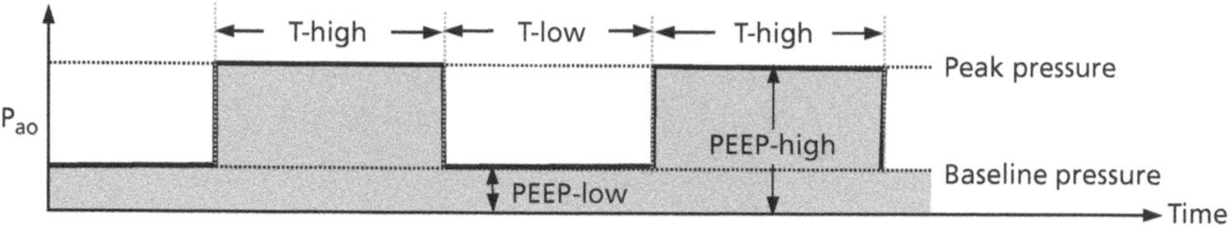

Fig. 8.27 Four unique control parameters to define baseline alternation in biphasic modes.

Currently, there are two biphasic ventilation modes: BiPAP (bilevel positive airway pressure) and APRV (airway pressure release ventilation). Although these might have very different origins, both can be realized with the same technical arrangement but different settings. This is the reason why some ventilators have separate BiPAP and APRV modes, whereas others have a single mode for both BiPAP and APRV (Table 8.17).

8.4.2 BiPAP

BiPAP stands for bilevel positive airway pressure. In this mode PEEP automatically alternates between the two set levels, and the patient can breathe freely at either level. This mode has its origins in non-invasive ventilation used to treat obstructive sleep apnoea, commonly in home care. Here we focus on the use of the BiPAP mode for intubated patients.

BiPAP is commonly used to mimic the pressure A/C mode (Fig. 8.28). Table 8.18 compares the settings used in both modes.

In BiPAP mode, all 'mechanical breaths' are quasi pressure control or pressure assist breaths. The word 'quasi' means that they are mimicked by PEEP alternation. PEEP-low serves as PEEP, and the difference between PEEP-high and PEEP-low serves as the inspiratory pressure. T-high serves as T_i, and T-low serves as T_e. The breaths are time or patient triggered, time cycled, and pressure controlled.

The patient can breathe spontaneously at either PEEP level, usually unsupported because PEEP-high already provides ventilatory support. Some intensive care unit ventilators let you add extra pressure support to spontaneous breaths, but be careful: pressure support is specified differently in different ventilators. Make sure you clearly understand how your ventilator defines pressure support before applying it.

In theory, the BiPAP mode is beneficial for active patients only. It can be also used for passive patients, but is no better than conventional volume A/C or pressure A/C modes.

8.4.3 APRV

APRV stands for airway pressure release ventilation, and can be regarded as a special form of BiPAP. It is characterized by a relatively long T-high and a very short T-low period (i.e. 0.5–0.8

Table 8.17 BiPAP and APRV modes may be merged into one mode

Ventilator model	GALILEO/HAMILTON-G5	Evita XL	AVEA	Puritan Bennett 840	SERVO-i	Care-station
Biphasic modes	DuoPAP, APRV	BiPAP	APRV/BiPhasic	BiLevel	Bi-vent	BiLevel

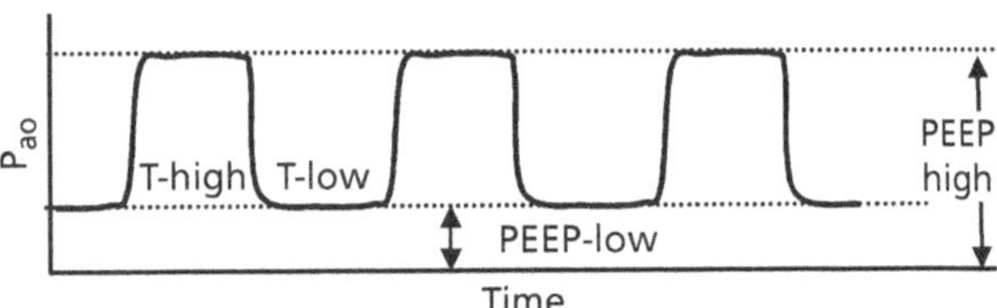

Fig. 8.28 The bilevel positive airway pressure (BiPAP) mode can be used to mimic pressure A/C mode.

second) in adult patients (Fig. 8.29). PEEP-high serves as the baseline pressure at which the patient breathes spontaneously. If we liken PEEP-high to inspiration and PEEP-low to expiration, then APRV is 'inverse ratio ventilation', although such a comparison is conceptually questionable.

As we discussed earlier, a pressure change in the ventilator system results in a corresponding change in lung volume. In most IPPV modes, the lung volume change is generated by an intermittently applied positive inspiratory pressure above PEEP. In APRV mode, however, the lung volume change is generated through the patient's spontaneous breathing activities and the baseline pressure drop.

APRV is mainly indicated for actively breathing patients with severe restrictive lung diseases, such as *acute respiratory distress syndrome (ARDS)* or *acute lung injury (ALI)*. In this patient population, lung-protective strategies are particularly beneficial. Lung-protective strategies include relatively small tidal volumes, a relatively high PEEP, and plateau pressures below 30 cmH_2O. What do you do, however, if CO_2 is rising and the plateau is already at 30 cmH_2O? In this case, APRV may be the best choice.

The APRV mode has two major advantages. First, it allows a combination of a relatively high pressure baseline (PEEP-high) and a relatively low plateau pressure. Second, the short pressure release with spontaneous breaths promotes CO_2 elimination.

APRV is contraindicated in passive patients. To date, no data is available on the use of APRV mode in patients with obstructive lung diseases such as chronic obstructive pulmonary disease or asthma. In theory it would not appear to benefit such patients.

The disadvantages of APRV mode include: (a) varying tidal volumes, (b) auto-PEEP and hyperinflation, (c) a possibly negative impact on haemodynamics, and (d) possible asynchrony during pressure release.

Table 8.18 Comparison of pressure A/C mode and BiPAP mode control settings

Pressure A/C mode controls	BiPAP mode controls
Rate and T_i (or I:E)	T-high and T-low
$P_{control}$ (inspiratory pressure)	The difference between PEEP-high and PEEP-low
Pressure/flow triggering	Pressure/flow triggering
PEEP	PEEP-low
Rise time	Rise time

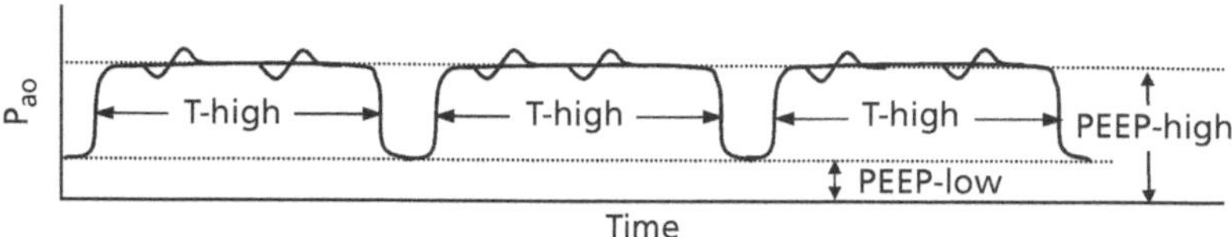

Fig. 8.29 Airway pressure release ventilation (APRV): Long inspiratory positive airway pressure (IPAP) and very short expiratory positive airway pressure (EPAP).

8.5 How to select a ventilation mode

Which is the best ventilation mode? This question is frequently asked. The answer is that there is no universally *best* mode, but there is the most *suitable* mode for an individual patient at the current moment.

Indeed, the choice of ventilation mode is just one of several important factors to consider when applying mechanical ventilation. These factors change over time, and we need to adapt the ventilator settings to these changes. In addition to mode, there are other control settings to consider; Chapter 9 will discuss these in detail.

We select a ventilation mode to define the mechanical breath types to be applied (Box 8.1). You will recall that a mode is a set of ventilator operations with one or more predefined mechanical breath types. Every ventilation mode has a unique set of control parameters to quantitatively define the essential variables of the breath types as well as to define other required parameters, such as F_iO_2.

In short, to operate properly, the ventilator requires both mode and control settings. Mechanical ventilation is optimal only when both mode and controls are set appropriately.

The following subsections provide four useful hints for determining the optimal mode.

8.5.1 Patient breathing activity

In selecting a mode, consider first and foremost the patient's breathing activity (Fig. 8.30). Ventilated patients can be categorized by spontaneous breathing activity, as follows:

- *Passive patients* who have no spontaneous breathing activity at all. The ventilator system must do all the work of breathing.
- *Partially active patients* who have weak or unstable spontaneous breathing activity. The ventilator system does most of the work of breathing.
- *Active patients* who have strong and stable spontaneous breathing activity. The patient and the ventilator system together provide the required work of breathing. Weaning and extubation are possible only when a ventilated patient is active.

Box 8.1 The relationship between ventilation modes and controls

Mode: Qualitatively defines the breath types permitted
Controls: Quantitatively defines the variables of the breath types

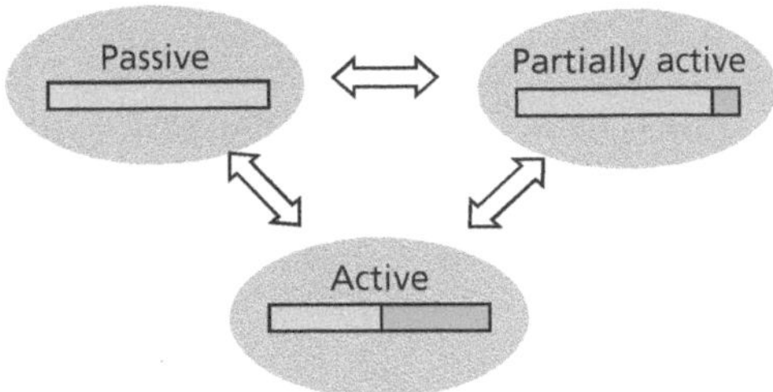

Fig. 8.30 Three categories of ventilated patients.

A ventilation mode may be appropriate for one or two or all three categories. When a ventilated patient's status changes, the operator should consider a mode change.

8.5.2 Staff familiarity

For a given patient status, there are several modes to select from; refer to Table 8.19. For instance, to ventilate an active patient, we can use PSV, volume support, SIMV modes, or APRV. Which one should we use?

Consider using the mode with which your staff are most familiar. The existing know-how of the staff and their confidence in using certain modes is a great asset that can reduce the incidence of human error.

8.5.3 Volume, pressure, or adaptive?

This is a controversial question.

Volume ventilation modes are the oldest and best known. Due to their inherent inflexibility, however, they have slowly but steadily lost their dominance to pressure modes. All modern and advanced modes are pressure based, including BiPAP, APRV, PRVC (*pressure regulated volume control*), ASV, PAV, SmartCare, and NAVA. Fig. 8.31 shows the changes in mode use over 25 years in a mixed intensive care unit in Switzerland.

Provided the ventilator system functions properly and control parameters are set and adjusted properly, the following guidelines may be useful:

- For passive patients, volume and pressure modes work equally well.
- For partially active patients, both volume modes and pressure modes are suitable. In theory, pressure modes may be a bit better.
- For active patients, only pressure modes should be used. Active patients cannot tolerate volume modes well.
- Adaptive modes and the corresponding pressure modes share the same indications. *If, and only if*, the target tidal volume is set and adjusted properly and promptly, an adaptive mode is superior to the corresponding pressure mode.

8.5.4 BiPAP and APRV?

The BiPAP mode, when used to mimic pressure A/C, is suitable for passive patients and partially active patients. It may be a bit superior to the pressure A/C mode in partially active patients.

The APRV mode may be a very good choice for active patients with severe restrictive lung diseases. It is contraindicated in passive patients.

Table 8.19 Common ventilation modes, permissible breath types, and suitable applications

Ventilation mode	Mechanical breath types								Application		
	Volume control breath	Pressure control breath	Adaptive control breath	Volume assist breath	Pressure assist breath	Adaptive assist breath	Pressure support breath	Adaptive support breath	Passive patients	Partially active patients	Active patients
Assist control modes											
Volume A/C mode	✓			✓					Suitable	Suitable	
Pressure A/C mode		✓			✓				Suitable	Suitable	
Adaptive A/C mode			✓			✓			Suitable	Suitable	
SIMV modes											
Volume SIMV mode	✓			✓			✓*		Suitable	Suitable	Suitable
Pressure SIMV mode		✓			✓		✓*		Suitable	Suitable	Suitable
Adaptive SIMV mode			✓			✓	✓*		Suitable	Suitable	Suitable
Support modes											
Pressure support mode							✓*				Suitable
Volume support mode								✓			Suitable
Biphasic modes											
BiPAP mode (mimicking A/C mode)							✓*		Suitable	Suitable	
APRV mode							✓*				Suitable

* The patient's spontaneous breaths may or may not be pressure supported.

APRV: airway pressure release ventilation; BiPAP: bilevel positive airway pressure; SIMV: synchronized intermittent mandatory ventilation.

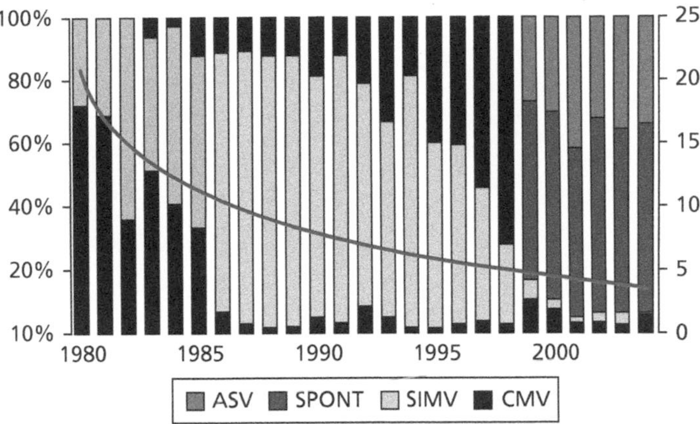

Fig. 8.31 The changes in ventilation mode selected in a mixed intensive care unit in Switzerland over the last 25 years.

Be aware that both BiPAP and APRV are relatively new modes. Adequate staff education is of paramount importance before the modes are introduced into clinical practice.

References

Chang DW (ed). *Clinical application of mechanical ventilation*, 3rd edn. 2006. Delmar Thomson Learning, New York, USA.

Chatburn RL. Classification of ventilator modes: Update and proposal for implementation. *Respir Care* 2007: 5; 301–23.

Hess DR, Kacmarek R. *Essentials of mechanical ventilation*. 2002, McGraw-Hill, New York, USA.

Iotti GA: *Mechanical ventilation: Skills and techniques*. 2003. Patient-centred acute care training (PACT) by ESICM.

Kacmarek R, Chapman D. 'Basic principles of ventilator machinery' in Tobin M (ed.) *Principles and practice of mechanical ventilation*, 2nd edn. 2006, McGraw-Hill, New York, USA, p.62.

Pilbeam SP. *Mechanical ventilation: Physiological and clinical applications*. 1998, Mosby, St Louis, USA.

Pilbeam SP. 'Introduction to ventilators' in Cairo JM, Pilbeam SP (eds.) *Mosby's respiratory care equipment*, 7th edn. 2004, Mosby, St Louis, USA, pp. 345–408.

Chapter 9

Ventilator Control Parameters

9.1 Controls in general

9.1.1 Definition

For mechanical ventilation, an operator must specify a ventilation mode. However, this in itself is not enough for a ventilator to function. The operator must also set the controls or *ventilator control parameters*. Fig. 9.1 shows a typical ventilator control window.

A control parameter defines a specific aspect of ventilator operation. For most controls, an operator quantitatively defines the magnitude (e.g. tidal volume). Less frequently the operator selects from one of several options provided (e.g. flow pattern in volume modes).

Every ventilation mode has a unique set of controls, depending on the mechanical breath type or types specific to the mode.

During mechanical ventilation, the operator should periodically check the mode and controls, and modify them when clinically necessary. Optimal mechanical ventilation is possible only when both mode *and* controls are appropriately set.

9.1.2 Terminology

As with other areas of mechanical ventilation, the terminology of ventilator controls is not globally standardized. It may be helpful to group the names according to their basic functions (Table 9.1).

9.1.3 A mode and its controls

You may notice that most controls seem to be related to those essential variables that we described in Chapter 7. Indeed they *are* related. For, as we know already, a ventilator mode is characterized by its mechanical breath types, which, in turn, are characterized by five essential variables. We also learned that an essential variable may have one or more mechanisms.

Ventilator controls can be either primary or secondary. Primary controls are directly related to essential variables. The sole exception is F_iO_2 (fraction of inspired oxygen). Secondary controls are used to define additional aspects of ventilator operation.

In some ventilators, a control, primary or secondary, may be set at the factory. If so, the control is not available on the ventilator. For instance, in Dräger Evita ventilators, flow cycling is fixed at 25%, so, you will not find a flow cycle control on these ventilators.

We know now that every mode has its unique set of controls. Can we roughly estimate the number of controls in a specific mode? Yes, we can: the number is directly related to the mechanical breath types in this mode.

Let's take a look at the volume SIMV (synchronized intermittent mandatory ventilation) mode with its three breath types, volume control breath, volume assist/control breath, and pressure support breath. The essential variables for these breath types are given in Table 9.2.

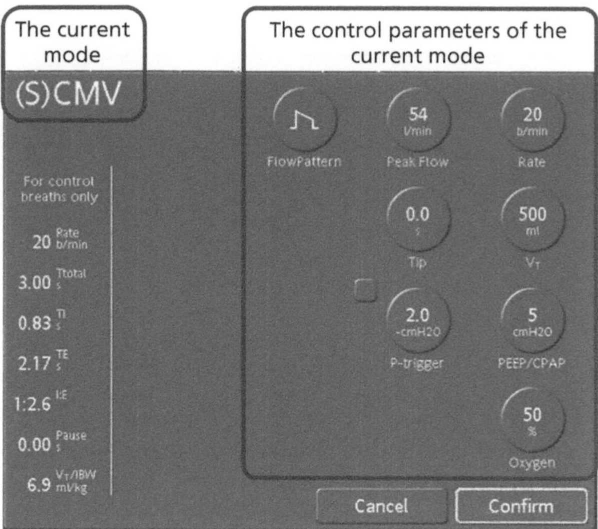

Fig. 9.1 A control window on the HAMILTON-G5 ventilator.

So, volume SIMV should have approximately ten controls. Of them, eight are primary controls, and two are secondary controls.

With this method, we can determine the controls for most common ventilation modes. Table 9.3 lists the number of controls commonly found in these modes. As you see, most ventilation modes have six to ten controls.

This method, however, does not fully apply to two special cases:

- Advanced adaptive modes, such as ASV (adaptive support ventilation) or PAV (proportional assist ventilation).
- TRC (tube resistance compensation), which is not regarded as a ventilation mode.
- F_iO_2, which is not related to any essential variable, but which is present in all ventilation modes.

9.2 **Common individual controls**

9.2.1 **Common controls for triggering**

Common triggering controls include the following.

Rate for time triggering

Terms: Mandatory rate, frequency (f), respiratory rate (RR)

Unit: Breaths per minute (b/min)

Mechanism: The set rate determines the duration of control breaths (breath cycle time). Refer to section 7.2.1.

Remarks: The rate setting is required in all modes except for pressure support and volume support. The ranges allowed differ in adult, paediatric, and neonatal patients. If rate and pressure/flow triggering settings coexist in a mode, the set rate serves as the backup. The set rate takes over only when no valid patient triggering is detected. Therefore, the actual or monitored total rate can be higher, but not lower, than the set rate. In SIMV modes, the set rate is also called the *SIMV rate*. It can be set much lower than in assist/control modes.

Table 9.1 Non-standardized terminology for ventilator controls

Group	Controls	Unit	Hamilton Medical	Dräger	Covidien/ PB	Maquet	GE	CareFusion
			GALILEO/ Hamilton G5	**Evita XL/ V500**	**840**	**SERVO-i**	**Care-Station**	**AVEA**
Triggering	**Mandatory rate**	b/min	**Rate**	**F/RR**	**F**	**RR**	**Rate**	**Rate**
	Pressure trigger	cmH_2O	**P-trigger**	—	P_{SENS}	**Trig. Pressure (setting < 0)**	**Trigger**	**Pres Trig**
	Flow trigger	L/min	**Flow trigger**	**(Flow) Trigger sensitivity**	V'_{SENS}	**Trigg. Flow (setting > 0)**	**Trigger**	**Flow Trig**
	Base flow	L/min	—	—	—	Bias flow	Bias flow	Bias Flow
Cycling	Inspiratory pause	% or s	Pause	Insp. pause*	T_{PL}	Tpause	Insp. pause	Insp Pause
	Inspiratory time	s	T_i	**Tinsp or/**T_i	T_i	T_i	**Tinsp (including pause)**	**Insp Time**
	I:E ratio	—	**I:E**	—	**I:E ratio**	**I:E**	**I:E**	—
	Percent inspiratory time	%	**%**T_i	—	—	—	—	—
	Peak inspiratory flow	L/min	**Peak flow**	**Flow**	V'_{MAX}	—	—	**Peak Flow**
	Flow cycle	%	**ETS**	—	E_{SENS}	**Inspiratory cycle-off**	**End Flow**	**Flow Cycle or PSV cycle**
	Maximum inspiratory time	s	TImax	—	$\bar{\uparrow} T_{I\,SPONT}$	—	—	PSV Tmax
	Expiratory time	s	—	—	T_E	—	—	—
Limiting	**Tidal volume**	ml	V_T	V_T/V_T	**Tidal volume**	V_T	**TV**	**Volume**
	Target tidal volume	ml	**Vtarget**	V_{Ti}	**Target volume**	**Tidal Volume**	**TV**	**Volume**
	Pressure control	cmH_2O	**Pcontrol**	**Pinsp**	P_I	**PC**	**Pinsp**	**Insp Pres**
	Pressure support	cmH_2O	**Psupport**	**PASB/**P_{supp}	P_{SUPP}	**PS**	**Psupp**	**PSV**
	Inspiratory pressure limit	cmH_2O	—	P_{max}	—	—	Pmax	—
	Volume limit	ml	—	—	—	—	—	Vol Limit

(continued)

Table 9.1 Continued

Group	Controls	Unit	Hamilton Medical	Dräger	Covidien/ PB	Maquet	GE	CareFusion
			GALILEO/ Hamilton G5	**Evita XL/ V500**	**840**	**SERVO-i**	**Care-Station**	**AVEA**
Inspiratory profile	Rise time	ms*	Pramp	Ramp/ Slope	P%	T inspiratory rise	Rise time PSV rise time	Insp Rise or PSV Rise
	Flow pattern	—	Flow pattern	—	Flow pattern	— (square)	—(square)	Waveform
Baseline	**Positive expiratory end pressure**	cmH_2O	**PEEP**	**PEEP**	**PEEP**	**PEEP**	**PEEP**	**PEEP**
Oxygen	**F_iO_2**	%	**F_iO_2**	**F_iO_2**	**O_2%**	**O_2 conc.**	**F_iO_2**	**%O_2**
Biphasic modes only	**PEEP high time**	s	**T_{high}**	**T_{high}**	**T_H**	**T_{High}**	**T_{high}**	**Time High**
	PEEP low time	s	**T_{low}**	**T_{low}**	**T_L**	**T_{PEEP}**	**T_{low}**	**Time Low**
	PEEP High	cmH_2O	**P_{high}**	**P_{high}**	**$PEEP_H$**	**P_{High}**	**P_{high}**	**Pres High**
	PEEP Low	cmH_2O	**P_{low} or PEEP**	**P_{low}**	**$PEEP_L$**	**PEEP**	**P_{low}**	**Pres Low**

Note: The terms in bold are primary control parameters.

Table 9.2 How many controls does the volume SIMV mode have?

Type	Control	Volume control	Volume assist	Pressure support	Number
Triggering	Time triggering (Rate)	✓			1
	Patient tripper (pressure/flow)		✓	✓	2
Cycling	Time cycling (T_i or I:E ratio)	✓	✓		3
	Flow cycle			✓	4
Limiting/control	Tidal volume	✓	✓		5
	Inspiratory pressure (Pressure support)			✓	6
	Inspiratory pressure (pressure control)				
	Target tidal volume (adaptive limiting/ control)				
Baseline	Baseline pressure (PEEP)	✓	✓	✓	7
Oxygen	F_iO_2	✓	✓	✓	8
Secondary	Rise time for pressure support breath			✓	9
	Flow pattern for volume breaths	✓	✓		10

Table 9.3 Estimated number of controls in common ventilation modes

Assist/control modes		SIMV modes		Support modes		Biphasic modes	
Volume A/C mode	7	Volume SIMV mode	10	Pressure support mode	6	BiPAP mode	9
Pressure A/C mode	7	Pressure SIMV mode	10	Volume support mode	6	APRV mode	9
Adaptive A/C mode	7	Adaptive SIMV mode	10				

Pressure trigger type and sensitivity

Terms: P-trigger, P_{sens}, Trigg. pressure, Pres. Trig
Unit: Centimetres of water (cmH_2O)
Mechanism: When the airway or circuit pressure drops below the set sensitivity threshold during the triggering window, the ventilator immediately starts inspiratory gas delivery. Refer to section 7.2.1.
Remarks: You can make the pressure trigger more or less sensitive through the sensitivity setting; the smaller the absolute value of the setting, the more sensitive the triggering. Not all ventilators provide pressure triggering. Note that the pressure trigger responds to the pneumatic signals not only from the patient's inspiratory efforts, but also possibly from such artefacts as a gas leak or circuit rainout.

In general, pressure triggering is harder for the patient than flow triggering.

Flow trigger type and sensitivity

Terms: Flow trigger, V'_{sens}, Trigg. flow, Flow Trig.
Unit: Litres per minute (L/min)
Mechanism: When the inspiratory airway flow meets or exceeds the set sensitivity threshold during the triggering window, the ventilator immediately starts inspiratory gas delivery. Refer to section 7.2.1.
Remarks: You can make the flow trigger more or less sensitive through the sensitivity setting. The smaller the absolute value of the setting, the more sensitive the triggering. Note that like the pressure trigger, the flow trigger responds to the pneumatic signals not only from the patient's inspiratory efforts, but also possibly from such artefacts as a gas leak or circuit rainout.

In general, flow triggering is slightly easier for the patient than pressure triggering.

Flow triggering is based on a special technical feature called *base flow*, which is activated during late expiration.

9.2.2 Common controls for cycling

Common cycling controls include time cycling and flow cycling. Time cycling has several mechanisms, such as inspiratory time (T_i); inspiration to expiration ratio (I:E ratio); and peak flow.

Inspiratory time

Terms: T_i, T_{insp}, Insp Time
Unit: Seconds (s)

Mechanism: T_i is a time cycling control. The ventilator switches to expiration when the set T_i is over.

Remarks: T_i is the simplest way to define inspiratory time. It applies to all breath types. Breath cycle time is the sum of inspiratory time and expiratory time. After rate and T_i are set, the expiratory time (T_e) is given. With a given rate, an increased T_i causes a decreased T_e, and vice versa.

I:E ratio

Terms: I:E ratio, I:E

Unit: None

Mechanism: I:E ratio is another way to define time cycling. The relationship between inspiratory time and expiratory time is expressed as a ratio. In clinical practice the commonly used I:E ratios include: 1:1, 1:2, 1:3, and 1:4. The assigned inspiratory portion is on the left of the colon, and the assigned expiratory portion is on the right. The I:E ratio control applies to all breath types.

Remarks: This control influences both inspiratory time and expiratory time at any given rate or breath cycle time.

Peak inspiratory flow

Terms: Peak flow, V'_{MAX}

Unit: Litres per minute (L/min)

Mechanism: Peak flow is yet another way to define time cycling. Its application is limited to volume control and volume assist breaths with a constant inspiratory flow. In these breaths, tidal volume is the product of inspiratory time and peak inspiratory flow (i.e. $V_T = T_i \times$ peak flow). At a given tidal volume, an increased peak flow causes a decreased T_i, and vice versa.

Remarks: The use of peak flow is limited to volume breaths with constant flow. This mechanism may be confusing, because the relationship between peak flow and T_i is not obvious. Over time, peak flow is losing ground, so that newer ventilators may not implement this mechanism at all.

Flow cycle

Terms: Flow cycle, ETS (for expiratory trigger sensitivity), E_{SENS}, Inspiratory cycle-off, End flow, PSV cycle

Unit: Percent (%)

Mechanism: As its name implies, flow cycle is a cycling mechanism based on the inspiratory flow. During inspiration, inspiratory flow typically rises quickly to its peak and then gradually drops to zero. This peak is considered to be 100%. The ventilator switches to expiration when inspiratory flow drops to a defined threshold, such as 5%, 25%, or 50%. The flow cycle control is available only for pressure support breaths or adaptive support breaths.

Remarks: The flow cycle control lets the operator influence the T_i of spontaneous breaths. If set properly, it improves patient comfort in active patients.

The flow cycle mechanism may fail if the control is set very low and a significant gas leak is present.

9.2.3 Common controls for targeting

The controls in this category define the size of a mechanical breath. They are tidal volume, inspiratory pressure, and target tidal volume.

Tidal volume

Terms: V_T, tidal volume, Volume
Unit: Millilitres (ml)
Mechanism: Tidal volume is the intended volume of gas that a ventilator delivers during inspiration. It relates exclusively to volume breaths (i.e. mechanical breaths with volume controlling). Typically the tidal volume is delivered at a constant flow rate during inspiration.
Remarks: When using volume modes, pay attention to circuit compliance. This consumes a part of the gas volume that the ventilator delivers, so the patient receives less volume than what the ventilator actually delivers. Refer to section 5.3.4 for details.

In some ventilators, you may also need to set the flow pattern. Refer to the section 7.2.3.

If the ventilator system has a gas leak, the patient may receive a tidal volume that is much less than the set tidal volume.

Pressure control

Terms: $P_{control}$, P_{INSP}, P_I, PC, Insp Pres
Unit: Centimetres of water (cmH_2O)
Mechanism: This control defines the inspiratory pressure above positive end-expiratory pressure (PEEP) in pressure control and pressure assist breaths. Inspiratory pressure generates the desired tidal volume.
Remarks: Pressure control is relative to PEEP. Pressure control and PEEP together make the peak airway pressure. This is very different from PEEP high in biphasic modes.

A secondary control, rise time, may be used with pressure control.

Pressure support

Terms: $P_{support}$, P_{SUPP}, PSV, PS
Unit: Centimetres of water (cmH_2O)
Mechanism: This control defines the inspiratory pressure above PEEP in pressure support breaths. Inspiratory pressure generates the desired tidal volume.
Remarks: Pressure support and pressure control have the same mechanism, yet are used in different pressure breath types.

Target tidal volume

Terms: V_{target}, Target volume, TV, Volume
Unit: Millilitres (ml)
Mechanism: Target tidal volume is used exclusively in adaptive breaths (i.e. adaptive control breaths, adaptive assist breaths, and adaptive support breaths). The ventilator automatically regulates the inspiratory pressure to match the resultant tidal volume to the target. Refer to section 7.2.3 for details.
Remarks: Target tidal volume is used exclusively in adaptive modes, while tidal volume is used in volume modes.

9.2.4 Common controls for baseline pressure

PEEP (positive end-expiratory pressure)

Terms: PEEP
Unit: Centimetres of water (cmH_2O)

Mechanism: PEEP defines the intended baseline pressure. Positive airway pressure is applied intermittently above the baseline. This control applies to all ventilation modes. Refer to section 7.2.5.

Remarks: PEEP can strongly influence oxygenation.

PEEP can keep the alveoli open and restore a decreased functional residual capacity (FRC). A moderate PEEP (3–5 cmH_2O) is considered beneficial for all ventilated patients. A relatively high PEEP may be needed to treat patients with restrictive lung diseases, such as acute respiratory distress (ARDS) or acute lung injury. PEEP can be set to zero, but zero PEEP (known as *ZEEP*) should be avoided.

In a pressure support breath, a patient can breathe spontaneously at PEEP without pressure support.

A stable PEEP is critical for pressure triggering.

9.2.5 **Common controls for oxygenation**

Fraction of inspired oxygen (F_iO_2)

Terms: F_iO_2, O_2%, %O_2, O_2 conc., Oxygen

Unit: Percent (%)

Mechanism: F_iO_2 defines the intended oxygen concentration in the inspiratory gas. It can be set from 21% to 100%. F_iO_2 is available in all ventilation modes.

Remarks: Obviously, F_iO_2 relies on the oxygen supply, which can greatly affect oxygenation.

9.2.6 **Common secondary controls**

Rise time

Terms: Rise time, Pramp, Slope, P%, T inspiratory rise, Insp Rise

Unit: Percent (%), seconds (s), or milliseconds (ms)

Mechanism: Rise time defines the intended speed at which the circuit or airway is pressurized (Fig. 9.2). It applies to pressure breaths and adaptive breaths, but not volume breaths.

Remarks: Not all ventilators have a rise time control, because this control is fixed in some ventilators.

Rise time has value mainly for active patients, especially those who have a strong drive. If set appropriately, it can improve patient comfort.

A super-fast rise time can cause pressure overshooting, an unwanted complication of mechanical ventilation.

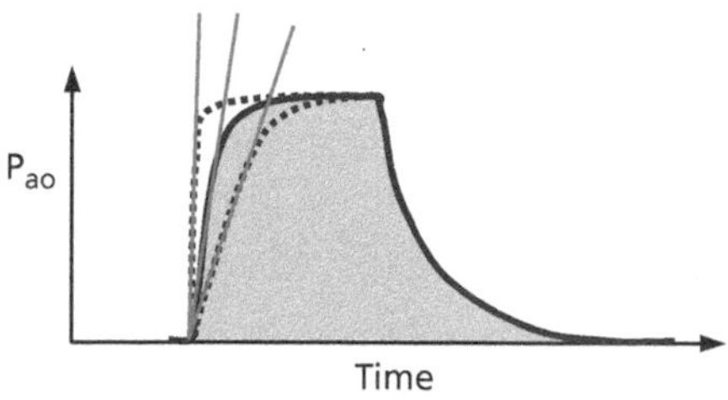

Fig. 9.2 By adjusting the rise time setting, the operator influences the speed at which inspiratory pressure increases.

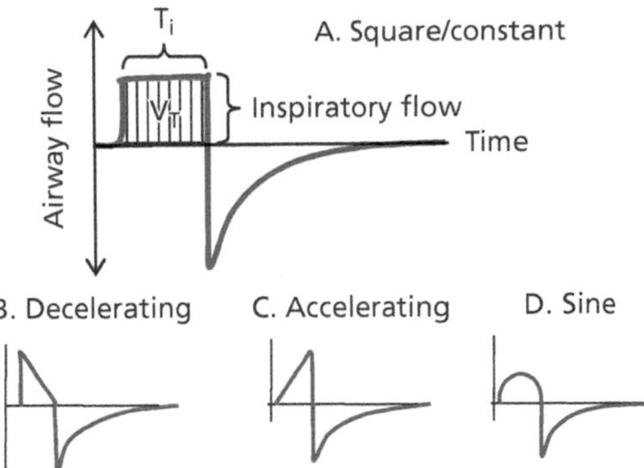

Fig. 9.3 Volume breaths have four common inspiratory flow patterns.

Flow pattern

Unit: None

Mechanism: The flow pattern control defines the intended profile of inspiratory flow. It applies exclusively to volume breaths. The most common pattern is square, also known as 'constant flow'. Other possible flow patterns are decelerating, accelerating, and sine (Fig. 9.3).

Remarks: Many ventilators do not have this control, because they use a single pattern, the square pattern.

9.2.7 **Common controls for biphasic modes**

The key feature of biphasic modes is the automatic alteration of the baseline pressure. Four controls are typically set to define this alteration: high PEEP, low PEEP, PEEP high time, and PEEP low time (Fig. 9.4).

PEEP high

Terms: P high, P_{high}, P_H, P_{HIGH}, Pres High

Unit: Centimetres of water (cmH_2O)

Mechanism: PEEP high defines the intended high level of PEEP.

Remarks: Another term for PEEP high is IPAP (inspiratory positive airway pressure).

PEEP at a high level is still PEEP. Like PEEP, it is relative to atmospheric pressure. This differs from inspiratory pressure, which is relative to PEEP.

The patient can breathe spontaneously at (high) PEEP.

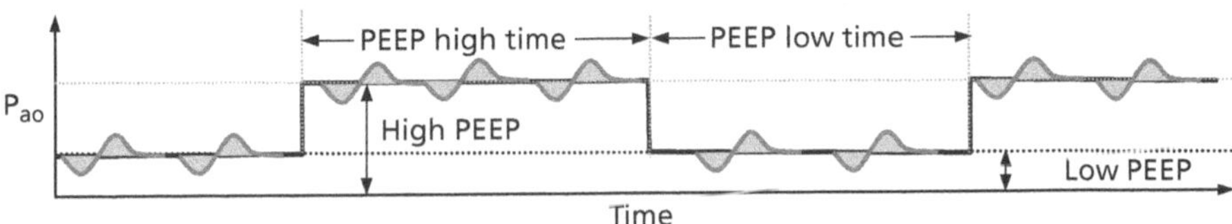

Fig. 9.4 Biphasic modes have four special controls to define automatic alternation of baseline pressure.

PEEP low

Terms: P low, P_{low}, P_L, P_{LOW}, Pres Low
Unit: Centimetres of water (cmH_2O)
Mechanism: PEEP low defines the intended low level of PEEP.
Remarks: Another term for PEEP low is EPAP (expiratory positive airway pressure).

PEEP low is comparable to PEEP in conventional or adaptive ventilation modes. It is relative to atmospheric pressure.

T high

Terms: T high, T_{high}, T_H, Thigh, Time High
Unit: Seconds (s)
Mechanism: PEEP high time defines the intended duration of PEEP high.
Remarks: Typically PEEP high time is relatively short in BiPAP (bilevel positive airway pressure) mode and quite long in APRV (airway pressure release ventilation) mode.

T low

Terms: T low, T_{low}, T_L, Tlow, Time Low
Unit: Seconds (s)
Mechanism: PEEP low time defines the intended duration of low PEEP.
Remarks: Typically PEEP low time is short in BiPAP mode and very short in APRV mode for pressure release purposes.

Chapter 10

Special Ventilation Functions

10.1 **Introduction**

In addition to ventilation modes and controls, ventilators typically have several other functions. These are not easy to classify, because they may be active in some or all modes. They are among the most frequently used functions. In this book, we call these features 'special ventilation functions'.

This chapter introduces six of these common functions: standby, sigh, oxygen enrichment, apnoea backup, and tube resistance compensation.

10.2 **Standby**

Standby is an intentional suspension of mechanical ventilation. This is necessary from time to time in clinical practice. A typical example is open tracheal suctioning in ventilated patients.

What would happen if we simply disconnected the airway while the ventilator system was running? The ventilator would not know that the disconnection was intentional. In non-volume modes, the ventilator would maximize gas delivery, attempting to compensate for the leak. The staff would face a potentially dangerous 'secretion shower', annoying and persistent alarms, and unnecessary and excessive gas consumption.

As an alternative, we could shut down the ventilator, for example for suctioning, and then switch it on afterwards. The problem is that it may take up to a minute for the ventilator to reboot, just like a computer. Restarting a ventilator every four hours is, for practical reasons, unacceptable.

Standby is designed so that we can easily stop and resume mechanical ventilation while the ventilator stays on.

Standby is frequently used, so a ventilator may even have a dedicated key on the front panel for direct access (Fig. 10.1). This key may be labelled with a standardized power symbol or the term 'STANDBY' or 'STBY'. In some ventilators, the standby key is also used to power the device on or off.

Standby may be activated in any mode at any time during mechanical ventilation.

10.2.1 **Standby in two steps**

To prevent the unintentional termination of ventilation, standby is often activated in two steps (Fig. 10.2).

Step 1: Pre-standby state

The pre-standby state is a temporary state before standby actually starts.

Typically, the operator presses the standby key to initiate the pre-standby state. The ventilator responds by opening the pre-standby window. Note that mechanical ventilation continues while in the pre-standby state. The operator then decides to enter standby or to cancel the pre-standby state. The pre-standby state typically has a time limit.

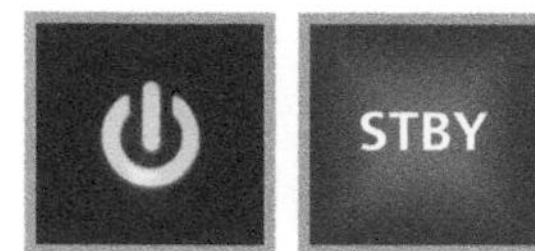

Fig. 10.1 Standby symbols.

Step 2: Standby state

As soon as the operator confirms their intention, the ventilator enters standby, which means mechanical ventilation is discontinued. The ventilator clearly indicates that it is in standby. Most alarms are suppressed to prevent acoustic disturbance.

Caution: If you are using an active humidifier, you must deactivate it before entering standby; otherwise, the circuit may overheat. Be sure to reactivate the humidifier after standby.

10.2.2 Terminating standby

You should be able to resume mechanical ventilation at any time during standby. There are a number of ways to do so. The most common one is to press the standby key again. The ventilator should immediately resume mechanical ventilation with the same settings as before.

Some ventilators can resume mechanical ventilation automatically when they detect that you have reconnected the patient. Such ventilators deliver a continuous, low 'detecting' flow (i.e. 2–6 L/min) during standby, and then monitor the airway or circuit pressure. If the circuit or airway is disconnected, the monitored pressure is close to zero. When the circuit or airway is reconnected, the circuit pressure rises. Mechanical ventilation resumes automatically if a predefined pressure threshold is reached.

This mechanism is convenient, but it has two major drawbacks. First, it is not as reliable as manual termination and resumption. Second, this automatic mechanism consumes gas continuously. Assuming that the detecting flow is 6 L/min, this feature uses 360 litres of gas per hour or 8640 litres of gas per day!

10.3 Sigh

A *sigh* is a deep breath. A healthy adult sighs six to eight times per hour to prevent microatelectasis.

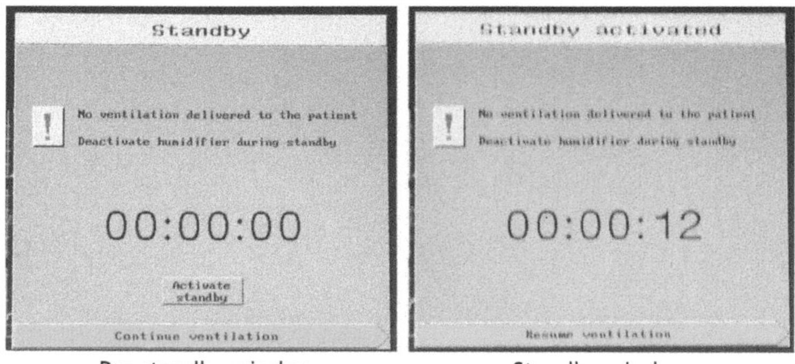

Fig. 10.2 Activating standby in two steps (GALILEO ventilator).
Modified from http://www.suru.com/

In mechanical ventilation, a sigh is a function where the ventilator periodically delivers a larger-than-normal mechanical breath throughout the entire course of mechanical ventilation.

Some believe that periodic insertion of a deep breath into the regular mechanical breathing pattern may serve as a simple lung recruitment manoeuvre. The use of sighs in mechanical ventilation became popular in the 1960s and 1970s, and interest in this function has recently been revived. The promised clinical benefits of the sigh include improved oxygenation and decreased atelectasis. The actual clinical benefits of sigh, however, are controversial.

The sigh function is generally defined by two parameters: frequency of delivery and breath size. However, this function is not standardized across ventilators.

The frequency of sigh breaths is typically defined either as:

- one sigh breath per 50 or 100 breaths, or
- the number of sigh breaths per hour (e.g. 4 or 6 sigh breaths per hour).

The size of a sigh breath may be defined differently for different modes. For example, in volume modes, a sigh may have a tidal volume that is 1.5 times the currently set V_T. In pressure modes, a sigh may have an inspiratory pressure that is 10 cmH_2O greater than the currently set pressure control or pressure support. To prevent overdistension, the sigh function is not recommended if the set tidal volume is between 10 and 12 ml/kg, or for neonates.

The sigh function must be manually turned off and on.

10.4 Temporary oxygen enrichment

All ICU (intensive care unit) ventilators allow an operator to set and adjust F_iO_2 throughout the range of 21% to 100%. The F_iO_2 stays constant after it is set.

In addition, most ICU ventilators have a special function that allows you to temporarily elevate F_iO_2 to meet the clinical need for short-term oxygenation. A typical use is for oxygenation before and after open tracheal suctioning.

The *oxygen enrichment* function can be activated manually at any time during mechanical ventilation regardless of mode, control settings, and patient population. A common way to activate this function is by pressing a front key labelled '100% O_2', 'Oxygen enrichment', 'O_2 breaths', or 'Increase O_2'.

This function is characterized by two parameters: the target F_iO_2 level and the duration of oxygen enrichment (Fig. 10.3). Once it is activated manually, the ventilator

a. increases F_iO_2 quickly from the current F_iO_2 level to the target level,
b. keeps F_iO_2 at the target level, and
c. decreases F_iO_2 to the set level after the defined duration ends.

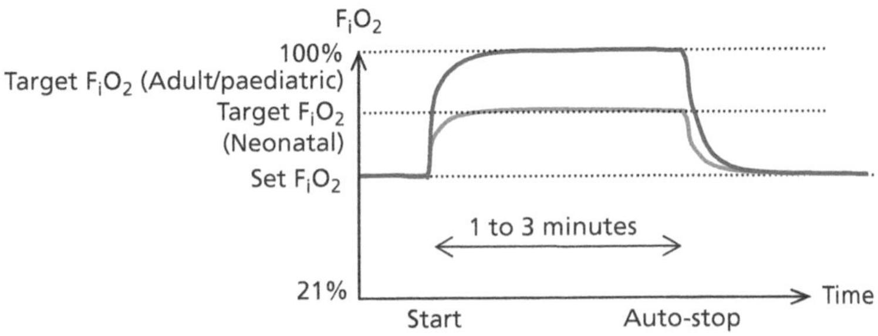

Fig. 10.3 Temporary oxygen enrichment.

The oxygen enrichment function typically has a target F_iO_2 level of 100% in adult and paediatric patients. Due to concerns about oxygen toxicity in neonates, the target for neonates may be less than 100%. For instance, in the HAMILTON-C2 ventilator, the target is 1.25 times the set F_iO_2.

The duration of temporary oxygen enrichment is between 1 and 3 minutes, depending on the ventilator brand and model.

Oxygen enrichment is automatically terminated when the defined duration ends. The operator can also terminate it manually during the enrichment time.

10.5 **Apnoea and apnoea backup ventilation**

An apnoea alarm and apnoea (backup) ventilation are safety features of ICU ventilators. In this section, we will discuss apnoea, apnoea detection, apnoea alarm, and apnoea (backup) ventilation in depth.

10.5.1 **Different definitions of apnoea**

In medical physiology, *apnoea* is defined as 'a temporary suspension of breathing'.

In mechanical ventilation, however, apnoea has a different definition. Here, apnoea occurs when the ventilator fails to detect the patient's breathing activity for a period longer than the set *apnoea time.*

There are two additional criteria used to define apnoea in a ventilator: (a) the ventilated patient must currently be breathing spontaneously, and (b) apnoea must be possible in the current mode; that is, it must be a support mode or a synchronized intermittent mandatory ventilation mode (SIMV) with a very low set rate.

We can derive four important conclusions from this definition:

- Apnoea in mechanical ventilation relies entirely on ventilator monitoring. Apnoea detection may fail if the monitoring is problematic for any reason. This explains why a ventilator may alarm for apnoea while the patient is apparently breathing.
- Apnoea detection depends on the set apnoea time, which is an important alarm setting.
- Apnoea is a relevant issue for actively breathing patients only.
- Apnoea cannot occur in an assist/control mode or an SIMV mode with a high set rate.

10.5.2 **Apnoea detection and alarm**

A ventilator is a machine. It does not know whether the ventilated patient is actively breathing.

Here we need to explain two key concepts or terms: *breath cycle time* and the *set apnoea time.*

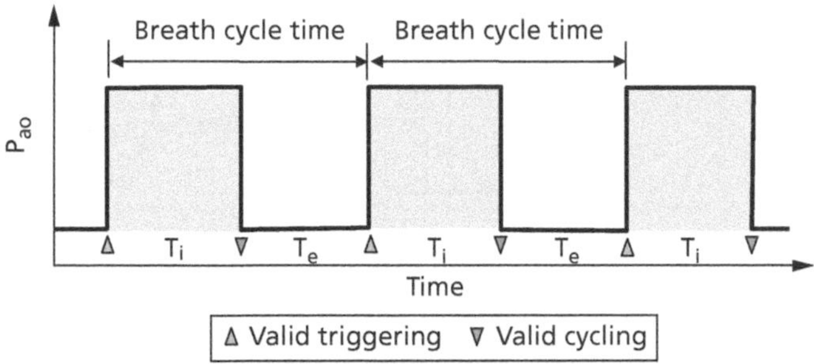

Fig. 10.4 Timing of a mechanical breath is defined by valid triggering and cycling.

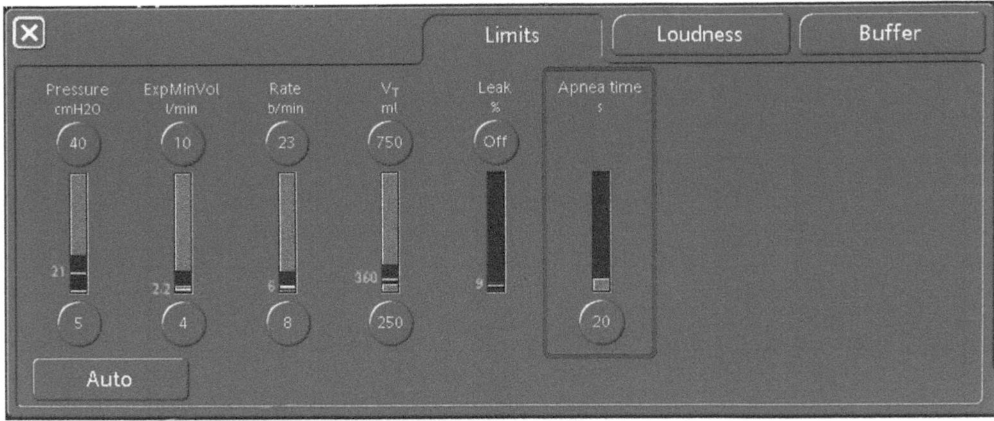

Fig. 10.5 In the HAMILTON-G5 ventilator, the apnoea time is set in alarm window.

Breath cycle time (BCT) is the duration of a mechanical breath, which contains T_i and T_e portions. For a ventilator, it is the interval from one valid triggering point to the next valid triggering point (Fig. 10.4). Refer to section 7.2 for details.

A critical word is 'valid', because for various reasons a patient's inspiratory effort may not necessarily trigger the next mechanical breath, resulting in the triggering effort being considered invalid.

Apnoea time is an alarm parameter to define the maximum acceptable interval between any two consecutive mechanical breaths. The apnoea time setting is in seconds, and it should differ in adult, paediatric, and neonatal patients. Fig. 10.5 shows the apnoea time setting in the alarm window of the HAMILTON-G5 ventilator.

During mechanical ventilation, the set apnoea time is used as a 'time ruler' (Fig. 10.6). The ventilator compares the BCT of every mechanical breath with the ruler. The rules of apnoea detection are rather simple:

- Apnoea detection is negative if BCT is shorter than the set apnoea time.
- Apnoea detection is positive if BCT reaches the set apnoea time, that is, it does not detect a valid triggering within the defined apnoea time.

10.5.3 Apnoea alarm

The *apnoea alarm* is a standard feature in ventilators. For safety reasons, it typically cannot be deactivated.

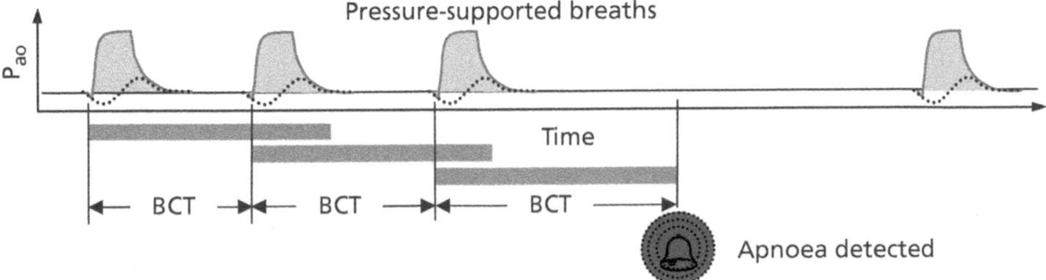

Fig. 10.6 The set apnoea time is used as a time ruler to measure the actual duration of every mechanical breath. The apnoea alarm is activated if a breath takes a longer time than the ruler.

Whenever apnoea is detected (i.e. the current BCT reaches the set apnoea time) the ventilator immediately announces this with an audible and visual apnoea alarm.

10.5.4 Apnoea (backup) ventilation

To maximize patient safety, most, if not all, ventilators have an automatic mechanism—*apnoea ventilation, apnoea backup ventilation*, or *apnoea backup*. Apnoea ventilation enables the ventilator to switch automatically between a support mode and a backup mode.

This mechanism relies completely on apnoea detection, as described above. Typically, an operator can turn it on or off.

Support mode and backup mode

A *support mode* is a ventilation mode intended for spontaneous breathing, patients with or without pressure support. It is usually very comfortable for active patients. However, an apnoea alarm can occur if it does not detect the patient's inspiratory effort. A typical example of a support mode is pressure support ventilation (PSV) mode.

A *backup mode* is a mandatory mode intended for passive patients. In such a mode, a ventilator delivers intermittent mechanical breaths according to ventilator settings. In a backup mode, patient triggering is acceptable but not required. Apnoea cannot occur in a backup mode, because the maximum BCT should be shorter than the minimum apnoea time setting. Typical backup modes are volume and pressure assist/control modes.

Support-backup mode coupling

There are several support modes and several backup modes. To achieve apnoea backup ventilation, ventilators couple support modes with backup modes. This coupling can be either 'all-to-one' or 'one-to-one'.

'All-to-one' means that all support modes share a common backup mode. This approach is simple, but mode switching may be disturbing if the support mode is pressure controlled and the backup mode is volume controlled.

'One-to-one' means that support modes and backup modes are individually coupled according to their controlling types (i.e. volume to volume, pressure to pressure, and adaptive to adaptive). One-to-one coupling is widely applied.

Support-backup mode coupling is a fixed aspect of ventilator design. The operator cannot control it, but needs to understand it.

Apnoea ventilation activation and control setting

When you activate apnoea ventilation, you not only turn it on, but you also check and adjust the control settings specific to the backup mode. The control settings specific to the backup mode may be only a subset of the settings you set when you use that same mode as a support mode. For example, if the support and backup modes are one-to-one coupled, you may need to set only the three controls that are essential to a control breath:

- Time triggering (the rate setting),
- Time cycling (I:E ratio, T_i, or $\%T_i$),
- Targeting (tidal volume or $P_{control}$).

The backup mode shares with the current support mode the remaining controls, such as F_iO_2 and PEEP (positive end-expiratory pressure).

Fig. 10.7 shows the apnoea backup controls on the HAMILTON-G5 ventilator. The current support mode is P-SIMV and the backup mode is P-CMV (or P-A/C). The yellow frame encloses

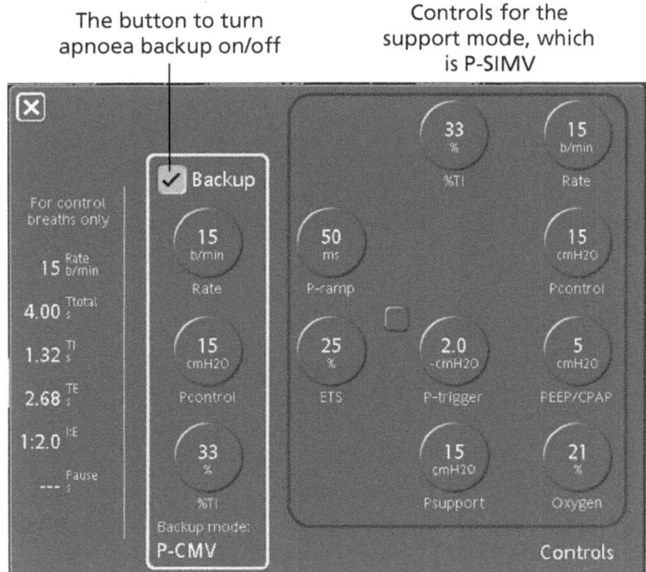

Fig. 10.7 Apnoea backup controls on the HAMILTON-G5 ventilator.
CMV: continuous mandatory ventilation; SIMV: synchronized intermittent mandatory ventilation.

the three control settings for apnoea backup ventilation. The controls shared by the current support mode and the backup mode include PEEP, Oxygen, P-trigger, and Pramp.

Automatic mode switchover

The mechanism of apnoea backup ventilation is simple: Whenever apnoea is detected, the ventilator announces this with an apnoea alarm, and it immediately and automatically switches from the current support mode to its backup mode. There is no need for any human intervention.

Traditionally, mechanical ventilation stays in the backup mode unless the operator manually switches the ventilator back to the support mode. If the operator does not switch the mode before the patient resumes their breathing activity, patient-ventilator asynchrony can occur. This arrangement is called *unidirectional apnoea backup* (Fig. 10.8).

A *bidirectional apnoea backup* design resolves this potential problem. If apnoea is detected, the ventilator automatically switches from the support mode to its backup mode. If a patient trigger is detected, the ventilator automatically switches from the backup mode to the support mode. The mode switchover is fully automatic. Bidirectional apnoea backup benefits both ventilated patients and clinicians, particularly the nursing staff.

10.5.5 A confusing apnoea alarm

As we have seen, apnoea detection is based on a comparison of the BCT to the defined apnoea time. BCT is the interval between two consecutive valid triggers.

Problematic trigger detection leads to an incorrect BCT definition and apnoea detection. An apnoea alarm can then be activated unexpectedly.

In one case, a newborn was intubated and mechanically ventilated in a support mode. The patient was apparently breathing hard, but the apnoea alarm was activated. 'This ventilator is unresponsive to the patient's efforts. How can apnoea occur when the patient is breathing intensely?' The operator was confused and angry.

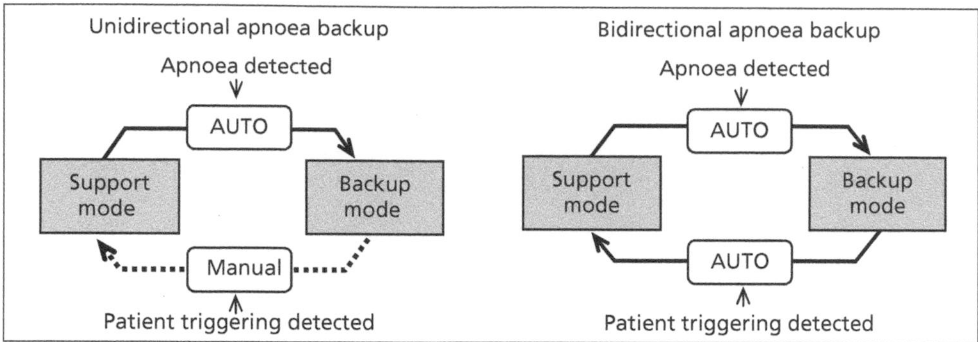

Fig. 10.8 Unidirectional apnoea backup (left) and bidirectional apnoea backup (right).

Two coexisting problems were identified in the following investigation (Fig. 10.9):

- The neonatal endotracheal tube (ETT) was uncuffed and too thin to seal the airway. The positive pressure applied caused a significant gas leak between the trachea and the ETT.
- The thin ETT was partially kinked, generating an excessive airway resistance against the gas flow in both directions. It also hindered the transmission of pneumatic signals generated by the patient.

The apnoea alarm was activated, because the ventilator did not detect valid patient triggering and cycling as expected. Therefore, the BCT was longer than the set apnoea time.

All abnormalities disappeared immediately after the ETT was replaced with a thicker one—this was the only correct solution in this case.

As you can see, apnoea can occur at any time in a support mode. Apnoea may or may not be possible in an SIMV mode, depending on the set rate. It cannot occur in a backup mode. This new way to classify modes is important for our understanding of apnoea backup ventilation.

10.6 Tube resistance compensation (TRC)

10.6.1 Tube resistance

Tracheal intubation is the placement of a tube, either an *endotracheal tube* (ETT) or a *tracheostomy tube* (TT), in the trachea (Fig. 10.10). In fact, we may regard the trachea as just another tube.

To be placed into another tube, the inner tube must have an outer diameter that is smaller than the inner diameter of the outer tube (Fig. 10.11). Because the inner tube has its own wall, the inner diameter of the inner tube must be much smaller than the inner diameter of the outer tube, causing a significant difference in their cross sections.

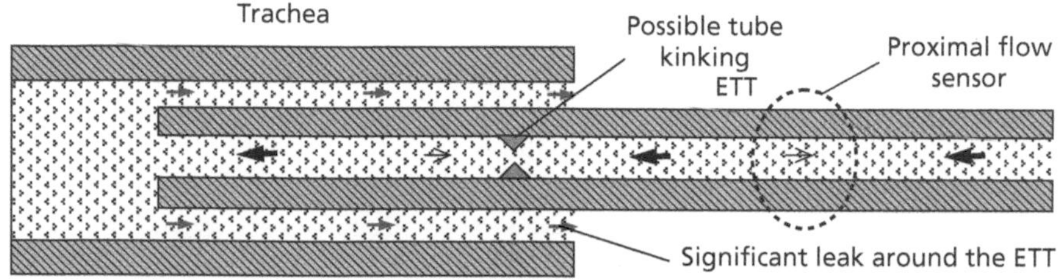

Fig. 10.9 Airway leakage and/or partial airway occlusion can occur, resulting in unwanted consequences.

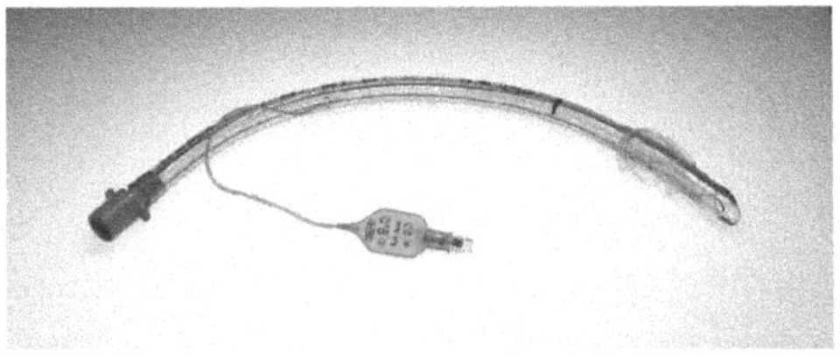

Endotracheal tube (ETT)

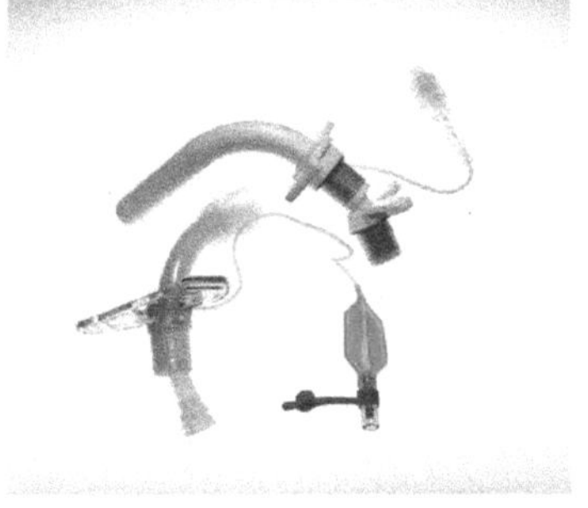

Tracheostomy tube (TT)

Fig. 10.10 Two typical tracheal tube types.

The trachea is a part of the natural airway, while the tracheal tube is an artificial airway. Different internal diameters or different cross sections mean different levels of resistance to the passing gas flow.

Poiseuille's law tells that if the diameter of a tube is halved, the resistance is 16 times as great!

$$R = \frac{8nl}{\pi r^4}$$

where: R = resistance, n = viscosity, l = length, and r = radius.

After intubation, the total airway resistance contains two parts, the natural airway resistance and the *tube resistance* imposed by the tracheal tube. The tube resistance is always present, and is independent of the ventilator brand, ventilation mode, and controls in use.

To minimize tube resistance, you should always choose the largest possible tracheal tubes.

You can easily feel the tube resistance yourself by breathing through an ETT. To get the air though the tube, you have to breathe slightly harder, or much harder, than normal. This indicates a higher 'patient' work of breathing (WOB) to overcome the tube resistance.

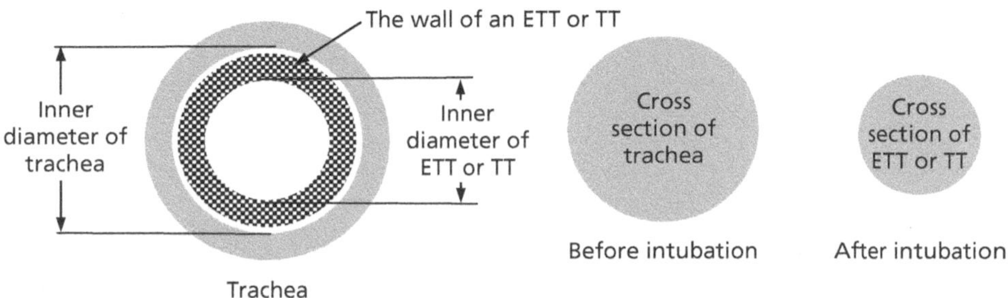

Fig. 10.11 Intubation decreases the cross section of the airway, leading to higher airway resistance.

10.6.2 What is tube resistance compensation?

Tube resistance compensation (TRC) is a relatively new ventilator feature that automatically offsets the tube resistance.

It has different names in different ventilators, such as:

- Automatic tube compensation (ATC);
- Tube compensation (TC);
- Airway resistance compensation (ARC);
- Artificial airway compensation (AAC).

The purpose and operating principle of these different implementations are identical, although their technical details may differ slightly.

Typically TRC is an option (sometimes called a 'mode addition'), which can be enabled or disabled in most or all ventilation modes. TRC is not a ventilation mode.

10.6.3 When is tube resistance compensation indicated?

Tube resistance compensation is indicated in ventilated patients who are actively breathing (Fig. 10.12). Typically the stronger the patient's the breathing efforts, the more beneficial this function.

If a ventilated patient is passive, you can enable TRC, but it has no patient benefit, because the ventilator system does all the work of breathing anyway, including the extra work to overcome the tube resistance.

TRC is contraindicated in non-invasive ventilation, simply because there is no tracheal tube in use.

10.6.4 How does TRC work?

Extra tube resistance

As we learned already, gas flow is dependent on two factors: resistance and the pressure gradient. Their relationship is described by the Ohm's law, when the flow is laminar:

$$I = V/R$$
or
$$Flow = Pressure\ gradient\ /\ Resistance$$

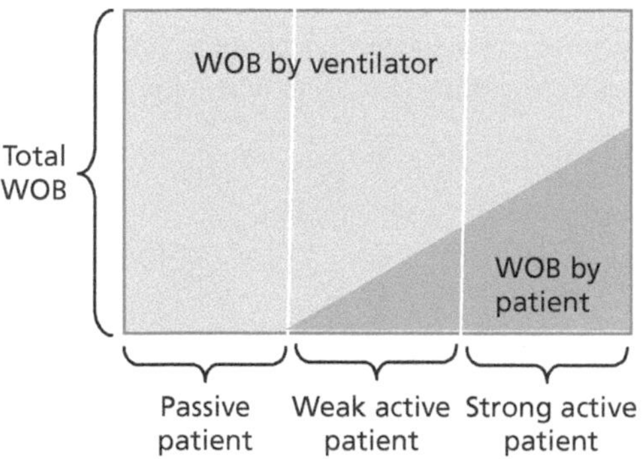

Fig. 10.12 Tube resistance is indicated in active patients, especially those with strong breathing activities.
WOB: work of breathing.

Table 10.1 Four ways to generate pressure gradients between P_{alv} and P_{ao}

Type of breathing	Inspiration ($P_{ao} > P_{alv}$)	Expiration ($P_{ao} < P_{alv}$)
Natural breathing	Decreased P_{alv}	Increased P_{alv}
IPPV in a passive patient	Increased P_{ao}	Decreased P_{ao}
IPPV in an active patient	Increased P_{ao} and possibly decreased P_{alv}	Decreased P_{ao} and possibly increased P_{alv}

This means that, in order to secure the same gas flow, a small pressure gradient is required if the resistance is low, and a large pressure gradient is required if the resistance is high.

During invasive mechanical ventilation, a tracheal tube connects the ventilator and the patient's respiratory system. The pressure at the patient end is alveolar pressure (P_{alv}), and the pressure at the ventilator end is airway opening pressure (P_{ao}).

The gradient (P_{ao}–P_{alv}) and the resistance together determine the direction and rate of the gas flow.

The pressure gradient is generated by varying P_{alv} during normal breathing and by varying P_{ao} during mechanical ventilation in a passive patient. The situations are summarized in Table 10.1.

To better understand the principle of tube resistance compensation, let's look at the situation where a healthy adult breathes normally and then breathes through an ETT.

When we breathe normally, the P_{ao} is constant and equals atmospheric pressure, while the P_{alv} varies. During inspiration, contraction of the inspiratory muscles generates a negative P_{alv}, sucking air into the lungs. During expiration, the inspiratory muscles relax. The elastic recoil force of the lungs and chest wall generates a positive P_{alv}, driving gas out of the lungs.

When we breathe through an ETT, we must breathe harder to secure the same gas flow. We must generate a larger variation in the P_{alv} to overcome the tube resistance.

In Fig. 10.13, the small P_{alv} variation, shown as the continuous curve, represents the work required to overcome the natural airway resistance. The large P_{alv} variation, shown as the dotted curve, represents the work required to overcome both airway and tube resistances. The

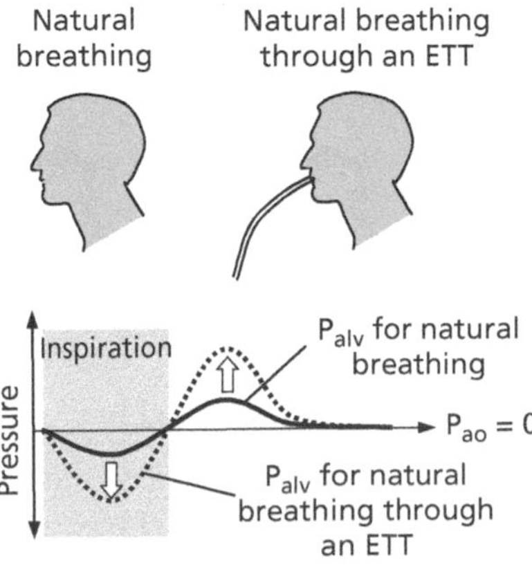

Fig. 10.13 Variation in alveolar pressure (P_{alv}) during natural breathing, with and without an ETT (endotracheal tube).

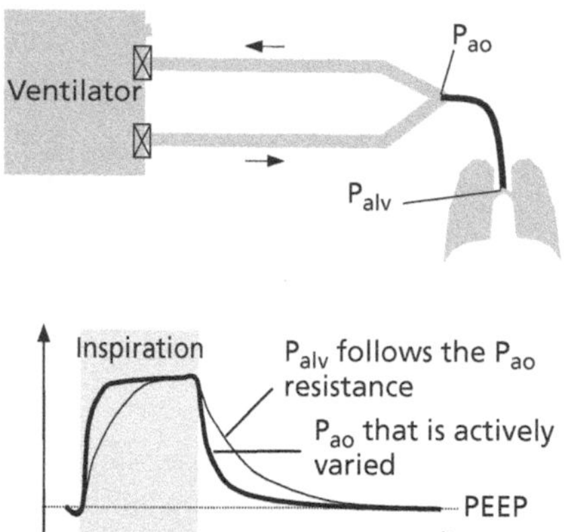

Fig. 10.14 Airway opening pressure (P_{ao}) and alveolar pressure (P_{alv}) variations during mechanical ventilation.

difference between the two curves, indicated by the white arrows, represents the extra work required to overcome the tube resistance. Note that the additional P_{alv} varies over time.

Assume that we now have a device that can generate the extra P_{alv} variations on top of the normal P_{alv} variation. We could now breathe through an ETT as if the tube were not present, because the device does the extra work. In theory, this is how tube resistance is compensated.

However, this model above does not apply to mechanical ventilation where the ventilator generates a varying P_{ao} and the P_{alv} follows, as shown in Fig. 10.14. Note that the difference between P_{ao} and P_{alv} represents the effect of the tube resistance. The situation is complicated in an active patient who can change the P_{alv}.

We know that intubation imposes extra resistance, and we know we need to apply additional P_{ao} to overcome the tube resistance. However, one spontaneous breath is different from another, and different tracheal tubes have different dimensions. So exactly how much extra P_{ao} is required?

To resolve this issue, tube resistance compensation is based on standardization of tracheal tubes and instantaneous airway flow measurement.

Standardization of tracheal tubes

The good news is that all commercially available tracheal tubes are, or should be, produced according to the international standard ISO 5361 for endotracheal tubes and ISO 5366 for tracheostomy tubes. This means that the tracheal tubes are very similar, if not identical, in their lengths and inner diameters. See Table 10.2.

The resistance imposed by standardized ETTs and TTs has been intensively studied. It is summarized in Fig. 10.15, which shows the ΔP required to fully overcome the resistance imposed by these tubes.

From these two charts, we can see that:

- Tube resistance is flow dependent, and the flow-resistance relationship is nonlinear.
- Tube resistance is related to tube inner diameter. To drive the gas to move at a given flow rate, the thinner the tube, the greater the tube resistance is, and vice versa.
- An ETT has a higher tube resistance than a TT, if the inner diameters are the same.

Be aware that these graphs show the tubes' physical properties as measured in a laboratory. The tubes are new, clean, and dry. In clinical practice, however, tubes are wet, coated with

Table 10.2 Endotracheal tube specifications

FR	8	10	12	14	16	18	20	22	24	26	28	30	32	34	36	38	40
ID (mm)	2.0	2.5	3.0	3.5	4.0	4.5	5.0	5.5	6.0	6.5	7.0	7.5	8.0	8.5	9.0	9.5	10.0
OD (mm)	2.7	3.3	4.0	4.7	5.3	6.0	6.7	7.3	8.0	8.7	9.3	10.0	10.7	11.3	12.0	12.7	13.3
L (mm)	140	145	165	185	210	225	245	275	285	295	310	315	330	330	330	330	330

FR: French; ID: internal diameter; OD: outer diameter; L: tube length.

Modified from http://www.suru.com/

secretions, and possibly curved so that the actual tube resistance can be higher than the data on the charts.

Airway flow measurement

During mechanical ventilation, airway flow is ideally measured directly at the Y-piece. Alternatively, it is measured indirectly as the difference between inspiratory flow and expiratory flow. The following points are important to know:

- Airway flow changes regularly in its direction and rate.
- Measured airway flow is a good indicator of the patient's current ventilatory demand.
- Measured airway flow is influenced by the tube resistance in an intubated patient.

By combining the above flow-resistance charts and the measured airway flow, the ventilator can calculate and automatically and instantaneously apply the extra P_{ao} required to overcome the tube resistance at the current gas flow. TRC can be regarded as an airway flow amplifier, that is, the higher the measured airway flow, the greater the extra P_{ao}, and vice versa.

Fig. 10.16 shows the P_{ao} and P_{alv} curves with and without TRC. Carefully comparing these curves in both graphs, you may see two important differences. First, TRC causes the P_{ao} curve to have a 'camel hump' change in shape. This hump appears in early inspiration and early expiration, corresponding to the highest inspiratory flow and expiratory flow. Second, with TRC the P_{alv} curve rises and falls more sharply, indicating faster lung inflation and deflation because of intensified inspiratory and expiratory flows.

Operator inputs

The operator manually activates TRC and sets TRC-specific settings (Fig. 10.17). These include (a) tube type—ETT or TT; (b) tube size, in internal diameter; and (c) intended compensation level—full (100% in theory) or partial.

After TRC is enabled, both the measured P_{ao} and the calculated P_{alv} are displayed together. The double waveforms indicate that TRC is activated.

Required conditions

TRC functions properly only when the following conditions are satisfied:

a. Airway flow measurement is continuous and accurate.
b. The entire ventilator system is operating correctly, having no excessive gas leak or occlusion.
c. The TRC settings are appropriate.
d. The tracheal tube is standard and intact (e.g. not shortened).

If any of these conditions is not fully satisfied, avoid using TRC. It may create more problems than it solves.

(a)

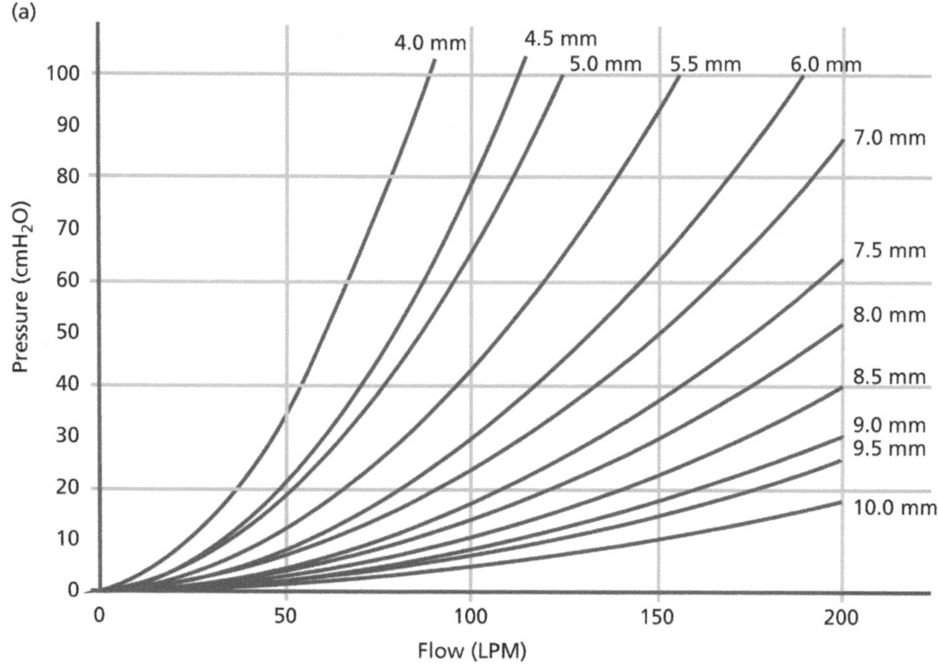

(b)

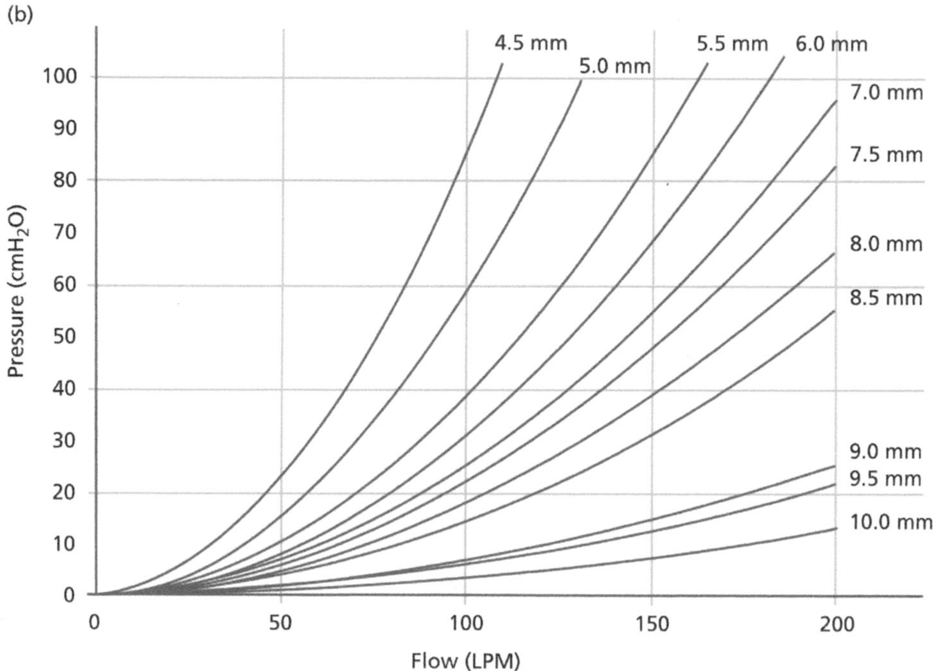

Fig. 10.15 The relationship between the intended flow and the required pressure gradient to move gas through a standard ETT (a) or TT (b). (a) This chart shows the resistance that a standard ETT imposes against passing flow. The resistance is expressed as the intended flow and the pressure gradient (ΔP) required. Every ETT has a representative curve. (b) This chart shows the resistance that a standard TT imposes against passing flow. The resistance is expressed as the intended flow and the pressure gradient (ΔP) required. Every TT has a representative curve.

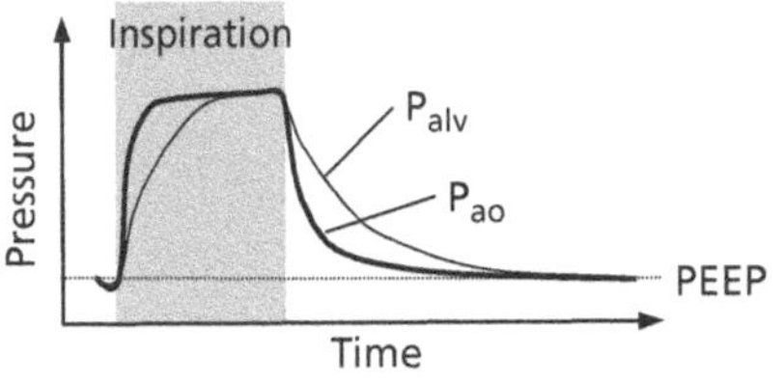

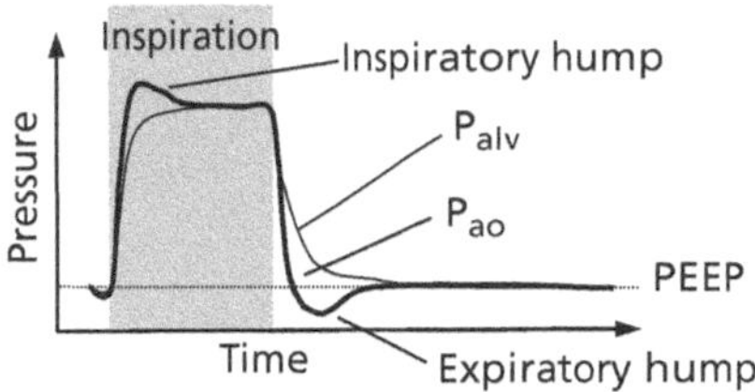

Fig. 10.16 Airway opening pressure (P_{ao}) and alveolar pressure (P_{alv}) curves without tube resistance compensation (TRC) (left), and with TRC (right).

Special remarks

TRC is designed to compensate tube resistance, but not natural airway resistance.

Note that tube compensation is an approximation. In the real world, we are dealing with a dynamic system, not a laboratory model.

There is an inevitable delay of some tens of milliseconds from capture of airway flow signal to appearance of the corresponding pneumatic effect. Therefore, compensation is always slightly delayed.

In a volume mode, TRC is typically inactive, because TRC operation conflicts with the predefined or fixed inspiratory flow and pattern of a volume breath.

In some ventilators, TRC is active during inspiration only. In other ventilators, TRC is active during both inspiration and expiration.

Expiratory TRC causes a downward 'camel hump'. The range for expiratory TRC is between the current PEEP and the zero line (i.e. atmospheric pressure). Therefore, expiratory TRC may be inadequate if PEEP is set low.

The inspiratory TRC hump increases the peak pressure slightly.

10.6.5 The effects of TRC

The four graphs in Fig. 10.18 and Fig. 10.19 show the effects of TRC in an adult volunteer with the following settings: mode = PSV, pressure support = 10 cmH_2O, PEEP = 4 cmH_2O, flow trigger sensitivity = 2 L/min, flow cycling or ETS = 50%, and rise time (P_{ramp}) = 50 ms.

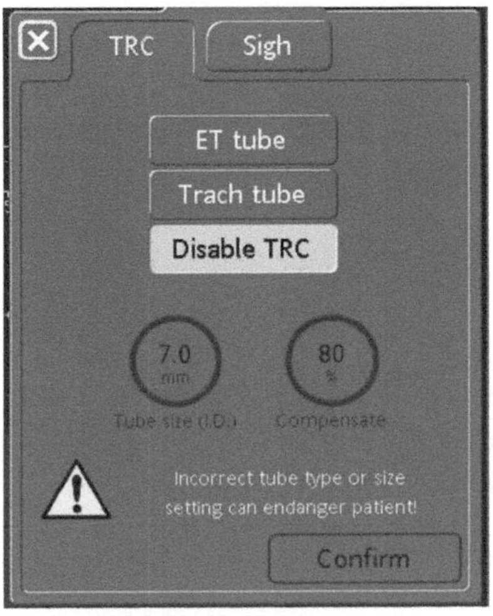

Fig. 10.17 TRC setting window (HAMILTON-G5 ventilator).

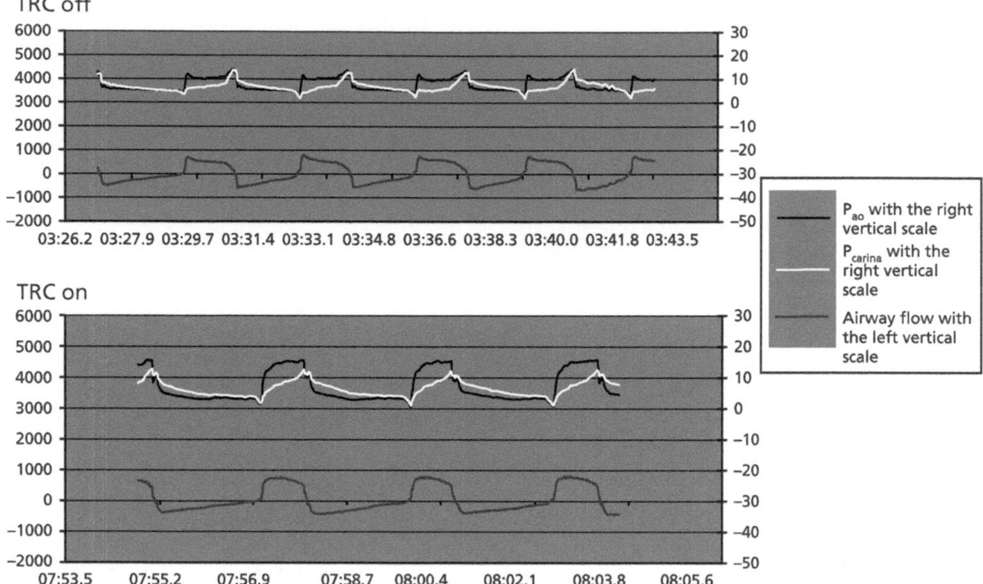

Fig. 10.18 Pressure and flow waveforms of peaceful spontaneous breathing with TRC off and on.

During peaceful spontaneous breathing, both inspiratory and expiratory flows are low, and both the tube resistance and its compensation are weak. The only visible difference is that P_{ao} (black curve) during inspiration is slightly concave without TRC, but convex with TRC.

When spontaneous breathing becomes intense, both inspiratory and expiratory peak flows increase significantly, as does the tube resistance. The direct consequence is a phenomenon called 'flow starvation', shown in the upper graphs. The P_{ao} (the black curve) fails to rise as

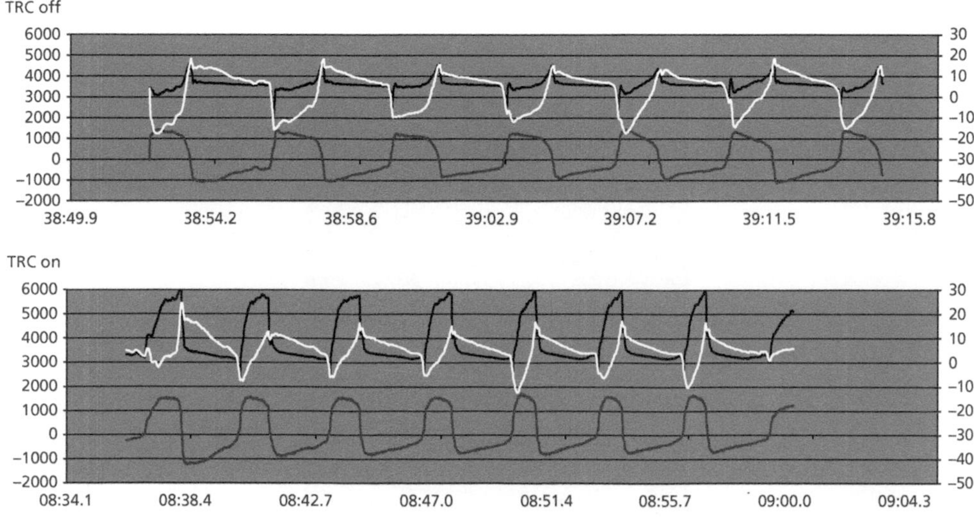

Fig. 10.19 Pressure and flow waveforms of intensive spontaneous breathing with and without TRC.

expected during inspiration, indicated by the pink inspiratory flow. The calculated P_{alv} (the white curve) drops significantly, indicating substantial patient work in breathing.

After TRC is activated, its effect is reflected by:

a. The reappearance of the expected shape of P_{ao};
b. A reduction of the P_{alv} drop, indicating a reduced patient work of breathing;
c. A slight increase in both inspiratory and expiratory peak flows.

Chapter 11

Ventilator Monitoring

11.1 Introduction

During mechanical ventilation, gas pressure, volume, and flow in the ventilator system fluctuate. We cannot see the pneumatic signals directly with our eyes, but we can observe them with special *monitoring* devices.

Ventilator monitoring refers to a group of specific ventilator functions that involves measuring the pneumatic and non-pneumatic signals at defined locations and displaying them in various ways.

Ventilator monitoring devices may be as old as the ventilator itself. Fig.11.1 shows the monitoring devices integrated in ventilators that are 150, 65, and 5 years old. The red frames show the displayed monitoring results.

Ventilator monitoring is also one of the fastest evolving areas of ventilator technology. It has expanded in three directions. First came the monitoring of new signal types, such as O_2, $P_{et}CO_2$ (end-tidal partial pressure of CO_2), gas temperature, and SpO_2; second, new monitoring information that is extracted from directly monitored signals; and third, the improved visualization of the monitoring for easier understanding.

A good example of the third is the 'dynamic lung' on the HAMILTON-G5 ventilator (Fig.11.2). Monitored respiratory compliance and airway resistance are typically presented numerically. This new feature shows the monitoring results graphically. The user gets much valuable information at a glance from the shape of the airway tree and the lungs.

This chapter will focus on the basics of ventilator monitoring, including:

- General monitoring concepts;
- The ventilator monitoring system;
- Conditions required for monitoring;
- Presentation of monitoring results;
- Common ventilator monitoring parameters.

11.2 General monitoring concepts

Before beginning our discussion of ventilator monitoring, let's clearly define a few general concepts related to monitoring technology.

11.2.1 Definition of four common terms

When talking about monitoring, the technical staff often use some special terms:

- The monitoring is *accurate*;
- The monitoring is *reproducible*;
- The monitoring has a high *resolution*;
- The monitoring is *precise*.

What do they really mean? Are they the same or different? Let's discuss them one by one.

(a)

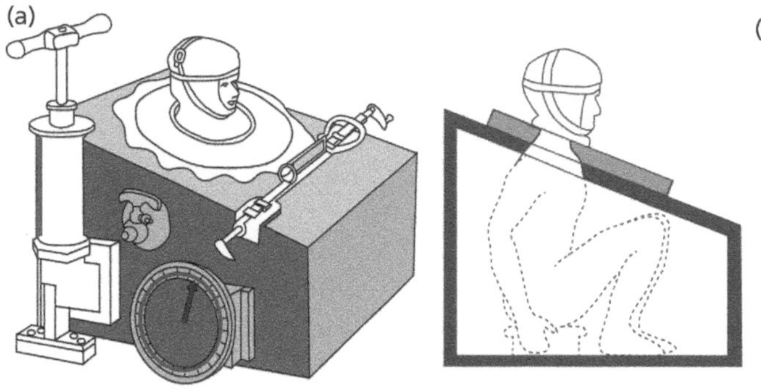

A barometer measures and indicates the tank pressure

(b)

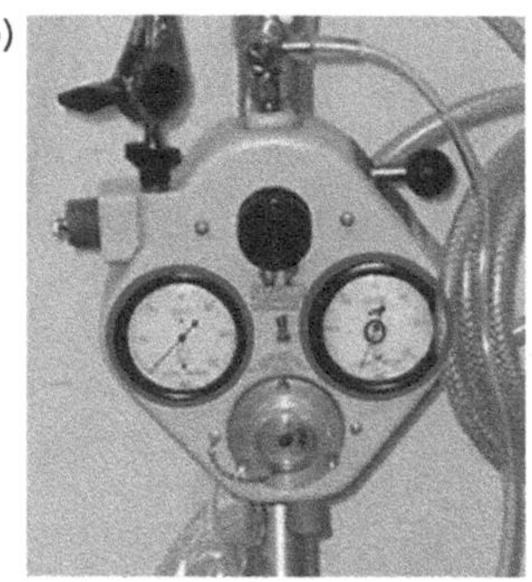

The Bennett TV-2P ventilator was released in 1948. It may be the first industrially produced ventilator.

(c)

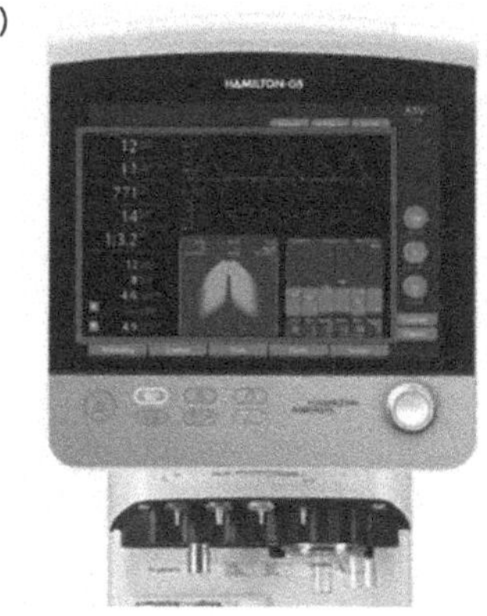

The user interface panel of the HAMILTON-G5 ventilator, which was released by HAMILTON MEDICAL in 2007

Fig. 11.1 Evolution of ventilator monitoring.

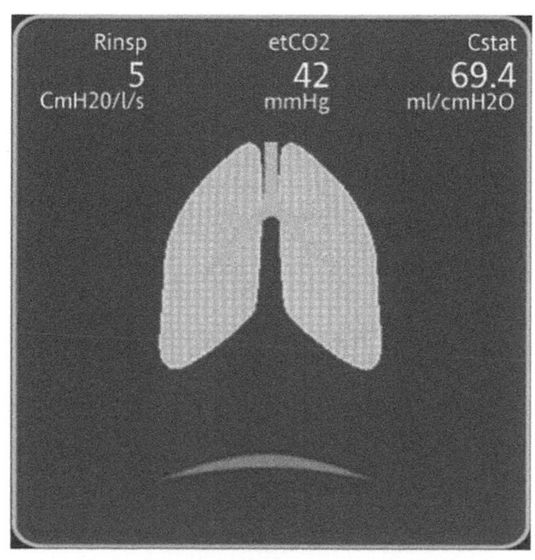

Fig. 11.2 The dynamic lung graphic on the HAMILTON-G5 ventilator.

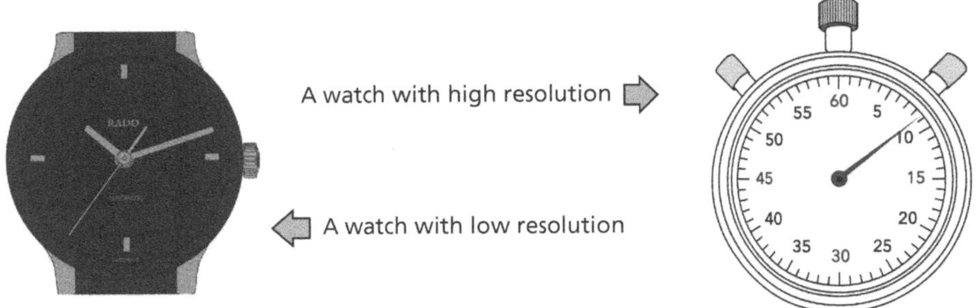

Fig. 11.3 Two examples to show the meaning of resolution.

Accuracy

Accuracy refers to the deviation between the truth and the monitored results. If the deviation is sufficiently small, the monitoring is accurate. Otherwise, the monitoring is not accurate.

Reproducibility

If we measure the same object repeatedly under the same conditions, we may still get different results. *Reproducibility* refers to the variability of the measurement results. The smaller the variability, the more reproducible the measurements are.

Precision

Precision is generally synonymous with reproducibility. A measurement system can be (a) accurate but not precise, (b) precise but not accurate, (c) neither accurate nor precise, or (d) both accurate and precise.

Resolution

Resolution is the ability to 'resolve' the differences of measurement results. A measurement device with higher resolution uses more gradations to report its measured results. A good way to understand resolution is to look at the scale of a watch (Fig.11.3). Resolution is unrelated to accuracy—a watch with low resolution can be very accurate, while a watch with high resolution can be inaccurate.

We can see the differences between accuracy, reproducibility or precision, and resolution by using a game of darts as an example (Fig.11.4). The blue centre represents the truth, while the red dots represent the measurement results.

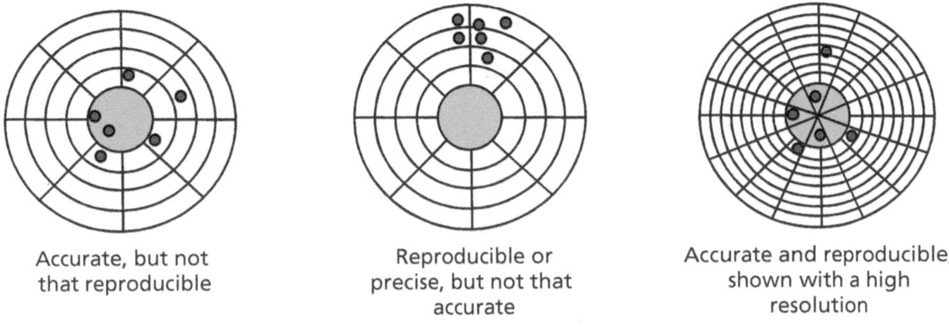

Fig. 11.4 The relationship between accuracy, reproducibility, and resolution.

11.2.2 Technical tolerance

Ideally, measurements should always be absolutely accurate and precise. In many cases, however, absolute accuracy is unfeasible, unaffordable, and unnecessary. For instance, if the true tidal volume of a breath is 500 ml, yet the monitored result is 501 ml or 499 ml, does the tiny difference matter clinically? In practice, 'sufficient' accuracy is typically satisfactory. The term 'tolerance' or *technical tolerance* refers to an acceptable range of values within which a measurement is considered to be accurate.

Let's look at an example. A ventilator manual states that the pressure monitoring tolerance is '±2 cmH_2O or ±10%, whichever is greater'. What does this mean?

In Fig.11.5, the x-axis shows actual airway pressure, and the y-axis shows measured airway pressure. The light blue line represents the absolute accuracy.

The tolerance described in the manual is the combination of two ranges, ±2 cmH_2O and ±10%. The range of ±2.0 cmH_2O is defined by two red lines parallel to the blue line. The range of ±10% is shown by the two yellow lines. The range widens as the pressure increases.

The light blue area is the tolerance defined by the two ranges. All measurements inside the light blue area are considered to be sufficiently accurate. The measurements outside that area are not considered to be sufficiently accurate.

When we discuss tolerance, we need to consider the relevant range of the measurement. For instance, the normal range of airway pressure is 0 to 40 cmH_2O. Here, the tolerance of ±2 cmH_2O may be appropriate. However, this same tolerance may be inappropriate for the measurement of a gas cylinder where the pressure range is between 0 and 200 bars.

The concept of tolerance applies not only to ventilator monitoring, but also to gas delivery by a ventilator system.

11.2.3 Calibration

A ventilator has various sensors, such as flow sensors, an oxygen sensor, and a CO_2 sensor. They measure the magnitude or concentration of intended signals in specific locations.

Ventilator manufacturers often recommend periodic calibration of these sensors in order to ensure monitoring accuracy. What is calibration? Why is it necessary?

Calibration is the act of checking or adjusting the accuracy of a measuring instrument. Calibration involves comparing the measuring instrument with a standard. Proper calibration

The light blue line indicates the absolute accuracy. The red lines indicate tolerance defined as an absolute number (2.0 cmH_2O). The yellow lines indicate tolerance defined in percent (10%).

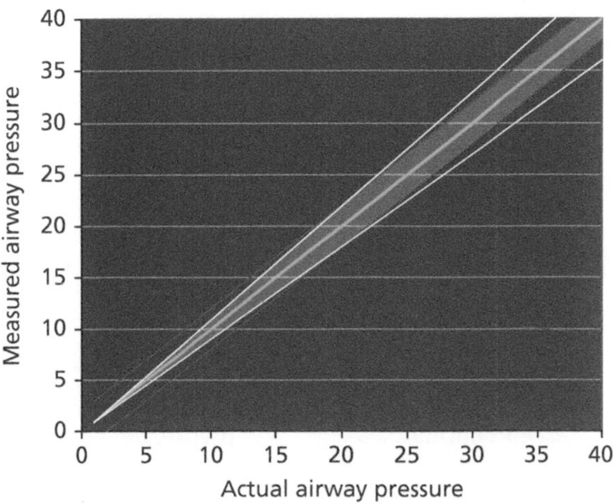

Fig. 11.5 Absolute accuracy and technical tolerances.

can improve the monitoring accuracy of a ventilator system, so it is sensible to conduct calibration as recommended.

11.3 **Ventilator monitoring system**

Inside a ventilator, the monitoring system should be functionally independent from the pneumatic operations so that the displayed readings tell the truth.

The material foundation of ventilator monitoring is a subsystem with three parts: (a) a sensor, (b) a signal processing device, and (c) a display device. They are typically connected in series.

11.3.1 **Sensor**

A sensor is a device to sense the magnitude of an intended signal, to convert it into an electronic signal, and to feed the converted signal to the signal processing device.

Conventionally, gas pressure, flow, and oxygen concentration are measured in all ventilators. A modern intensive care unit (ICU) ventilator may measure even more types of signal, such as $P_{et}CO_2$, gas temperature, and SpO_2. The Maquet SERVO-i ventilator uses a newer technique called NAVA (neutrally adjusted ventilatory assist), where a special oesophageal catheter sensor captures neural (bioelectric) signals.

A *flow sensor* is a common device to measure pneumatic signals, typically gas flow and pressure, in the gas passageway of a ventilator system. Flow sensors may use various operating principles, such as a fixed or variable orifice, a heating wire, or ultrasonic techniques. Each operating principle has its own strengths and weaknesses. As clinical ventilator operators, we may not need to know these sensor principles in detail. A wealth of information is available elsewhere for anyone who wants to know more.

What we do need to know, however, is that a sensor may behave very differently under laboratory conditions than under clinical conditions. For instance, a flow sensor can operate perfectly when the passing gas is clean and dry. However, if the passing gas contains moisture, secretions, and medication aerosols, the same flow sensor may not work as well or at all. This explains why monitoring quality worsens over time for a flow sensor installed in the airway or the expiratory limb of the circuit.

In most cases, a sensor has a specific location. For instance, for F_iO_2 monitoring the *oxygen sensor* (*cell*) should be in the inspiratory limb, and for $P_{et}CO_2$ monitoring the CO_2 sensor should be at the airway.

Typically, a ventilator has two flow sensors. The inspiratory flow sensor is always in the inspiratory limb. The second may be positioned at the expiratory valve or the airway (Fig. 11.6). Conventionally, a flow sensor at the expiratory valve is called a distal flow sensor and a flow

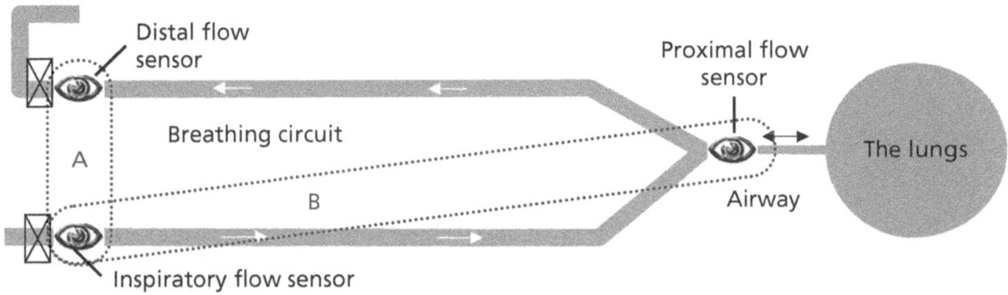

Fig. 11.6 Flow sensor positions.

Table 11.1 Comparison of distal and proximal flow sensors

Distal flow sensor		Proximal flow sensor
Applications	Most ventilators	Most neonatal ventilators and Hamilton Medical ventilators
Advantages	◆ Integrated into the ventilator ◆ No need for a proximal flow sensor, which is perceived as an extra accessory with associated potential problems	◆ Directly measures airway flow and pressure ◆ Much better signal-to-noise ratio ◆ Less sensitive to circuit leaks ◆ In volume modes, V_T monitoring is minimally affected by circuit compliance
Weaknesses	◆ Airway flow is not directly measured, but is calculated from the difference between the simultaneously measured inspiratory flow and expiratory flow ◆ Inferior signal-to-noise ratio under comparable conditions ◆ Susceptible to circuit leaks ◆ In volume modes, the patient may receive a lower V_T than that delivered, due to circuit compliance (refer to section 5.3.4). Additional correction is necessary	◆ Perceived to be an extra accessory ◆ Increased probability of airway disconnection ◆ Increased airway dead space (refer to section 5.3.5)

sensor at the airway is a proximal flow sensor. The position of the second flow sensor may noticeably affect the monitoring. Table 11.1 summarizes the differences.

A flow sensor can only measure the flow of the gas that passes through it at its assigned location, which may confuse the clinician. For instance, let's say we are ventilating a neonate in P-SIMV mode. There is a leak around the endotracheal tube (ETT), which is typically uncuffed in neonates. The ventilator reports that the monitored V_T is a surprisingly low 5 ml, and it activates a low V_T alarm. We expected a V_T of approximately 20 ml, and we fear that the baby cannot survive with such a low tidal volume. Then we start to question whether the ventilator is defective.

To our surprise, our technician tells us that the ventilator is working properly. The reported V_T is so low, because much of the exhaled gas has leaked, while only a fraction passed through the flow sensor and was (correctly) measured (Fig.11.7). In this case, the ventilator monitoring is functioning properly, but the sensor senses only a part of the flow, not the whole. The flow and volume readings return to normal after the gas leak is eliminated.

11.3.2 Signal processing device

A modern ICU ventilator displays a number of monitoring parameters. These may be grouped into three categories:

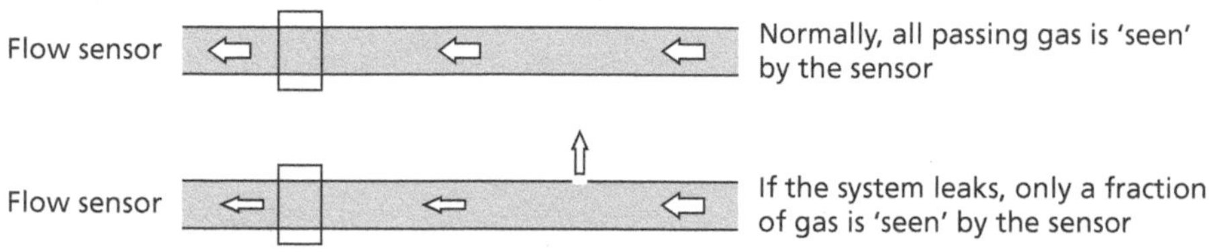

Fig. 11.7 A flow sensor can only detect the gas flow that passes through it.

a. Direct measurements;
b. Monitoring parameters that are extracted from direct measurements;
c. Monitoring parameters that are calculated from direct measurements.

There are just a small number of signal types that are directly measured. These commonly include gas flow, gas pressure, and the O_2 concentration of the inspiratory gas. Other possible signal types include $P_{et}CO_2$, gas temperature, and SpO_2. This direct measurement is continuous and in real time. The results may be displayed graphically, such as in waveforms. The original signals are often weak and full of noise, so that signal amplification and filtering are often the first steps required.

The ventilator processes these direct measurements to create additional monitoring parameters through extraction and calculation (Fig.11.8):

- For extracted parameters, the ventilator takes certain pieces of information from the measured results in defined ways. A typical example is peak airway pressure.
- For calculated parameters, the ventilator computes results using special mathematical models. A typical example is expiratory tidal volume.

The extracted and calculated parameters are typically displayed numerically.

11.3.3 Display device

A display device is designed to visualize the monitoring data. The device can be a gauge scale, a digital display, or liquid crystal display (LCD) in various shapes, colours, and sizes. In rare cases, the monitoring data takes the form of audible signals.

A modern ventilator typically has an LCD screen, which provides versatility for the data display. In section 11.5, we will discuss in depth the presentation of monitoring results.

11.4 Required conditions for ventilator monitoring

Ventilator monitoring is conditional: it functions as expected only when all required conditions are fully satisfied. If the displayed monitoring results are outside the expected range, there are three possibilities:

A. The monitoring system is malfunctioning, because:
  - One or more components are missing, incompatible, or inoperative;
  - Components are incorrectly or insecurely connected;
  - The sensor is positioned incorrectly;

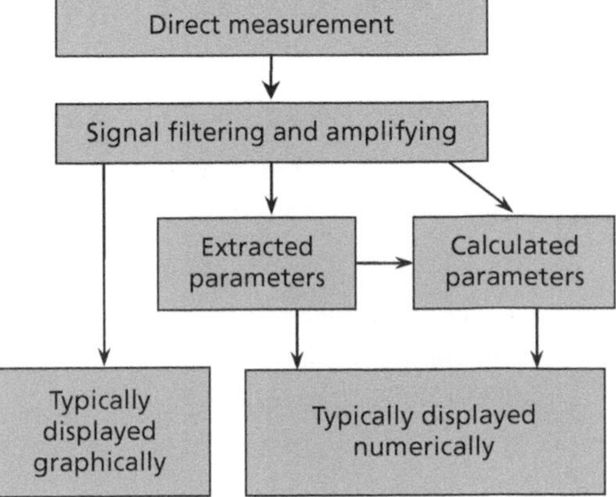

Fig. 11.8 Overview of signal sensing, processing, and displaying.

- The inner surface of a flow sensor is coated with moisture, secretions, or aerosolized medication;
- The monitoring system is not calibrated as recommended.

B. The monitoring system is functioning properly, but the ventilator system is malfunctioning, because:

- One or more required parts are missing, incompatible, or inoperative;
- Components are incorrectly or insecurely connected;
- The system has a noticeable leak;
- The system has a noticeable occlusion in its gas passageway.

C. Both A and B

11.5 **Presentation of monitoring results**

The results of ventilator monitoring must be presented so that a human being can see and understand them. Conventionally, ventilator monitoring results are presented numerically and graphically.

11.5.1 **Numerical parameters**

Numerical parameters are the most common way to present monitoring results. The displayed parameters are extracted or calculated from direct measurements. Parameters are typically updated after every mechanical breath.

For each monitoring parameter, there are three components: the term, the unit of measurement, and the current value (the signal magnitude or concentration), as shown in Fig.11.9.

The major advantage of the numerical presentation is digital precision, which does not necessarily mean high accuracy.

Its major disadvantage is that it is difficult to link the displayed value to the patient's clinical condition. Furthermore, a numerical parameter is just a snapshot: it does not show change over time. For instance, a tidal volume of 500 ml in an adult might appear to be normal or acceptable.

Monitor
SIMV
Operating hours: 79 h
2004-02-25 15:42
32 Ppeak cmH20
517 VTE ml
20 fTotal b/min
---- Pplateau cmH20
9.3 ExpMinVol l/min
5 fSpont b/min
13 Pmean cmH20
39 VLeak ml
1.29 TI s
5.4 PEEP/CPAP cmH20
34.6 Insp Flow l/min
3.65 TE s
5.1 Pminimum cmH20
86.8 Exp Flow l/min
1:2.8 I:E
---- AutoPEEP cmH20
10 Rinsp cmH20/l/s
0.21 RCinsp s
---- P01 cmH20
9 Rexp cmH20/l/s
0.26 RCexp s
0.00 WOBimp J/l
19.8 Cstat ml/cmH20
0.0 PTP cmH20*s
39 RSB 1/(l*min)
21 Oxygen %
Close

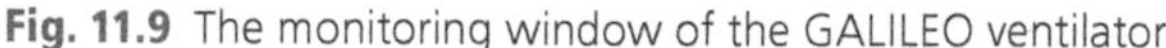

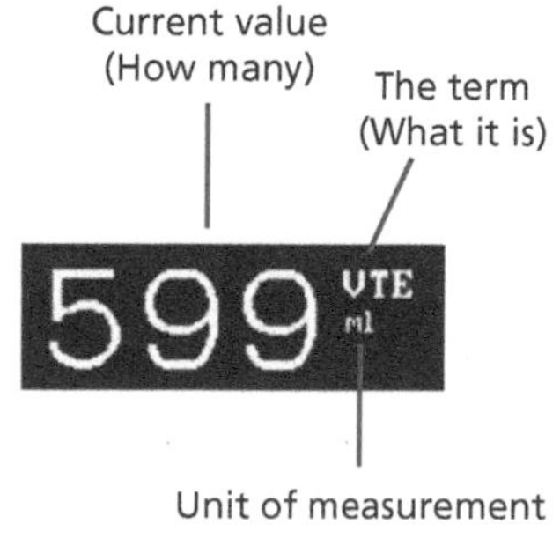

Fig. 11.9 The monitoring window of the GALILEO ventilator.

It can signal a problem if it was 800 ml 10 minutes ago, provided that the ventilator settings were not changed.

Be aware that some ventilator controls and monitoring parameters share the same terms (e.g. PEEP, F_iO_2, rate, and tidal volume). V_T as a control parameter means the desired or targeted tidal volume, while V_T as a monitoring parameter means the actual tidal volume. For this reason, if someone tells you that the tidal volume for a patient is 600 ml, always ask whether they are referring to the *set* tidal volume or the *monitored* tidal volume.

11.5.2 Graphic presentations

Graphic presentations of monitored data take three common forms: waveforms, dynamic loops, and trend curves.

Waveforms

Waveforms are the most common way to graphically display directly measured parameters. A typical ventilator displays waveforms of gas pressure, flow, and (calculated) volume (Fig.11.10). $P_{et}CO_2$, SpO_2, gas temperature, and others may optionally be displayed.

The waveform is a running curve on a chart with time as the x-axis and the monitored parameter as the y-axis. Typically, two or three waveforms share the same time scale so that we can observe them simultaneously.

To read and understand a waveform, we must identify four basic elements: (a) the displayed parameter; (b) the unit of measure; (c) the x and y-axes; and (d) the scales of these axes.

By comparing these side by side, we can identify four differences between the waveforms:

- The graphical presentations are different, with different colour schemes and with the waveforms in the Evita 4 filled in.
- The two ventilators display these same three parameters in different orders.
- The volume waveform of the Evita 4 is in litres (L), while that of the GALILEO waveform is in millilitres (ml).
- The two waveforms have slightly different time scales: 16 s for the Evita 4, and 10 s for the GALILEO.

Note that scaling of the x or y-axis may cause the same waveforms to look very different. The two waveforms shown in Fig.11.11 are identical, but have different y-scales. The y-scales of the left-hand graph range from 0–16 cmH_2O, while that of the right-hand graph range from 0–64 cmH_2O.

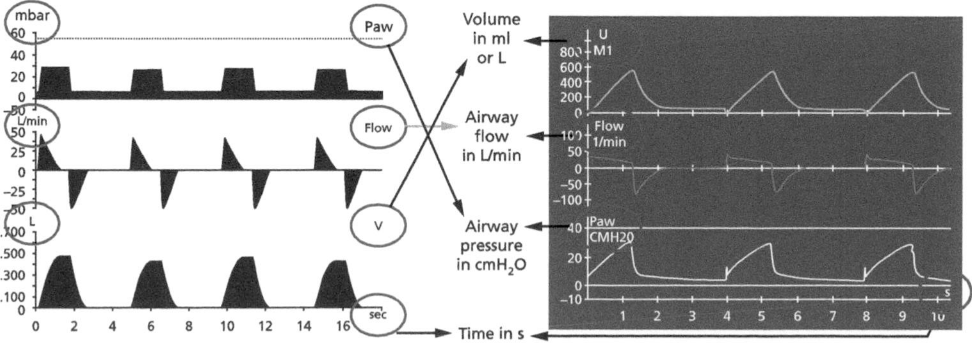

Fig. 11.10 Pressure, flow, and volume waveforms displayed on the Evita 4 ventilator from Dräger (left) and the GALILEO ventilator (right).

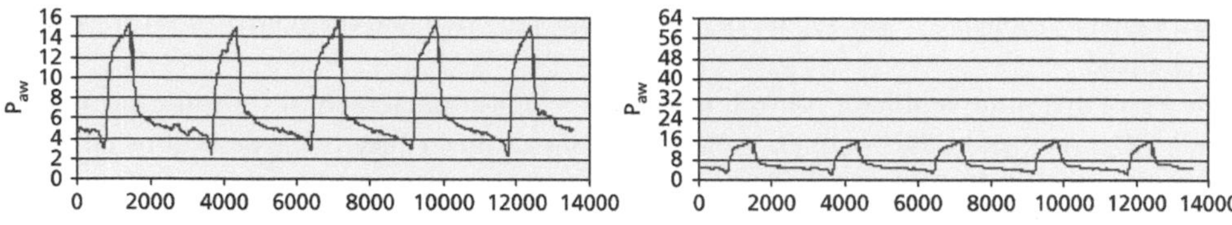

Fig. 11.11 A waveform can look very different with different Y scales.

Provided that the monitoring is accurate, the shape or profile of a waveform is mainly determined by four factors:

- The patient's respiratory mechanics (e.g. respiratory compliance and airway resistance);
- The functional status of the ventilator system;
- The ventilator settings, mainly the ventilation mode and control parameters;
- The patient's breathing activities.

Any change in the four factors results in a corresponding change in the waveforms.

Waveforms are a rich source of useful information. Waveform analysis and interpretation require deep understanding of mechanical ventilation, the ventilator system, and their interactions. Details on waveform analysis are beyond the scope of this book, but they can be found in many readily available information sources.

Waveforms are running curves. They are constantly updated, and the old waveform data is continuously discarded unless it is saved with special equipment.

Shapes of normal waveforms To recognize an abnormality in a waveform, we must be truly familiar with the shapes of normal waveforms. These shapes are directly related to the types of mechanical breaths, which we discussed in section 7.3 and which are summarized in Table 11.2. Fig.11.12 shows some normal types of waveform.

Dynamic loops

Monitoring data, mainly directly measured parameters, can also be presented as dynamic loops (Fig.11.13). The common signal types shown include airway pressure, flow, and volume.

A *dynamic loop* is shown on a two-dimensional graph. One monitoring parameter is plotted as the x-axis, and another monitoring parameter as the y-axis. As the monitoring data continuously becomes available, the loop is dynamically displayed in real time.

Table 11.2 Eight breath types and their essential variables

Type	Basic breath type	Trigger variable	Cycle variable	Control variable
A	Volume control	Time	Time	Volume
B	Pressure control	Time	Time	Pressure
C	Volume assist	Patient	Time	Volume
D	Pressure assist	Patient	Time	Pressure
E	Pressure support	Patient	Flow	Pressure
F	Adaptive control	Time	Time	Adaptive
G	Adaptive assist	Patient	Time	Adaptive
H	Adaptive support	Patient	Time	Adaptive

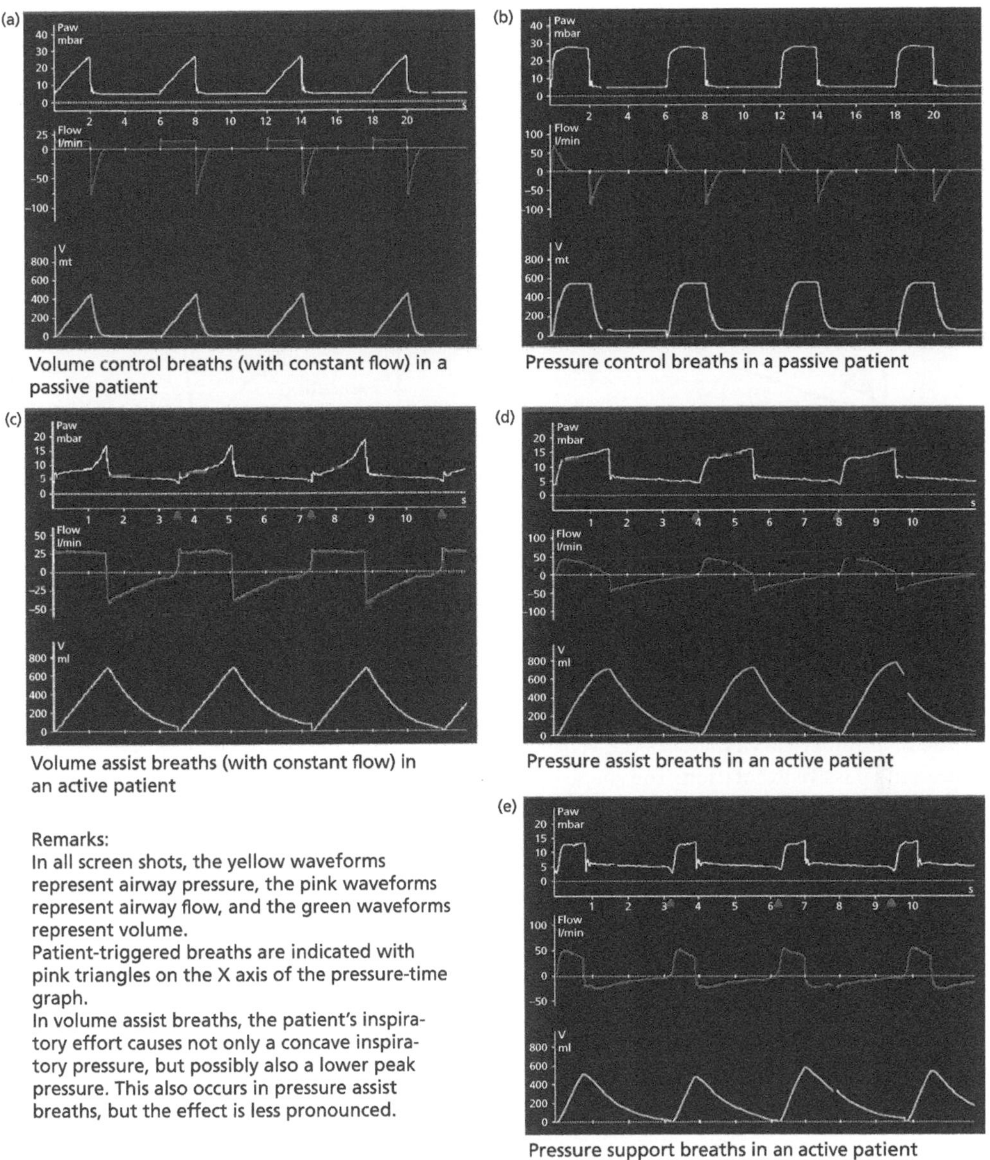

Fig. 11.12 Waveforms of normal breath types in passive and active patients.

There are several possible combinations of the three signals. In clinical practice, however, only two loop types are widely used and studied: pressure-volume loops and flow-volume loops.

Pressure-volume loop In a pressure-volume loop, monitored airway pressure is plotted on the x-axis, and volume is plotted on the y-axis. The inspiratory curve goes upward, and the expiratory curve goes downward.

Spontaneous breaths without pressure support go clockwise, and positive pressure breaths go counter-clockwise.

The bottom of the loop is at the set positive end-expiratory pressure (PEEP) level, which may be zero or a positive value. If we draw a line down the middle of the loop, the area

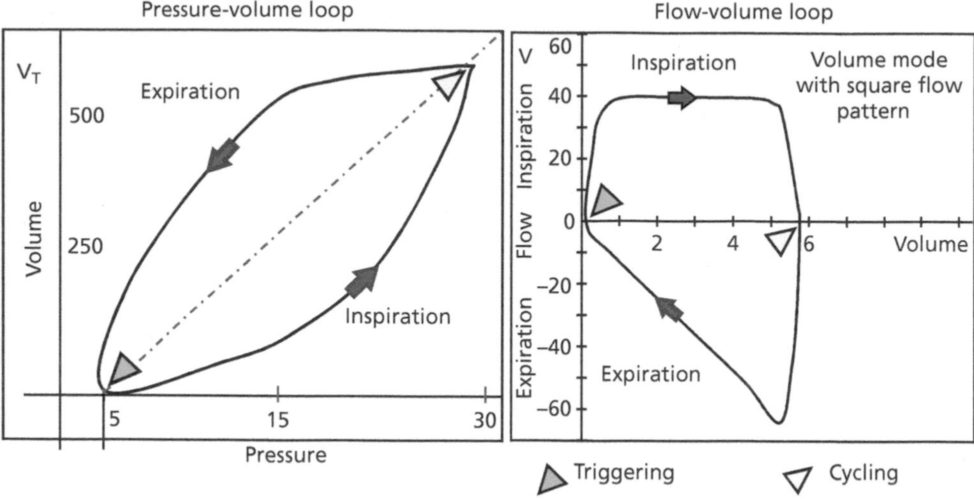

Fig. 11.13 Two common dynamic loop types.

to the right represents inspiratory resistance, and the area to the left represents expiratory resistance.

Flow-volume loop In a flow-volume loop, airway flow is plotted on the y-axis, and volume is plotted on the x-axis. Inspiration is above the horizontal line, and expiration is below. The shape of the inspiratory curve matches the ventilator settings. The shape of the expiratory flow curve represents passive exhalation. The shape of the pressure-volume loop differs in different breath types. With spontaneous breaths, the flow-volume loop looks circular.

Just like waveforms, dynamic loops are a rich source of useful information. Analysis and interpretation of the loops require deep understanding of mechanical ventilation and ventilators.

Trend curves

Both waveforms and dynamic loops are displayed for a short period of time: one breath or several breaths. By contrast, *trending curves* show events over a much longer period. However, they do not necessarily suggest with accuracy what will happen in the future.

As we have seen, a number of numeric monitoring parameters are displayed and updated after every breath. These parameters may or may not be identical to those of previous breaths.

A trend curve is a two-dimensional graph with time as its x-axis and the monitoring parameter as its y-axis. It contains numerous tiny bars (Fig. 11.14). Each bar represents one reading or the average of several consecutive readings of the monitoring parameter.

As new readings are continuously available, the trend curve moves very slowly but continuously from right to left. The right-most bar shows the most recent reading, while the left-most bar shows the oldest reading.

The trend curve shows how the monitoring parameter has changed over a defined period of time, such as 1 hour, 6 hours, 12 hours, or 24 hours.

Typically, you select and define a trend curve in four steps:

a. Activate the trend function;
b. Select the monitoring parameters to display as a trend curve;
c. Set the desired trending duration; and
d. Confirm the selection.

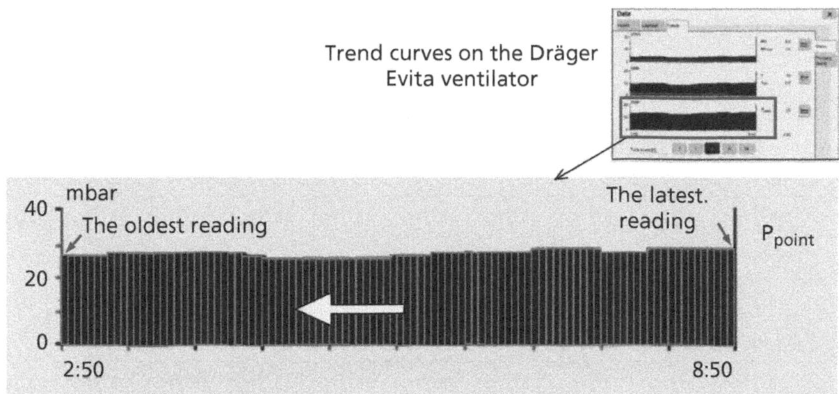

Fig. 11.14 A trend curve is composed of a number of vertical bars. Every bar represents the value of the monitoring parameter during that unit of time.

Some ventilators allow multiple trend curves to be displayed simultaneously.

Trend curves are particularly useful for a number of reasons. They allow a clinician to understand what happened to a ventilated patient the previous night. They provide hints about how the ventilator settings changed over the period of surveillance. They can also show how the patient responded to a special therapy (e.g. the effects of a bronchodilator or tracheal suction on respiratory mechanics).

Do not confuse trend curves with waveforms!

Freeze and cursor measurement

Waveforms and dynamic loops are continuously updated. The updating may happen so fast that you can barely take a close look at an interesting detail before it disappears forever.

The solution is freeze and cursor measurement functions, which are two interrelated technical features.

The *freeze function* lets you temporarily stop the running waveforms or loops while mechanical ventilation continues in the background. This allows you to study the waveforms at your leisure. The 'freezing' status can be cancelled manually or automatically.

Cursor measurement is a graphic tool primarily to analyse the frozen waveforms. The cursor is an indicator on the frozen waveforms, as shown in Fig.11.15. Once the cursor is activated, you can move it back and forth and read the numerical values of the waveform at selected time points.

The freeze and cursor measurement functions are strictly monitoring functions: they have no effect upon mechanical ventilation.

11.6 **Common pressure monitoring parameters**

Now let's shift our attention to common ventilator monitoring parameters.

Pressure parameters displayed on a ventilator are extracted or calculated from the continuously monitored circuit or airway pressure. Under normal conditions, both circuit pressure and airway pressure are almost identical, so that circuit pressure is often used as a synonym for airway pressure.

Common pressure monitoring parameters include peak inspiratory pressure (PIP), plateau pressure ($P_{plateau}$), PEEP, and mean airway pressure (P_{mean}); see Fig.11.16. These parameters are updated after every breath.

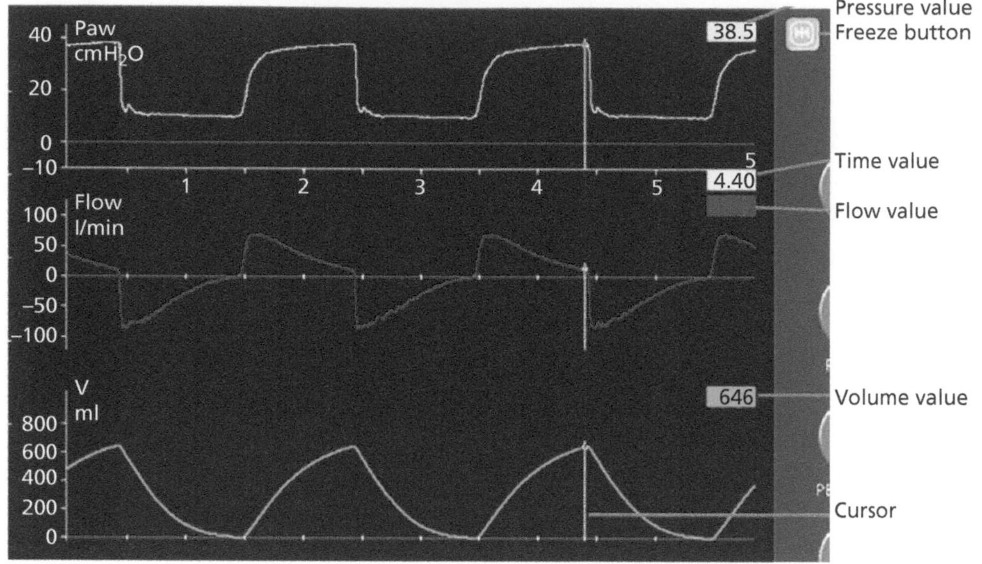

Fig. 11.15 Freeze and cursor measurement in the HAMILTON-G5 ventilator.

11.6.1 Peak inspiratory pressure (PIP)

Peak inspiratory pressure is the highest airway/circuit pressure measured during a mechanical breath. It is also called peak pressure, positive inspiratory pressure, maximum inspiratory pressure, maximum airway pressure, and peak circuit pressure. Common abbreviations are PIP and Ppeak.

Peak inspiratory pressure has three components:

- PEEP;
- The maximum inspiratory pressure applied by the ventilator;
- Abnormal pressure overshoot or spikes, if present.

PIP has a different clinical significance in pressure and volume breaths.

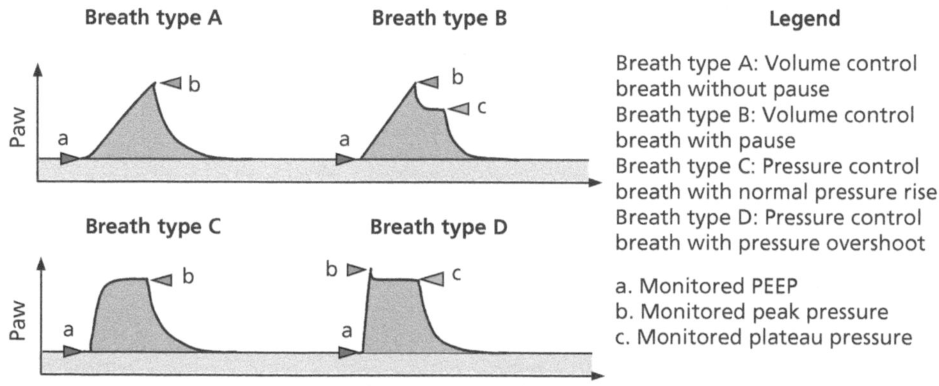

Fig. 11.16 Waveforms for peak inspiratory pressure, plateau pressure, and positive end-expiratory pressure (PEEP).

PIP in a volume breath

In a volume mode, the operator sets the tidal volume and the inspiratory flow or inspiratory time. The ventilator delivers the desired volume at the set inspiratory flow within the set T_i. PIP varies depending on (a) the settings (V_T, T_i, or peak flow), (b) the current respiratory mechanics, and (c) the patient breathing activity. A change to any of the three factors may cause a corresponding change to PIP, provided all other factors remain unchanged.

PIP in a pressure breath

In a pressure mode, the operator sets the inspiratory pressure, which is the difference between PIP and PEEP. The ventilator delivers the inspiratory gas into the circuit in order to achieve the set target pressure. The tidal volume varies depending on (a) the set inspiratory pressure, (b) the current respiratory mechanics, (c) the patient's breathing activity, and (d) in rare cases, the set T_i. Any change in the four factors can cause a corresponding change in the resultant tidal volume, provided that other factors remain unchanged.

An abnormally high PIP takes two forms: pressure overshooting and a pressure spike (Fig.11.17). Pressure overshooting appears at the beginning of inspiration due to circuit pressurization that is too fast. A pressure spike occurs at the end of inspiration, in active patients only. It is a form of patient-ventilator asynchrony.

Common causes of increased or decreased PIP are summarized in Table 11.3.

11.6.2 Plateau pressure ($P_{plateau}$)

Plateau pressure is the end-inspiratory pressure at zero flow. Under this condition, the P_{ao} and the P_{alv} equilibrate. The unit of measurement for $P_{plateau}$ is cmH_2O or millibars. Plateau pressure is also called Ppause, end-inspiratory pressure, Pplat, $P_{plateau}$, $P_{I\ END}$, and P_{PL}.

Plateau pressure is clinically important because it represents the alveolar pressure when the lungs are inflated. It can be used to estimate the current static respiratory compliance.

Plateau pressure can be monitored in passive patients only. Conventionally, plateau pressure is measured in volume modes during an inspiratory pause (Fig.11.18). Less conventionally, plateau pressure can also be measured in pressure breaths if the inspiratory time is sufficiently long so that the airway flow reaches zero. In this case, PIP is equal to the plateau pressure.

During mechanical ventilation, we should do everything possible to lower the plateau pressure in order to avoid barotrauma of the lungs.

11.6.3 PEEP

PEEP (positive end-expiratory pressure) is the monitored pressure at the end of expiration. It is expressed in cmH_2O or millibars.

It is important to clearly differentiate the set PEEP from the measured PEEP. The set PEEP is the intended or desired PEEP, while the latter is the actual PEEP. Under normal conditions, both should be equal or very close to each other.

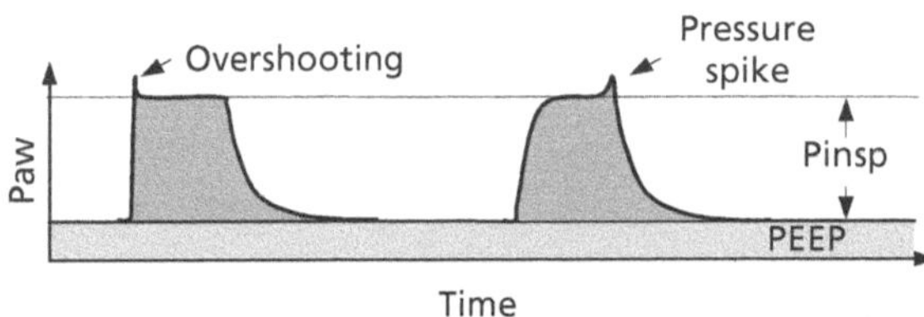

Fig. 11.17 Two forms of abnormally high peak inspiratory pressure (PIP).

Table 11.3 Common causes of increased and decreased PIP

	In a volume breath	In a pressure breath
What causes PIP to increase	◆ The set PEEP increases ◆ The set tidal volume increases ◆ The airway resistance increases ◆ The respiratory compliance decreases ◆ The set inspiratory time decreases ◆ The set inspiratory flow increases ◆ The patient is active	◆ The set PEEP increases ◆ The set inspiratory pressure ($P_{control}$ or $P_{support}$) increases ◆ A pressure overshoot or pressure spike occurs ◆ Tube resistance compensation (TRC) is active ◆ The patient is active
What causes PIP to decrease	◆ The gas passageway has a leak or disconnection ◆ The set PEEP decreases ◆ The set tidal volume decreases ◆ The airway resistance decreases ◆ The respiratory compliance increases ◆ The set inspiratory time increases ◆ The set inspiratory flow decreases ◆ The patient is active	◆ The gas passageway of the ventilator system has a noticeable gas leak or disconnection ◆ The set inspiratory pressure decreases ◆ The set PEEP decreases ◆ The patient is active

PEEP: positive end-expiratory pressure; PIP: peak inspiratory pressure.

If the measured PEEP differs significantly from the set PEEP, troubleshooting is indicated. The common causes for the difference include a significant gas leak, patient-ventilator asynchrony, or a ventilator malfunction.

11.6.4 Mean airway pressure (MAP)

Mean airway pressure is the average pressure applied over one mechanical breath. It is expressed in cmH_2O or millibars. It is also called mean pressure, mean circuit pressure, P_{mean}, PMEAN, and mPaw.

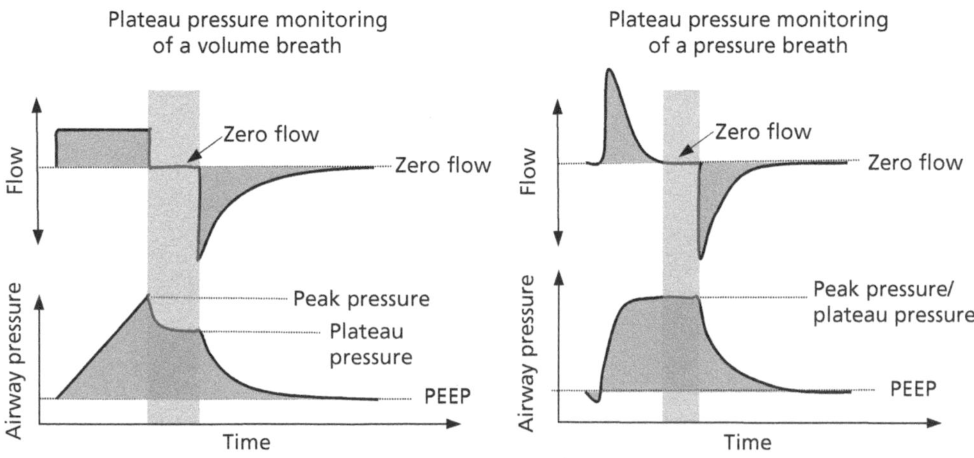

Fig. 11.18 Plateau pressure is typically monitored in a volume breath during an inspiratory pause (left). However, it is also possible in a pressure breath if T_i is long enough (right).

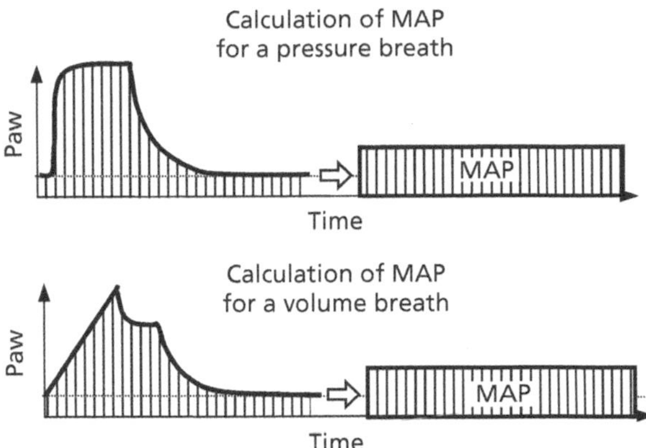

Fig. 11.19 Mean area pressure (MAP) is the average airway pressure throughout a mechanical breath.

Mean airway pressure is calculated in two steps (Fig.11.19). First, the breath cycle time (i.e. the duration of one breath) is divided into a number of equal slices. Second, the pressure values for all time slices are totalled, and this total is divided by the number of the slices. In other words, peak airway pressure is the average of the applied pressure over a breath. PEEP is part of the mean airway pressure.

The heart, large blood vessels, and the lungs are soft structures sitting inside the thoracic cavity. A positive pressure applied to the airway and lungs compresses the circulatory organs. A high MAP can cause elevated pulmonary vascular resistance, decreased cardiac output, and even decreased system blood pressure. Mean airway pressure is a good indicator of how much these intrathoracic structures are compressed. To minimize this unwanted effect, mean airway pressure should be kept as low as clinically acceptable.

In the past, mean airway pressure was manually calculated in volume modes. This tedious work is automated in modern ventilators. The displayed mean airway pressure is updated after every breath.

11.7 **Common flow monitoring parameters**

When we talk about 'flow' monitoring in ventilation, we are referring to the airway gas flow. As we discussed earlier, airway flow is either measured directly by a proximal flow sensor or calculated from the difference in the simultaneously measured flows through the inspiratory and expiratory limbs of the breathing circuit.

Monitored airway flow is often displayed as a flow-time waveform. In rare cases, peak inspiratory and expiratory flows are shown as numeric parameters. Both parameters are expressed in litres per minute or L/min, and updated after every breath. Airway flow monitoring is also the basis for calculating tidal volume.

Peak inspiratory and expiratory flows are useful and sensitive indicators of changes in the ventilator system pneumatics, and are especially useful for troubleshooting. The trend curves for *peak flow* are the most helpful, because they show how the peak flow has changed over time.

Fig.11.20 shows pressure and flow waveform displays.

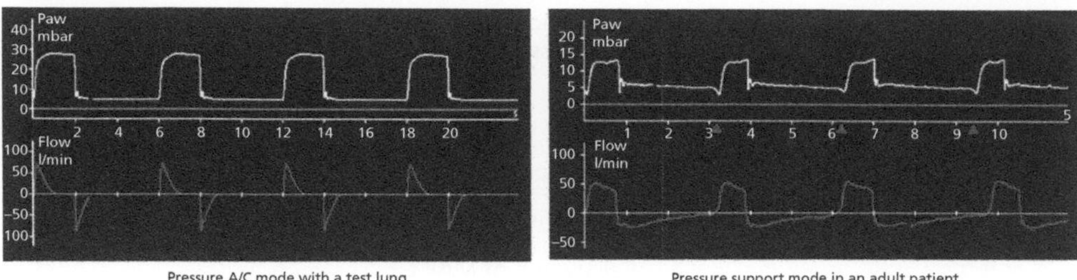

Fig. 11.20 Typical pressure-time waveform (yellow) and flow-time waveform (pink).

11.7.1 **Peak inspiratory flow (Insp flow)**

Peak inspiratory flow refers to the highest (most positive) reading of the inspiratory flow monitored over a mechanical breath. Peak inspiratory flow rate and inspiratory flow pattern are predefined in a volume breath, but variable in a pressure breath. In pressure breaths, peak inspiratory flow is determined by several factors:

- The set inspiratory pressure;
- The set rise time;
- The patient's current airway resistance and respiratory compliance;
- The patient's breathing activities;
- Inspiratory limb or airway occlusion;
- Any large gas leak in the ventilator system;
- Tube resistance compensation.

11.7.2 **Peak expiratory flow (Exp flow)**

Peak expiratory flow refers to the lowest (most negative) reading of the monitored expiratory flow over a mechanical breath.

In a passive patient, expiration is usually a passive process, driven by the elastic recoil force of the chest wall and lungs. Expiratory flow typically drops sharply to its negative maximum and then exponentially returns to zero. The process is the same for both volume and pressure breaths.

If a ventilated patient is active, the patient can influence expiration by use of the expiratory muscles, resulting in variable peak expiratory flows.

Peak expiratory flow can be influenced by:

- The actual tidal volume or the inspiratory pressure;
- The patient's current airway resistance and respiratory compliance;
- The patient's breathing activities;
- Airway or expiratory limb occlusion;
- Any large gas leak in the ventilator system;
- Tube resistance compensation.

Clinically, peak expiratory flow is an excellent indicator of airway patency. Its reading is much lower than normal in patients with obstructive diseases such as chronic obstructive pulmonary disease (COPD) and asthma. Trending this parameter may prove more helpful than simply reading the values for single breaths.

11.8 Common volume monitoring parameters

As we know, lung ventilation is achieved by moving a certain volume of gas into and out of the lungs in a series of natural or artificial breaths.

Monitored tidal volume is just one of several key parameters of lung ventilation. Fig.11.21 shows the relationship between tidal volume, respiratory rate, dead space, alveolar tidal volume, (minute) alveolar ventilation, and minute ventilation.

CO_2 removal is directly related to alveolar ventilation. Under normal conditions, increased alveolar ventilation leads to decreased $PaCO_2$, and vice versa.

Common volume monitoring parameters include tidal volume and minute volume.

11.8.1 Expiratory tidal volume (VTE)

In respiratory physiology, tidal volume refers to the volume of gas that one inhales (inspiratory tidal volume) or exhales (expiratory tidal volume) during one breath. Normally, both tidal volumes are almost identical. The tidal volume displayed by the ventilator is an estimation of this physiological tidal volume. This monitored tidal volume can be very close to the actual tidal volume if all required conditions are satisfied; otherwise, they may differ considerably. An example of this situation is shown in Fig. 11.7.

There are two types of monitored tidal volume: inspiratory tidal volume and expiratory tidal volume.

Inspiratory tidal volume (VTI) is the monitored volume of gas going into the lungs. It represents the maximum tidal volume that the ventilated patient can possibly receive.

Expiratory tidal volume (VTE) is the monitored volume of gas leaving the lungs. It represents the minimum tidal volume that the ventilated patient can possibly receive.

VTE is commonly displayed, because it is considered to be more clinically relevant.

Designators for expiratory tidal volume include VTE, V_{TE}, and TVexp. It is expressed in millilitres (ml) or litres (l or L).

Tidal volume, both VTI and VTE, is not directly measured, but calculated from the measured airway flow over time, as shown in Fig.11.22.

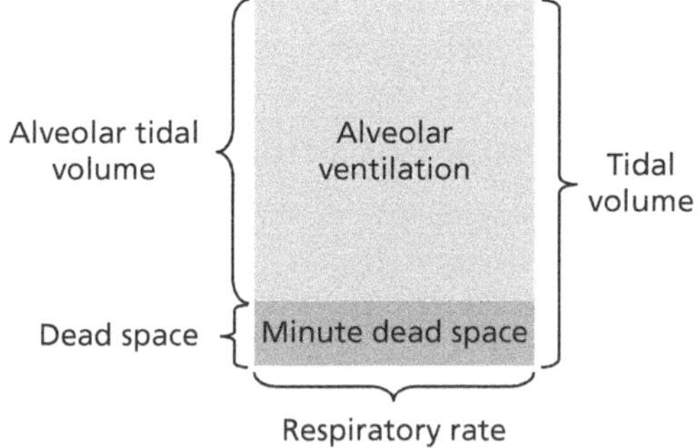

Fig. 11.21 The relationship between tidal volume, rate, and dead space. Note: Minute volume is represented by the combined light and dark grey areas.

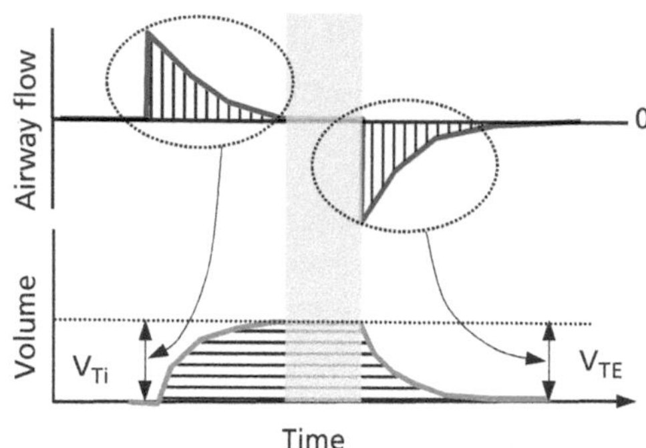

Fig. 11.22 Tidal volume is typically calculated from measured flow over time.

If a ventilator system leaks, the displayed VTE can be much lower than expected, because (a) the leak lowers the applied positive pressure, and (b) the flow sensor may detect just a part, but not all, of the exhaled gas, as shown in Fig.11.7. In this case, both the low tidal volume alarm and the low airway pressure alarm may be activated as the direct consequence.

11.8.2 Expiratory minute volume (MVexp)

Expiratory minute volume is the sum of the monitored VTE of all mechanical breaths within one minute. It represents the minimum cumulative volume that the patient exhales within that minute. Technically, MVexp is a moving average of the monitored VTE of the last 5 to 10 consecutive breaths, extrapolated to a minute volume. The display of MVexp is updated after every breath.

Designators for expiratory minute volume include ExpMinVol, VE TOT, MV, Ve, MVe, and MVexp. It is expressed in litres per minute (L/min).

Expiratory minute volume indicates the minimum level of the patient's lung ventilation. In a passive patient, expiratory minute volume is the product of monitored expiratory tidal volume and the respiratory rate. In an active patient, the monitored expiratory minute volume may vary as both the respiratory rate and the expiratory tidal volume can change dynamically.

Like tidal volume, the monitored expiratory minute volume also contains an ineffective portion due to dead space, which is not involved in gas exchange. Do not forget this portion when interpreting the monitored expiratory minute volume.

11.9 Common time-related monitoring parameters

During mechanical ventilation, all pneumatic parameters, such as pressure, flow, and volume, change over time. Common time-related parameters include total rate, inspiratory time, expiratory time, I:E ratio, and spontaneous breath rate.

It is important for us to distinguish the time parameters used as controls from the monitoring parameters. Both may share the same name, such as rate, I:E ratio, and T_i. The former are the operator's commands to the ventilator system, while the latter are the monitored results. For this reason, if we hear 'a rate of 15', we need to ask whether this refers to a ventilator setting or a monitored value.

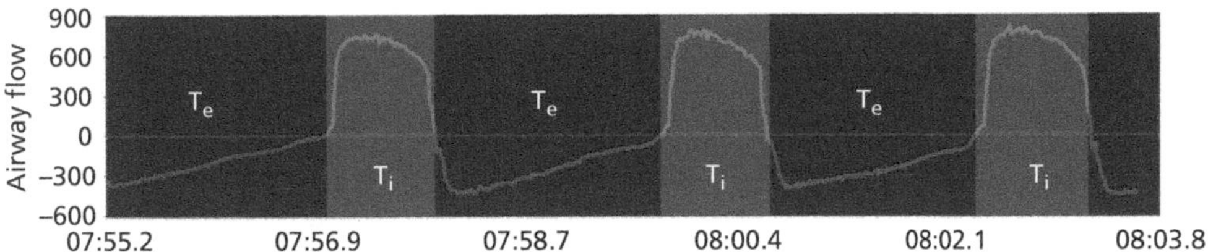

Fig. 11.23 In spontaneous breaths, we can recognize T_i and T_e more easily on a flow waveform rather than a pressure waveform.

11.9.1 Inspiratory time (T_i) and expiratory time (T_e)

As with other parameters, it is also important to differentiate T_i and T_e settings from T_i and T_e monitored values. In this discussion, we are referring to the monitored values only. In mechanical ventilation, monitored T_i is defined as the time between a valid triggering point and the following valid cycling point, while T_e is the time between a valid cycling point and the following valid triggering point. Both T_i and T_e are expressed in seconds.

The best way to identify T_i and T_e is with a flow-time waveform where T_i is the part with positive flow and T_e is the part with negative flow (Fig.11.23). Identifying these parameters on a pressure-time waveform may be confusing or misleading when the ventilated patient is active.

Lung inflation and lung deflation take time. If T_i is too short, inspiration is incomplete. In a pressure mode, this results in a lower-than-expected tidal volume. Similarly, if T_e is too short, the expiration cannot complete, resulting in autoPEEP.

In a *natural breath*, T_i is always longer than T_e. During mechanical ventilation, we can also intentionally set T_i longer than T_e. This strategy, known as inverse ratio ventilation (IRV), is thought to improve oxygenation in patients with acute respiratory distress syndrome (ARDS).

11.9.2 Total frequency (fTotal)

The monitored *total breath rate* is sometimes called total frequency (*fTotal*) to distinguish it from the set rate. Other designators for total frequency include RR, Rate, and fTOT.

The total frequency, expressed in breaths per minute, is typically calculated as a moving average over the latest 8 to 10 breaths, updated after every breath.

In an actively breathing patient, the monitored total breathing frequency is often higher than the set rate.

The monitored frequency may be abnormally low if the ventilator fails to detect the patient's inspiratory efforts in a (pressure or volume) support mode. It may be abnormally high if autotriggering is present.

11.9.3 Spontaneous breath rate (fSpont) and mandatory breath rate (fControl)

The mandatory breath rate (fControl) is the number of control breaths and assist breaths in one minute. It is calculated from a moving average of 8 to 10 breaths.

The spontaneous breath rate (fSpont) is the number of support breaths in one minute. It is also calculated from the moving average of 8 to 10 breaths. Other designators include RRspont and Spon Rate.

$$fTotal \approx fControl + fSpont$$

In a passive patient, fTotal and fControl are equal, and fSpont is zero.

In an active patient, fTotal equals fSpont, and fControl is zero.

In a partially active patient, fTotal is the sum of fSpont and fControl. Both are greater than zero.

Fig.11.24 shows the relationship between total breath frequency, spontaneous breath frequency, and mandatory breath frequency.

Clinically, fSpont is an excellent indicator of the patient's breathing activity and possibly also of ventilator demand. The displayed monitored breath frequencies may provide a false picture if (a) auto-triggering is present, (b) the patient signals are too weak, or (c) the ventilator monitoring is problematic.

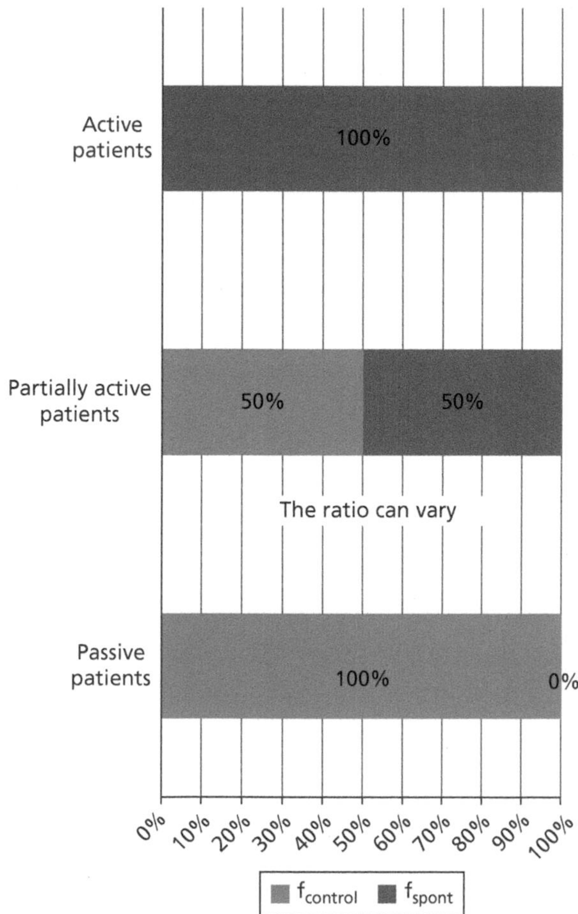

Fig. 11.24 The relationship between total breath frequency, spontaneous breath frequency, and mandatory breath frequency.

11.10 Oxygen concentration

Oxygen concentration refers to the oxygen concentration of the gas that the patient is inhaling. It is also called F_iO_2, O_2, or O_2%. It is expressed as a percentage.

Again, we need to differentiate the set F_iO_2 from the monitored F_iO_2. Normally, both are, or should be, very close to each other, if not identical. They may differ temporarily immediately after the F_iO_2 setting is readjusted.

The key component of F_iO_2 monitoring is an oxygen cell or sensor, which has a limited lifetime. Calibrate the oxygen cell periodically to assure its accuracy, and replace it if the calibration fails more than once. Note that pure oxygen gas is required for oxygen cell calibration.

Chapter 12

Alarms and Safety Mechanisms

12.1 Introduction

Ventilator *alarms* are a group of important functions that every ventilator must have. These functions are designed to safeguard the ventilated patient. Ventilator alarms rely entirely on ventilator monitoring which is functioning properly; this was introduced in Chapter 11.

For many clinicians, ventilator alarms represent a puzzling and annoying black box. A clinician may have little idea why a device alarms and what to do when it does. This unfortunate situation is caused by a lack of basic education on ventilator alarms as well as a general lack of readily available information regarding the different types of alarms (high volume, low volume, etc.), common reasons for the alarms, and what interventions are needed.

This chapter will reveal the truths about ventilator alarms. It starts by describing the basics of ventilator alarms, and then moves on to describe common individual alarms. After reading this chapter, you should have a clear understanding of the most common ventilator alarms and of alarms in general.

12.2 Ventilator alarm system

12.2.1 General principle of ventilator alarms

Ventilator alarms are based on a fairly simple wish: we clinicians want the ventilator to alert us whenever a ventilated patient faces potential danger associated with the mechanical ventilation.

Accomplishing this involves working out the following:

1. The alarm conditions—those under which a ventilated patient may be uncomfortable, injured, or even die;
2. How an alarm condition will be detected, including (a) which monitored parameters are used, and (b) what the normal ranges (non-alarm zones) for those parameters are;
3. Timing—when the alarm should be activated if the alarm condition is detected (i.e. immediately or with a slight delay);
4. The alarm message to be displayed.

As an example, let's take a look at the high peak pressure alarm, which we call simply the 'high pressure' alarm.

It is well known that excessive airway pressure can cause barotrauma to the lungs. So we want the ventilator to alert us if the peak pressure is dangerously high. Clearly, the monitored peak airway pressure should be used as the foundation of this alarm. In ventilator alarm design, we also recognize that a threshold is necessary to differentiate between normal and high peak airway pressure. The threshold may differ under various clinical conditions, so it should be set individually by the clinicians in charge. To prevent the alarm from being oversensitive, we decide that the alarm 'high peak pressure' should be activated only when the monitored peak pressure exceeds the threshold for two consecutive breaths.

Table 12.1 Two categories of ventilator alarm

Technical alarms	Application alarms
◆ Technical problems of ventilator and accessories (design, production, and maintenance) ◆ Electrical supply problems ◆ Gas (air and oxygen) supply problems	◆ Leak or occlusion of ventilator system in which ventilator and accessories are technically in order ◆ Problems with patient's pulmonary system, e.g. pneumothorax ◆ Improper ventilator setting

Being so designed, after every breath the ventilator compares the monitored peak pressure with the operator-set threshold. The alarm, with its visual and audible indications, is activated only when the defined alarm condition is detected. Otherwise, the alarm is inactive.

The principle is applicable to all ventilator alarms, simple or complex.

12.2.2 Technical alarms and application alarms

A ventilator can have a number of alarms. They can be roughly divided into two categories: *technical alarms* and *application alarms*. Refer to Table 12.1.

Technical alarms

Technical alarms are related to abnormalities of the ventilator itself, the electrical supply, or the gas (air and oxygen) supplies. Ventilator abnormalities can have various origins, such as problems with ventilator design and development, problems with production, and problems with device maintenance and service.

Application alarms

At this point, let's return to some fundamental points about mechanical ventilation. We know that the equipment required for mechanical ventilation is a ventilator system composed of six parts. A ventilator is just one of them. A ventilator system works properly only when all three conditions are satisfied:

1. All parts are present, functioning, compatible, and properly connected.
2. The gas passageway inside the ventilator system is neither leaking nor obstructed.
3. The operation of the ventilator system is adapted appropriately and individually to the patient's clinical conditions.

Obviously, it is important that we know when a ventilator system is not functioning properly. Application alarms are designed to signal such functional abnormalities. Note that with an application alarm, the ventilator itself is often technically in order.

Application alarms occur far more frequently than technical alarms. However, application alarms may be less understood.

Typically technical personnel (e.g. engineers from ventilator manufacturing firms and hospital technicians) deal with technical alarms. Ventilator operators (clinicians) deal with application alarms, so this chapter will focus on application alarms.

12.2.3 Non-alarm zone and limits

After a monitoring parameter is selected for a specific alarm, a *non-alarm zone* needs to be defined (Fig. 12.1). A non-alarm zone is the normal or clinically acceptable range for the selected monitoring parameter. As long as the value of the selected parameter falls within this range, the alarm is not activated.

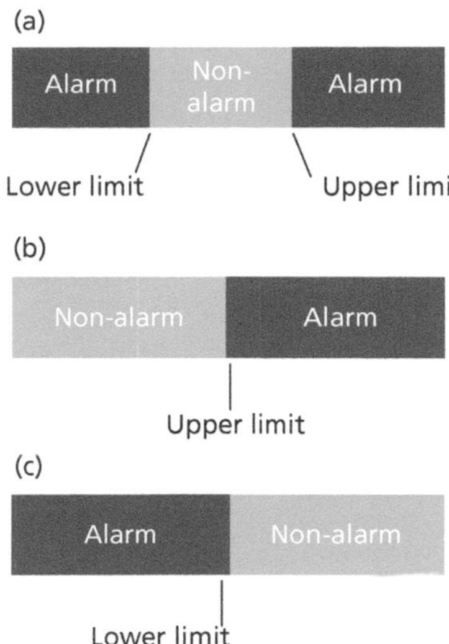

Fig. 12.1 Three ways to define non-alarm zones.

Non-alarm zone with two limits

In most cases, the non-alarm zone is defined by an upper limit and a lower limit. Both limits need to be quantitative. The ventilator alarms if the current value of the monitoring parameter is above the upper limit or below the lower limit. Simultaneously, the corresponding alarm messages are displayed.

For instance, let's say peak airway pressure is the parameter we measure for high peak pressure and low peak pressure alarms. We expect the peak pressure to be approximately 25 cmH_2O, so we set the upper limit to 40 cmH_2O and the lower limit to 15 cmH_2O. As long as the monitored peak pressure is between 15 and 40 cmH_2O, the ventilator does not alarm. The high peak pressure alarm is activated when the monitored peak pressure rises above 40 cmH_2O. The low peak pressure alarm is activated when the monitored peak pressure falls below 15 cmH_2O.

Non-alarm zone with one limit

Less frequently, a non-alarm zone may be defined by a single limit. If the non-alarm zone has an upper limit only, the ventilator alarms only when the monitored value is above the limit. A typical example is the apnoea alarm, which is based on the monitored time. If a non-alarm zone has a lower limit only, the ventilator alarms only when the monitored value is below the limit. A typical example is a low battery alarm, which is based on the capacity of the internal battery.

The limits for application alarms may be defined in three ways:

- Factory defaults: The alarm limits are preset in the factory and cannot be modified by the ventilator operator. These are *non-adjustable alarms.* All technical alarms and some application alarms fall into this group. An example is a low battery alarm.
- Operator settings: During mechanical ventilation, an operator can modify the limits of common application alarms. They are *adjustable alarms.*
- Configuration defaults: Some ventilators allow an operator to preset or *configure* alarm limits and other important ventilator settings. Whenever it is switched on, the ventilator starts with the configured alarm limit. Note that configuration defaults can be modified as part of device configuration, but cannot be changed during mechanical ventilation.

12.2.4 Alarm algorithms

The inputs used in ventilator alarms are monitored parameters. Updated inputs may be continuously provided, or they may be provided for each completed breath.

To check for an alarm condition, the ventilator software compares monitored values to set limits and then decides how to respond according to predefined rules or logic algorithms. These logic algorithms can be simple or complex.

The simplest and most common algorithm is: 'If A occurs or is detected, then do X'. In this case, *A* is a monitored value and *X* is a predefined reaction. For instance, if the current value of the monitored peak airway pressure exceeds the set upper alarm limit, then the ventilator annunciates the high peak pressure alarm.

A more complex form of the alarm algorithm may be: 'If A, B, and C are detected simultaneously, then do X, Y, and Z', or 'if A and C but not B occur, or are detected simultaneously, then do X and Z but not Y'. Here *A, B*, and *C* are violating events, and *X, Y*, and *Z* are the predefined reactions.

12.2.5 Alarm signals

When a predefined alarm condition is detected, a ventilator alerts the operator or other clinicians with audible and visual *alarm signals*.

Audible alarms

A ventilator commonly has an internal loudspeaker and a buzzer to generate audible alarm signals.

The loudspeaker sounds out programmed melodies, while a buzzer sounds out specific tones. The alarm volume can usually be adapted to the hospital environment (e.g. quieter for night-time use).

Visual alarms

An LED (light-emitting diode) is a simple way to visualize ventilator alarms. When an alarm is detected, the corresponding LED lights up or flashes. Fig. 12.2 shows the alarm panel of the AMADEUS ventilator from Hamilton Medical.

LCDs (liquid crystal displays) have become the most common visual alarm signalling device. Either coloured or monochrome, the displays show multiple types of information digitally and graphically. Fig. 12.3 shows the LCD screen on the HAMILTON-C2 ventilator.

The alarm message indicates what alarm condition or conditions are detected. If multiple alarms are active simultaneously, the alarm messages may be displayed alternately or in a special window.

The HAMILTON-G5 ventilator has an alarm lamp on top of a detachable panel (Fig. 12.4). The alarm lamp lights whenever an alarm is active. The alarm lamp helps the clinician easily identify which ventilator is sounding an alarm, if several ventilators are operating simultaneously in the same room.

12.2.6 Alarm silence

Alarm silence is arguably the most frequently used ventilator function in daily practice. It lets a clinician temporarily stop an alarm from sounding while the alarm remains active. This function prevents unnecessary disturbance to the clinician who is already at the patient's bedside. Typically, you activate and deactivate this function by pressing an alarm silence key or button. Fig. 12.5 shows some typical alarm silence symbols.

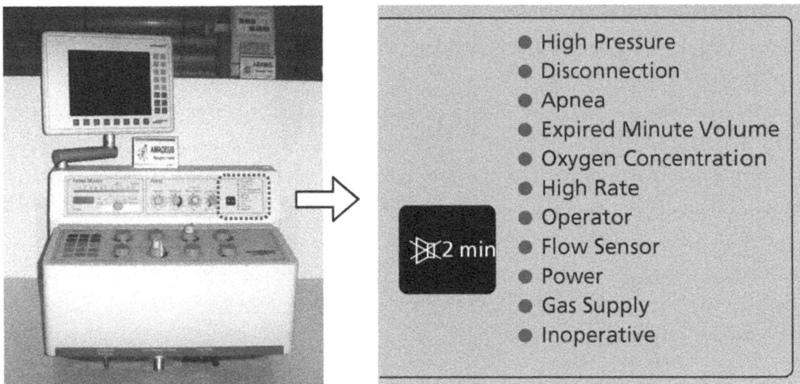

Fig. 12.2 The AMADEUS ventilator has a column of LEDs with predefined alarm messages.

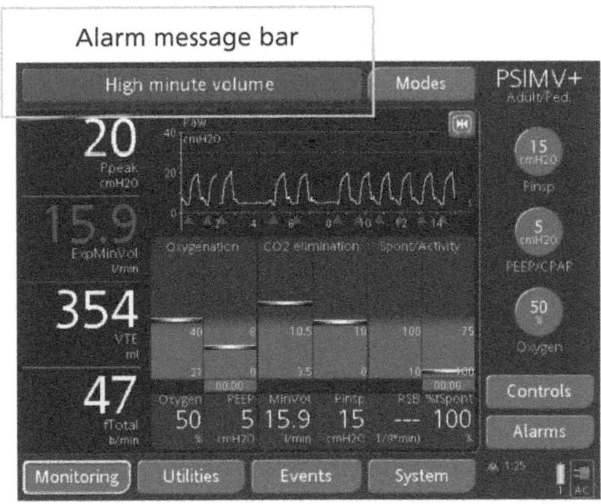

Fig. 12.3 The LCD screen of the HAMILTON-C2 ventilator. The alarm message bar is on the top left.

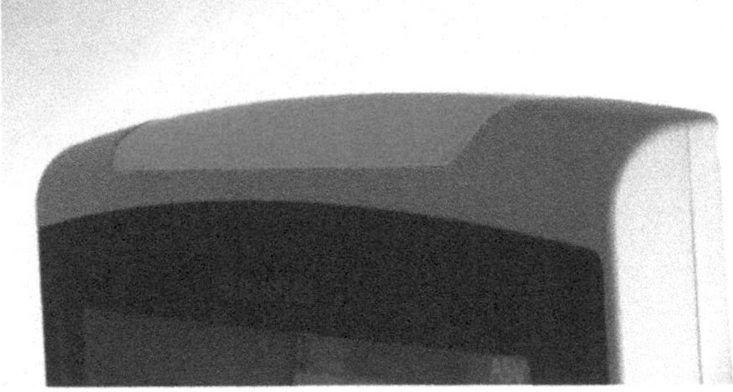

Fig. 12.4 The alarm lamp on top of the HAMILTON-G5 ventilator.

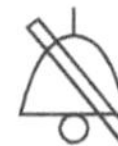
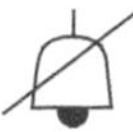

Fig. 12.5 Alarm silence symbols.

The duration of alarm silence ranges from one to three minutes, depending on the ventilator make. The audible alarm automatically resumes after the defined duration if the detected alarm condition remains.

Alarm silence is typically activated by the operator. Under some conditions it may also be activated automatically, to prevent unnecessary alarms while the ventilator system stabilizes. For example, automatic activation may occur (a) immediately after the ventilator is switched on, and (b) immediately after a mode change.

Note that a few critical alarms cannot be silenced, because the patient's life may be endangered.

Caution: The alarm silence function is often dangerously overused and misused. An alarm will stop on its own when the condition that caused it ceases. Silencing an alarm blindly and repeatedly does not remove the cause!

12.2.7 Alarm priorities

We know that ventilator alarms can be either technical alarms or application alarms. They can also be either adjustable alarms or non-adjustable.

The third way to classify ventilator alarms is by priority. If a defined alarm condition emerges, its consequences may be merely uncomfortable or they may be immediately life-threatening. The *alarm priority* relates to the estimated severity of the alarm condition.

Ventilator alarms may be of high, medium, or low priority. Each is annunciated in a specific way, so that the operator can recognize the priority of an active alarm. In practice, however, operators often cannot distinguish one priority from another.

Table 12.2 summarizes this prioritization scheme and shows how it is implemented in the GALILEO ventilator.

12.2.8 User messages

In addition to annunciating alarms of different priorities, a ventilator may also display user messages or user information, which indicate normal operation or situations. Typical examples are: 'Flow sensor calibration in process', 'Auto-zeroing', and 'O_2 cell calibration OK'.

Table 12.2 Alarm priorities in the Hamilton Medical GALILEO ventilator

Alarm priority	Meaning	Typical examples	Visual alarm signals	Acoustic alarm signals
High	The consequence may be serious injury or death	◆ Electrical power or gas failure ◆ Minute volume too low ◆ Apnoea ◆ Airway disconnection	Alarm message on red background	A series of 5 beeps in this sequence, repeated: □□□_□□____□□□_□□
Medium	The consequence may be serious if the abnormality persists	◆ High total rate ◆ Inappropriate PEEP/CPAP ◆ Inappropriate F_iO_2	Alarm message on yellow background	A series of 3 beeps in this sequence, repeated: □□□____□□□
Low	The consequence may be moderate if the abnormality persists	◆ Compliance/ resistance change ◆ High tidal volume	Alarm message on yellow background	A series of 2 beeps, not repeated: □□

CPAP: continuous positive airways pressure; PEEP: positive end-expiratory pressure.

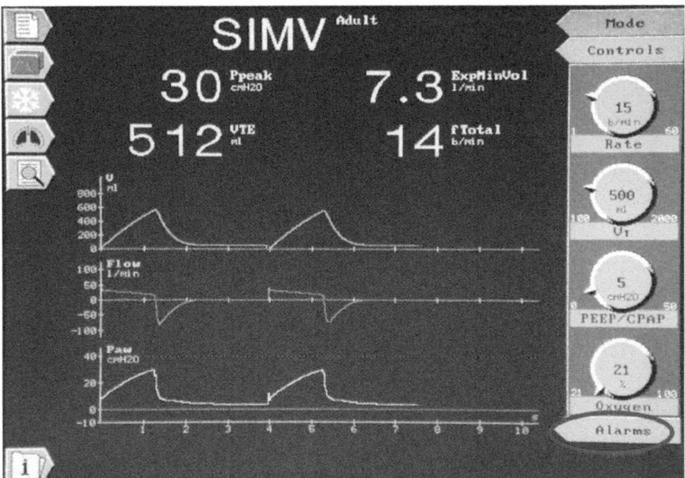

Fig. 12.6 The indicated arrow opens the alarm setting window in the GALILEO ventilator.

12.2.9 Alarm settings

The operator can set or modify the limits of adjustable alarms as well as other alarm-related parameters, such as the volume of audible alarm signals.

To modify an alarm limit, you typically open an *alarm settings* window. For instance, on the GALILEO ventilator you access that window through an arrow labelled 'Alarm' on the primary screen (Fig. 12.6).

In the alarm window, you should see all adjustable alarms, including:

- The alarm name and description;
- The unit of measurement;
- The current limits;
- The current monitored value.

Fig. 12.7 shows a typical alarm setting window.

Every alarm limit has a defined setting range and resolution. Resolution refers to the smallest step used to increment or decrement the setting.

When a new patient is placed on the ventilator, the alarm limits are automatically set to their default values, allowing mechanical ventilation to start immediately. Then, when it is clinically feasible, you can check the alarm limits and adjust them if necessary.

Typically, you adjust an alarm limit in three steps: (a) select and activate the intended alarm limit, (b) adjust the limit to the desired level, and (c) confirm the change.

Note that after the confirmation, the modified alarm limit may become effective immediately, even while the alarm window is still open.

12.3 True alarm or false alarm?

What do we expect from a ventilator alarm system? The ventilator should annunciate an alarm when—and only when—it detects the predefined alarm condition. Indeed, this is the ultimate goal of ventilator alarm design.

Alarm systems in modern intensive care unit (ICU) ventilators work as expected in most, but not in all cases. Although abnormal ventilator alarms are infrequent, they raise a new

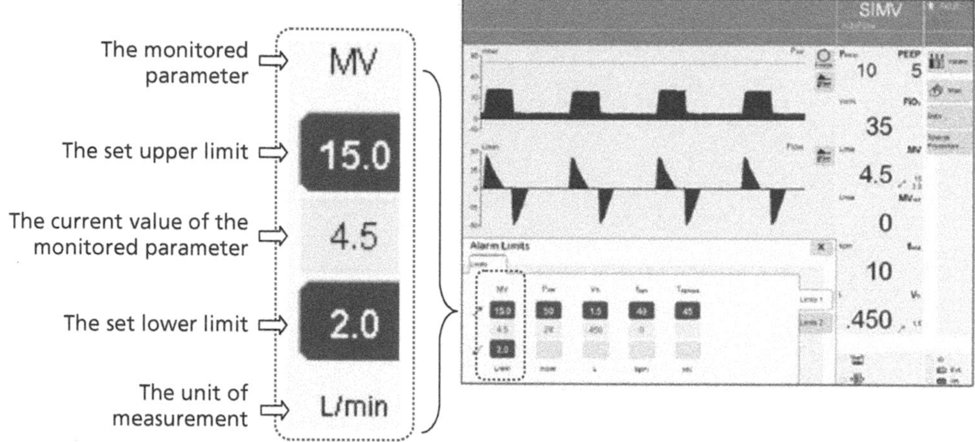

Fig. 12.7 Alarm setting window in the Evita XL ventilator.

question: How do we distinguish the few abnormal ventilation alarms from the ones that function as expected?

Abnormal ventilators alarms have two forms: those that annunciate when there is no valid alarm condition, and those that do not annunciate when there is a valid alarm condition. Table 12.3 shows the possible combinations.

Clearly, we cannot rely entirely on the ventilator alarm system to alert us to *all* abnormal situations. Close clinical observation or monitoring remains vital.

You may have experienced the frustrating situation where a ventilator alarmed repeatedly, but you simply could not find the root cause. In such a case, it is natural to suspect that the ventilator is malfunctioning.

Determining if the alarm is legitimate often requires thorough troubleshooting, which will be described in Chapter 13. The fact that we cannot identify the cause for the alarm condition does not mean that it does not exist. We simply may not know or understand it yet.

We should not blame the ventilator too quickly: true positives and negatives are far more likely than *false positives* and *negatives*. Instead, seek help from more experienced co-workers, hospital technicians, or the manufacturer.

Blindly silencing alarms is dangerous, and it does not solve the problem.

12.4 **Common ventilator alarms**

Most common ventilator alarms are application alarms. They are annunciated due to the complex interaction of five critical factors:

1. Problems with the integrity and functional status of the ventilator system;
2. A significant change in the patient's ventilatory demand (e.g. metabolic acidosis);

Table 12.3 True and false alarms

Alarm status	Presence of alarm condition	Absence of alarm condition
Alarm activated	True positive	False negative
Alarm not activated	False positive	True negative

Table 12.4 Common ventilator alarms grouped by category

Technical alarms		Application alarms
Gas supply	Failure of air supply	High/low (peak) pressure
	Failure of O_2 supply	High/low tidal volume
	Failure of air and O_2	High/low minute volume
	High/low F_iO_2	High/low respiratory rate
Power supply	Loss of AC power	Apnoea
	Low battery	Patient circuit/airway disconnection
Ventilator inoperative	Various technical alarms	Expiration occluded

3. A significant change in the patient's lung mechanics (i.e. airway resistance or compliance);
4. A significant change in the patient's spontaneous breathing activity;
5. Inappropriate ventilator settings (mode, controls, and alarms).

The first factor is the common cause of all technical alarms. It points out a basic prerequisite of mechanical ventilator therapy, but one that is often ignored: a properly functioning ventilator system. The most common equipment integrity problems stem from a significant gas leak or disconnection, occlusion of the gas passageway, and circuit rainout.

We can eliminate alarms triggered by factor 2, 3, or 4 above by adapting the ventilator settings to the current clinical conditions. In fact, this is precisely the optimization referred to in factor 5. Optimizing settings is the ventilator operator's routine work during mechanical ventilation.

Table 12.4 categorizes common ventilator alarms.

12.4.1 Technical alarms

A ventilator system requires stable and continuous supplies of pressurized oxygen and air for its proper functioning. The normal working pressure of both supplies is typically between 2 or 3 and 6 or 6.5 bars (between 200 or 300 and 600 or 650 kPa, or between 29 or 43.5 and 87 or 94 psi) (see Tables 12.5 and 12.6)

High/low F_iO_2 (concentration)

The oxygen supply failure alarm relates to supply pressure, while the F_iO_2 alarms indicate that the current inspiratory O_2 concentration is outside the set range (see Tables 12.7–12.10).

12.4.2 Application alarms

High/low tidal volume alarm

High and low tidal volume alarms are based on breath-by-breath tidal volume monitoring.

Tidal volume alarms are mainly relevant in pressure modes where tidal volume varies. Volume modes generally assure a tidal volume, so that tidal volume alarms should not be activated under normal conditions of use. However, the tidal volume can sharply decrease if the peak pressure reaches the limit of the high peak pressure alarm, causing premature cycling.

As we saw earlier, monitored tidal volume can be either inspiratory tidal volume or expiratory tidal volume. Inspiratory tidal volume is the maximum gas volume that the patient

Table 12.5 Failure of air or O_2 supply

Alarm message	Failure of air supply	Failure of oxygen supply
Other possible alarm messages	◆ Air supply loss ◆ Air supply failed ◆ Loss of air	◆ O_2 supply down ◆ O_2 supply failed ◆ Loss of O_2
Meaning	The supply pressure is less than the lower limit of 2 or 3 bars	The oxygen supply pressure is less than the lower limit of 2 or 3 bars
Type of alarm	◆ Non-adjustable alarm ◆ Gas supply alarm	◆ Non-adjustable alarm ◆ Gas supply alarm
Recommended setting	—	—
Common causes	The air supply pressure is too low because of: ◆ Unexpected interruption of central air supply ◆ A significant leak or disconnection in the air supply route, i.e. hose or fitting ◆ Nearly empty air cylinder ◆ Defective air compressor	The oxygen supply pressure is too low because of: ◆ Unexpected interruption of central oxygen supply ◆ A significant leak or disconnection in the oxygen supply route, i.e. hose or fitting ◆ Nearly empty oxygen cylinder
Corrective actions	◆ Have a hospital technician restore the air supply ◆ Remedy the leak or discon nection ◆ Replace the air cylinder ◆ Replace the air compressor	◆ Have a hospital technician restore the oxygen supply ◆ Remedy the leak or disconnection ◆ Replace the oxygen cylinder
Remarks	If an oxygen supply is available, mechanical ventilation should continue with 100% oxygen	If an air supply is available, mechanical ventilation should continue with air alone

Table 12.6 Failure of both air and oxygen supplies

Alarm message	Failure of air and O_2 supplies
Other possible messages	◆ Loss of gas supply ◆ Gas supply pressure: low
Meaning	Both air and oxygen supply pressures are less than 2 or 3 bars
Type of alarm	◆ Non-user-adjustable alarm ◆ Technical alarm
Recommended setting	—
Common causes	Both air and oxygen supply pressures are too low
Corrective actions	◆ Immediately remove the patient from the ventilator, and ventilate with an alternative means, e.g. a resuscitator ◆ Have a hospital technician restore normal air and oxygen supplies
Remarks	**WARNING**: if both gas supplies fail at the same time, a ventilator system cannot continue to function. The ventilator automatically switches to the ambient state. See section 12.6 for details.

Table 12.7 High/low fraction of inspired oxygen (F_iO_2) table

Alarm message	**High F_iO_2**	**Low F_iO_2**
Other possible alarm messages	◆ High delivered O_2% ◆ F_iO_2 high ◆ High oxygen ◆ O_2 concentration: high	◆ Low delivered O_2% ◆ F_iO_2 low ◆ Low oxygen ◆ O_2 concentration: low
Meaning	The monitored F_iO_2 is 5% to 7% above the set F_iO_2 for a defined duration, e.g. 30 s	The monitored F_iO_2 is 5% or 7% below the set F_iO_2 for a defined duration, e.g. 30 s
Type of alarm	Non-adjustable alarm	Non-adjustable alarm
Recommended setting	—	—
Common causes	◆ Faulty ventilator mixing function ◆ Faulty oxygen monitoring, e.g. defective or uncalibrated oxygen cell	◆ Faulty ventilator mixing function ◆ Faulty oxygen monitoring, e.g. defective or uncalibrated oxygen cell ◆ Low F_iO_2 due to use of an oxygen concentrator. Standard oxygen supplies provide pure oxygen. O_2 from a concentrator may be as low as 90%
Corrective actions	◆ Calibrate or replace the oxygen cell ◆ Call a hospital technician to troubleshoot	◆ Calibrate or replace the oxygen cell ◆ Call a hospital technician to troubleshoot ◆ Discontinue use of oxygen concentrator as oxygen supply
Remarks	—	—

can receive, while expiratory tidal volume is the minimum gas volume that the patient can receive. Typically, tidal volume alarms are based on *expiratory* tidal volume. If you are not sure how your ventilator's tidal volume alarm functions, clarify this with the manufacturer (see Table 12.11).

High/low expiratory minute volume

Expiratory minute volume alarms are based entirely on expiratory minute volume monitoring, which is the best possible indicator of the current level of lung ventilation (Table 12.12).

High/low respiratory rate alarms

High and low respiratory rate alarms are based on the monitored total rate of all valid mechanical breaths. Respiratory rate directly affects minute volume.

A mechanical breath can be triggered in two ways: time triggering and patient triggering (pressure of flow). Time triggering is reliable and rigid, while patient triggering is not 100% reliable. Missed triggering and auto-triggering are possible (see Tables 12.13 and 12.14).

Apnoea alarm

Refer to section 10.5.

Table 12.8 Electrical power supply alarms

Alarm message	Loss of AC power	Battery low
Other possible alarm messages	AC power loss	Limited battery capacity
Meaning	The ventilator is switched on, but no AC power is available	If AC power is interrupted, the ventilator is powered from the internal battery, and mechanical ventilation continues. This alarm is active if the remaining battery power can power the ventilator for only a few more minutes
Type of alarm	◆ Non-adjustable alarm ◆ Power supply alarm	◆ Non-adjustable alarm ◆ Power supply alarm
Recommended setting	—	—
Common causes	◆ AC power interrupted ◆ Ventilator accidentally unplugged ◆ Unpowered AC receptacle ◆ Failure to connect the ventilator to AC power	The AC power remains interrupted, and the internal battery is almost depleted
Corrective actions	◆ Always be prepared for unexpected power interruptions ◆ Make sure all ventilators are equipped with internal batteries ◆ Restore AC power as quickly as possible	If AC power cannot be restored at once, remove the patient from the ventilator, and ventilate with an alternative means, e.g. a resuscitator
Remarks	AC power interruptions do occur, however infrequently. The key is to be well prepared	◆ Make sure the internal battery is fully charged at all times. Keep the ventilator connected to AC power, even when it is not in use ◆ The operating time of the battery may be significantly reduced as the battery ages ◆ Have your ventilators serviced periodically. Replace older batteries according to the ventilator manufacturer's recommendation

Table 12.9 Ventilator inoperative alarms

Alarm message	Ventilator inoperative
Other possible messages	◆ Ventilator faulty ◆ Technical fault
Meaning	The ventilator has detected a serious technical problem that prevents normal operation
Type of alarm	◆ Non-user-adjustable alarm ◆ Technical alarm
Recommended setting	—
Common causes	Serious ventilator hardware or software problem
Corrective actions	◆ Immediately remove the patient from the ventilator, and ventilate with an alternative means, e.g. a resuscitator ◆ Have the ventilator serviced
Remarks	If this alarm is activated, the ventilator automatically switches to the ambient state. See section 12.6 for details.

Table 12.10 High/low peak (airway) pressure alarm

Alarm message	Peak airway pressure: High	Peak airway pressure: Low
Other possible alarm messages	◆ High circuit pressure ◆ Airway pressure high ◆ High Ppeak ◆ High Paw	◆ Low circuit pressure ◆ Airway pressure low ◆ Low Ppeak ◆ Low Paw
Meaning	The monitored peak pressure is above the upper limit of the peak pressure alarm	The monitored peak pressure is below the lower limit of the peak pressure alarm
Type of alarm	◆ User-adjustable alarm ◆ Application alarm	◆ User-adjustable alarm ◆ Application alarm
Recommended setting for adults	◆ For a passive patient, 10 cmH_2O above the expected peak pressure ◆ For an active patient, 15 cmH_2O above the expected peak pressure	◆ For a passive patient, 5 cmH_2O below the expected peak pressure ◆ For an active patient, 5 to 10 cmH_2O below the expected peak pressure
Common causes	◆ Patient coughing ◆ Patient-ventilator asynchrony ◆ In a volume mode: – Increased airway resistance, e.g. ETT kinked – Decreased lung compliance – Inspiratory flow set too high – T_i set too short ◆ Condensed water in the patient circuit ◆ Set alarm limit too close to the actual peak pressure	◆ Significant leak or disconnection ◆ Patient-ventilator asynchrony ◆ In a volume mode: – Decreased airway resistance – Increased lung compliance – Inspiratory flow set too low – T_i set too long ◆ Set alarm limit too close to the actual peak pressure
Corrective actions	◆ Identify and remove the root cause of: – High airway resistance – Low lung compliance – Water in the patient circuit ◆ Improve patient-ventilator synchrony ◆ Check and readjust mode and control settings ◆ Check and readjust alarm settings	◆ Identify and remove the root cause, e.g. gas leak or disconnection ◆ Improve patient-ventilator synchrony ◆ Check and readjust mode and control settings ◆ Check and readjust alarm settings
Remarks	This is a critical alarm in a volume mode. Excessive airway pressure, if persistent, can induce lung barotrauma. In an emergency, immediately remove the patient from the ventilator, and ventilate with an alternative means, e.g. a resuscitator	This is a critical alarm in a pressure mode. It often signals hypoventilation, especially when accompanied by a low tidal volume or low minute volume alarm. In an emergency, immediately remove the patient from the ventilator, and ventilate with an alternative means, e.g. a resuscitator

Table 12.11 High/low expiratory minute volume

Alarm message	**Expiratory tidal volume: High**	**Expiratory tidal volume: Low**
Other possible alarm messages	◆ High tidal volume ◆ Tidal volume high ◆ High V_T ◆ High expiratory tidal volume	◆ Low tidal volume ◆ Tidal volume low ◆ Low V_T ◆ Low expiratory tidal volume
Meaning	The monitored expiratory tidal volume is above the upper limit of the tidal volume alarm	The monitored expiratory tidal volume is below the lower limit of the tidal volume alarm
Type of alarm	◆ User-adjustable alarm ◆ Application alarm	◆ User-adjustable alarm ◆ Application alarm
Recommended setting for adults	◆ For a passive adult patient, 100 to 150 ml greater than the expected tidal volume ◆ For an active patient, 50% greater than the expected tidal volume	◆ For a passive adult patient, 100 to 150 ml less than the expected tidal volume ◆ For an active patient, 50% less than the expected tidal volume
Common causes	◆ In a pressure mode: ✍ The patient's actual demand is much greater than expected – Decreased airway resistance – Increased lung compliance – Patient-ventilator asynchrony ◆ High tidal volume alarm limit set too close to the actual tidal volume ◆ Faulty or inaccurate volume monitoring	◆ A significant leak ◆ In a pressure mode: – Increased airway resistance – Decreased lung compliance – Patient-ventilator asynchrony ◆ Low tidal volume alarm limit set too close to actual tidal volume ◆ Faulty volume monitoring
Corrective actions	◆ Improve patient-ventilator synchrony ◆ Check and adjust mode and control settings ◆ Check and adjust alarm settings ◆ Check the volume monitoring ◆ Check the flow measurement	◆ Ensure sufficient and effective lung ventilation ◆ Identify and remove the root cause of gas leakage and/or occlusion ◆ Improve patient-ventilator synchrony ◆ Check and adjust mode and controls ◆ Check and adjust alarm settings ◆ Check the flow measurement
Remarks	The high tidal volume alarm is meaningful in a pressure mode. It may indicate a potential risk of volutrauma of the lungs	The low tidal volume alarm is critical in a pressure mode. Hypoventilation is often the consequence

12.5 Responding to ventilator alarms

12.5.1 Be prepared

Like any other medical device, a ventilator and its alarm functions can fail. The consequence of a ventilator system malfunction can be fatal, because a ventilator system is a life supporting or sustaining medical device. Indeed a great variety of problems do occur throughout mechanical ventilation, so the question is not *whether* a problem will occur, but *what* and *when*.

The old adage that 'prevention is better than cure' applies perfectly to this situation. It is critical that you apply these three preventive measures, at a minimum:

Table 12.12 High/low expiratory minute volume

Alarm message	Expiratory minute volume: High	Expiratory minute volume: Low
Other possible alarm messages	◆ High minute volume ◆ MV high ◆ High Ve	◆ Low minute volume ◆ MV low ◆ Low Ve
Meaning	The monitored expiratory minute volume is above the set limit of high minute volume alarm	The monitored expiratory minute volume is below the set limit of low minute volume alarm
Type of alarm	◆ User-adjustable alarm ◆ Application alarm	◆ User-adjustable alarm ◆ Application alarm
Recommended setting for adults	◆ For a passive patient, 20% greater than the expected minute volume ◆ For an active patient, 50% greater than the expected minute volume	◆ For a passive patient, 20% less than the expected minute volume ◆ For an active patient, 50% less than the expected minute volume
Common causes	◆ In a volume mode: – The tidal volume setting is very high – The set respiratory rate is very high ◆ In a pressure mode: ✍ The patient has a high ventilatory demand, e.g. acidosis ✍ The set inspiratory pressure ($P_{control}$ or $P_{support}$) is high, especially in COPD or emphysema patients ◆ Auto-triggering ◆ Set alarm limit too close to the expected minute volume ◆ Faulty volume monitoring	◆ Patient-ventilator asynchrony ◆ In a volume mode: ✍ The tidal volume setting is very low ✍ The respiratory rate setting is very low ◆ In a pressure mode: – Inadequate inspiratory pressure ($P_{control}$ or $P_{support}$) – Inadequate T_i – Increased airway resistance – Decreased respiratory compliance, e.g. ARDS or ALI ◆ Significant leak ◆ Significant airway occlusion ◆ Set alarm limit too close to the actual minute volume ◆ Faulty volume monitoring
Corrective actions	◆ Check and adjust the mode and control settings ◆ Correct the auto-triggering ◆ Check and adjust the alarm settings	◆ Improve patient-ventilator synchrony ◆ Check the patient circuit and airway for leaks or occlusion ◆ Check and adjust the mode and control settings ◆ Check and adjust the alarm settings ◆ Check the volume monitoring
Remarks	This alarm is meaningful in a pressure mode. It may indicate a potential risk of volutrauma of the lungs	This alarm is critical in a pressure mode, indicating possible hypoventilation and requiring immediate corrective action. If hypoventilation cannot be resolved quickly, remove the patient from the ventilator and ventilate with an alternative means, e.g. a resuscitator

Table 12.13 High/low respiratory rate alarm

Alarm message	Respiratory rate: High	Respiratory rate: Low
Other possible alarm messages	◆ High rate ◆ High frequency	◆ Low rate ◆ Low frequency
Meaning	The monitored total respiratory rate is greater than the upper limit of the rate alarm	The monitored total respiratory rate is less than the lower limit of the rate alarm
Type of alarm	◆ User-adjustable alarm ◆ Application alarm	◆ User-adjustable alarm ◆ Application alarm
Recommended setting for adults	◆ For a passive patient, 10 breaths per minute greater than the expected total rate ◆ For an active patient, 15 breaths per minute greater than the expected total rate	◆ For a passive patient, 10 breaths per minute less than the expected total rate ◆ For an active patient, 15 breaths per minute less than the expected total rate
Common causes	◆ Auto-triggering ◆ Control rate set very high ◆ Upper limit of rate alarm set too close to the actual rate	◆ Apnoea ◆ Missed patient triggering ◆ Rate set unusually low ◆ Lower limit of rate alarm set too close to the actual rate
Corrective actions	◆ Check and adjust the rate and trigger sensitivity settings ◆ Check and adjust the alarm limit ◆ Troubleshoot auto-triggering, if present	◆ Check and adjust the rate and trigger sensitivity settings ◆ Check and adjust the alarm limit ◆ Identify and eliminate the root cause of the delayed trigger
Remarks	With a very high total rate, T_e may be too short for the patient to complete expiration, resulting in overdistention and autoPEEP	A very low total rate leads to hypoventilation, requiring prompt correction

- Have a resuscitator for every ventilated patient, and check its function regularly.
- Make sure all staff members involved in mechanical ventilation receive regular training on mechanical ventilation and the ventilator system. They should know how to prevent ventilator problems and how to correct them when they occur. This training should be highly practical and 'hands on'.
- Have your ventilators and accessories checked and serviced regularly by qualified technical personnel. Such a simple routine can save numerous lives!

12.5.2 Respond to ventilator alarms

Here are some general rules on how to respond to ventilator alarms (Fig. 12.8):

1. Immediately approach the ventilated patient and silence the audible alarm.
2. If the root cause for the alarm is obvious (e.g. airway disconnection) remove the root cause. After normal mechanical ventilation resumes, the ventilated patient should be relaxed.
3. If the root cause cannot be identified or removed quickly, check the ventilated patient for signs of severe acute respiratory distress.

Table 12.14 Circuit disconnection and expiratory limb occlusion

Alarm message	Circuit disconnection	Expiratory limb occlusion
Other possible alarm messages	Disconnection at vent	Expiratory route occluded
Meaning	The breathing circuit is disconnected, causing a massive gas leak. The PEEP and peak pressure are significantly lower than the settings	Normally, the circuit or airway pressures drop sharply at early expiration. If the expiratory limb is occluded, the pressure drops much more slowly or not at all
Type of alarm	◆ Non-adjustable alarm ◆ Application alarm	◆ Non-adjustable alarm ◆ Application alarm
Recommended setting	—	—
Common causes	◆ Actual circuit disconnection ◆ Massive circuit leak	◆ Expiratory valve malfunction or blockage ◆ Kinked expiratory limb ◆ Clogged expiratory filter
Corrective actions	◆ Reconnect the circuit ◆ Stop the circuit leak	◆ Replace the expiratory filter ◆ Check the expiratory valve ◆ Replace the expiratory limb
Remarks	A circuit disconnection is easy to identify	This is an emergency, because expiration is very difficult or impossible. If the root cause cannot be quickly found and corrected, immediately remove the patient from the ventilator, and ventilate with an alternative means, e.g. a resuscitator

4. If the patient exhibits severe respiratory distress, remove them from the ventilator immediately and ensure continuation of adequate lung ventilation with an alternative means (e.g. a resuscitator or another ventilator system). Then troubleshoot the ventilator offline with a test lung.
5. If you cannot quickly identify the root cause and the patient is not in severe respiratory distress, troubleshoot the problem with caution; alarm messages often provide useful hints about the root cause. Call for help. While troubleshooting, notice the patient's responses. Return to step 4 if the patient's condition deteriorates.

In all cases, if you successfully remove the true root causes, the alarm should stop within one or two minutes.

Troubleshooting ventilator alarms can be very easy in simple cases, but it can be extremely challenging in complicated cases, with the variables of equipment, patient, and settings to consider. Clearly, a thorough understanding of mechanical ventilation and the ventilator system is required to troubleshoot the complicated cases.

In Chapter 13 we will discuss at length these general rules about responding to alarms.

12.6 Ambient state

With intermittent positive pressure ventilation (IPPV), the patient must breathe, passively or actively, through the connected ventilator system—they are isolated from ambient air. What

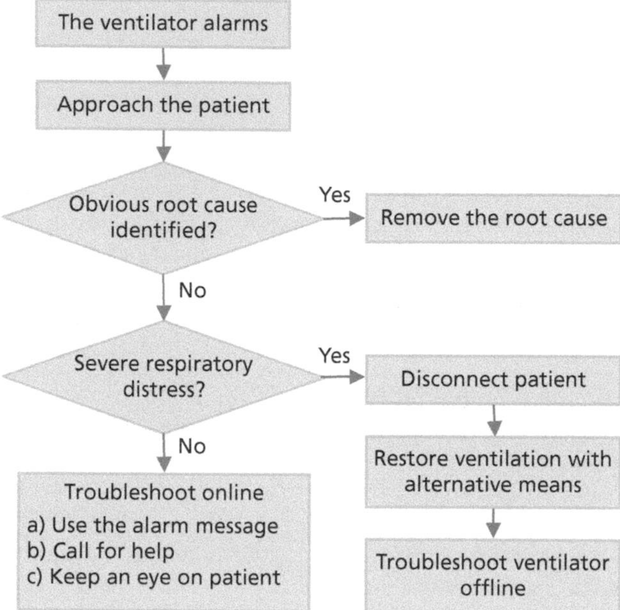

Fig. 12.8 How to respond to ventilator alarms.

happens to the patient, then, when the ventilator system fails completely? The patient cannot breathe! The *ambient state* is the answer to this predicament. It is a set of predefined actions that a ventilator automatically takes when it detects any of several predefined conditions.

12.6.1 Predefined actions

Typically, the ambient state involves four actions (Fig. 12.9):

a. The inspiratory valve is closed;
b. The expiratory valve is opened;
c. The *safety* or *ambient valve* is opened;
d. The alarm is annunciated audibly and visually.

During the ambient state, normal mechanical ventilation stops and the ventilator does not respond to the operator's commands. The opened safety valve connects the breathing circuit to room air. This valve, which is closed during normal operation, opens only in the ambient state. A spontaneously breathing patient can inhale room air through the safety valve and exhale through the opened expiratory valve.

12.6.2 Predefined conditions

There are catastrophic conditions under which normal ventilator operation is impossible. If one of these conditions is detected, the ventilator automatically switches to the ambient state. Typical examples are:

- Both gas supplies fail at the same time;
- The ventilator loses all electrical power from AC and the internal battery;
- The ventilator itself has a serious technical fault.

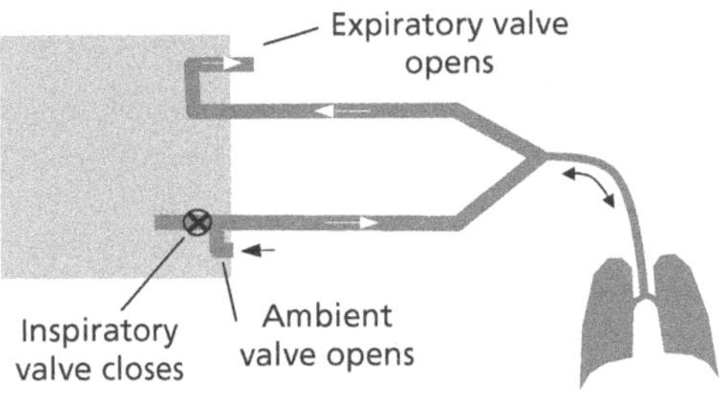

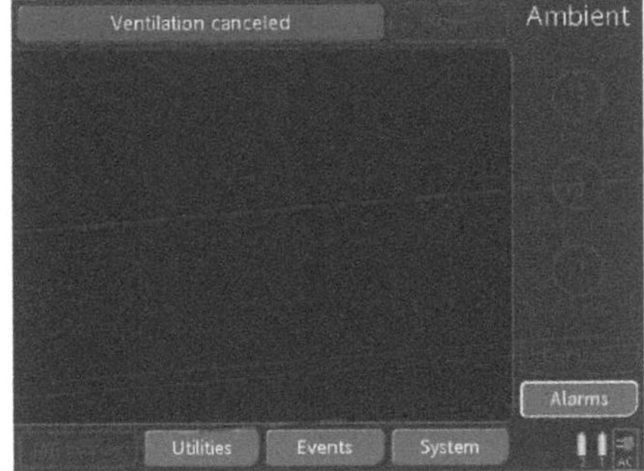

Fig. 12.9 The principle and graphic presentation of the ambient state in the HAMILTON-C2 ventilator.

WARNING: The ambient state is an emergency state. Immediately remove the patient from the faulty ventilator system, and ensure continuation of effective and sufficient lung ventilation with alternative means. Do not try to troubleshoot the system while the patient is still connected. Remove the affected ventilator from further clinical use and have it checked by qualified technical staff.

12-27	12:04:34	Alarms	High frequency	4007
12-27	12:04:33	Alarms	Low minute volume	5006
12-27	12:04:27	Alarms	Disconnection pat. side	5010
12-27	**12:04:27**	**Alarms**	**Low tidal volume**	**4008**
12-27	12:03:42	Special	Alarm silence On	516
12-27	**12:03:33**	**Alarms**	**High pressure**	**5020**
12-27	**12:03:32**	**Alarms**	**Low tidal volume**	**4008**
12-27	**12:03:24**	**Alarms**	**High pressure**	**5020**
12-27	**12:02:52**	**Alarms**	**High pressure**	**5020**
12-27	**12:02:49**	**Alarms**	**Low tidal volume**	**4008**
12-27	**12:02:42**	**Alarms**	**Low tidal volume**	**4008**
12-27	**12:02:41**	**Alarms**	**High pressure**	**5020**
12-27	**12:02:31**	**Alarms**	**Low tidal volume**	**4008**
12-27	**12:02:30**	**Alarms**	**High pressure**	**5020**
12-27	**12:02:00**	**Alarms**	**Low tidal volume**	**4008**
12-27	**12:01:58**	**Alarms**	**High pressure**	**5020**
12-27	**12:01:27**	**Alarms**	**Low tidal volume**	**4008**
12-27	**12:01:26**	**Alarms**	**High pressure**	**5020**
12-27	12:00:21	Setting	Flowtrigger 2.0 l/min	304
12-27	**12:00:16**	**Alarms**	**High pressure**	**5020**
12-27	12:00:15	Setting	P-trigger 2.0 -cmH2O	303
12-27	12:00:15	Alarms	Turn the Flow Sensor	4011
12-27	12:00:14	Alarms	Apnea	5009
12-27	12:00:14	Alarms	Low minute volume	5006

Fig. 12.10 A portion of an event log on a GALILEO ventilator.

12.7 Event logging

Event logging is a ventilator function designed to chronologically record all 'events'.

Events may include an alarm activation, a change in a ventilator setting, or another user action (e.g. enabling/disabling a special function, or executing a test or calibration and its result). From the time the ventilator is turned on, the defined events are recorded in the *event log* for later reviewing. This function lets you clearly see what occurred in the recent past, and when it occurred. For this reason, the event log can be very helpful when analysing an earlier issue.

A portion of the GALILEO event log is shown in Fig. 12.10. The patient was a spontaneously breathing adult, ventilated in the pressure assist/control mode. Alarms are highlighted with yellow or red depending on the alarm priorities.

Chapter 13

Troubleshooting and Error Reporting

13.1 Introduction

Mechanical ventilation therapy is highly complex. Any number of problems can occur at any time and in any patient. The bad news is that these occur more often than we would like to believe, but the good news is that most do not end in catastrophe. It helps to remember that we are likely to face such issues, although we may not know when and how they will manifest.

This chapter focuses on troubleshooting or the process of identifying root causes and eliminating them. It covers the following topics:

- Troubleshooting basics
- Emergency management
- Troubleshooting common problems
- Error reporting.

13.2 Mechanical ventilation problems in general

For the sake of simplicity, we will shorten the phrase 'mechanical ventilation problems' to 'MV problems.'

13.2.1 Risks, problems, and consequences

Firstly, we need to distinguish between the three terms used to describe any MV problem—risks, problems, and consequences. These represent three stages of an unwanted event (Fig. 13.1):

- A *risk* is a potential problem. It has not occurred yet, but it may occur at any time.
- A *problem* is an unwanted event that is occurring now.
- A *consequence* is the result of a problem. A consequence can harm the patient. The severity of a problem's consequence can vary widely, from being minor to catastrophic, depending largely on our response.

For instance, airway disconnection is a common problem in mechanical ventilation. Potentially, it could occur in every ventilated patient. If a nurse discovers a disconnected tube and reconnects it immediately, the consequence to the patient will most likely be negligible. However, an airway disconnection in a passively ventilated patient can be deadly without such a prompt response.

To err is human. In reality, it is impossible to eliminate all risks or potential problems of mechanical ventilation. In many cases, however, we can stop a risk from escalating to a problem through effective preventive measures. Catastrophic consequences can be drastically reduced by proper and prompt reactions.

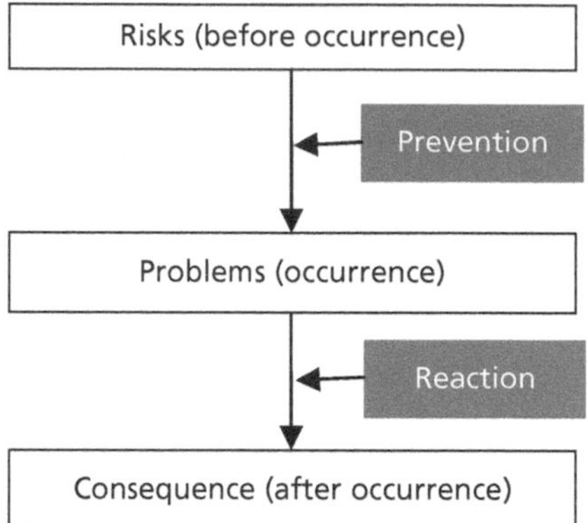

Fig. 13.1 Two approaches to dealing with a problem: prevention and reaction.

Prevention

In theory, the importance of prevention is self-evident. In practice, however, institutions often ignore the need for preventive measures due to financial or resource shortages. These are the most basic preventive measures, which apply universally:

- All staff involved in mechanical ventilation should be sufficiently trained so they know how to respond to MV problems. Staff training should be repeated periodically.
- Spare ventilator accessories should be prepared (e.g. spare circuits, connectors, filters, masks, and valves).
- An alternative ventilation device should be available for each ventilated patient, at the minimum a resuscitator with necessary accessories. The functioning of these devices should also be checked periodically. In this way, mechanical ventilation can continue should the current ventilator system fail.
- Spare, filled air and oxygen cylinders should be available in every intensive care unit (ICU).
- An alternative electrical source (e.g. a backup diesel generator), should be available in an emergency.

13.2.2 Root causes—single and multiple

Every MV problem has a root cause(s) and consequence(s). An MV problem goes away if its root cause is successfully removed.

Root causes and their resultant problems have three possible relationships (Fig. 13.2). Most MV problems have a single cause. Causes *A*, *B*, and *C* result in problems *x*, *y*, and *z*, respectively. *A* causes *x*, but it does not cause *y* and *z*, and so on.

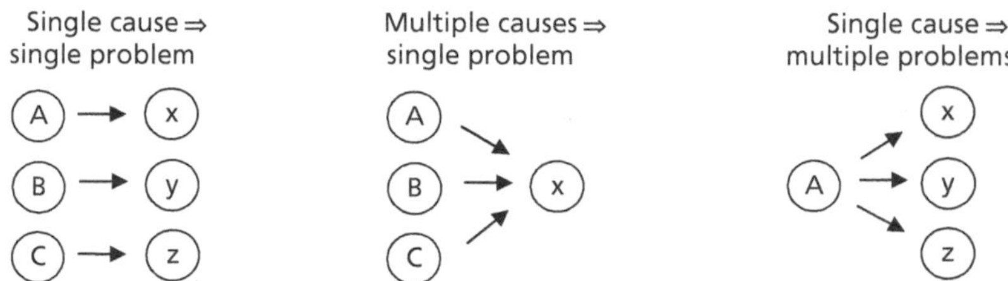

Fig. 13.2 Three possible relationships between cause and consequence.

In rare cases, however, a problem may have more than one cause. For instance, problem *x* occurs only when causes *A*, *B*, and *C* coexist. In other words, this problem does not appear if only one cause is present. In difficult troubleshooting cases, we need to consider this possibility. Fig. 13.2 illustrates these relationships.

A single cause may also result in multiple problems. For instance, a disconnection at the patient airway can trigger several alarms such as loss of PEEP (positive end-expiratory pressure), low peak pressure, low tidal volume, and low minute volume. All alarms should disappear after reconnection.

13.2.3 MV problem classification

MV problems can be roughly divided into three categories:

Equipment problems The ventilator system fails to function as it should. The root cause can be a missing, malfunctioning, or incompatible part, or other interference with the system's proper functioning. Recall again that the ventilator is just one of six required parts!

***Operation problems* (also known as user errors)** These are related to the indications for and timing of intubation, mechanical ventilation, and extubation; ventilator settings; and responses to ventilator alarms. In this case, the ventilator system is typically functioning properly.

Clinical problems A ventilated patient is not a passive physical model. Patient changes are inevitable during mechanical ventilation. For this reason, ventilator settings need to be adjusted. For instance, the assist/control mode works for a passive patient, but not for an active patient. So as you can see, clinical problems are closely related to operation problems. In ventilator terminology, both 'operation problems' and 'clinical problems' are known as 'application problems.'

Fig. 13.3 presents a structured overview of MV problems. A thorough understanding of this overview is the first step in systematic MV troubleshooting.

Most MV problems are application (operation and clinical) problems, or are related to the setup of the ventilator system. True ventilator malfunctions are relatively infrequent.

13.3 Emergency management

The intubated patient has to inhale and exhale exclusively through the connected ventilator system. In other words, the patient is isolated from the atmosphere.

This arrangement has an inherent risk: the patient is endangered if the ventilator system malfunctions for any reason. For patient safety, all clinicians directly involved in this therapy must be trained to react immediately and appropriately in an emergency.

The general rules of emergency management (summarized in Fig. 13.4) are:

1. **Approach the patient immediately**: Every ventilated patient should be closely observed even when the ventilator alarms have not been triggered. When a ventilator alarm is triggered, approach the patient without delay. Silence the audible alarm, and then determine two critical points: (a) whether the cause of the alarm is obvious, and (b) whether the patient is in *sudden and severe respiratory distress (SSRD)*.
2. **Correct the obvious problem(s)**: In some cases, the problems that activate ventilator alarms are obvious (e.g. unintended airway disconnection). In such a case, correct the problem at once. The alarms should stop shortly after the root cause is removed.
3. **Determine whether the patient has SSRD**: MV problems, regardless of nature and category, result in hypoventilation. An active patient reacts by intensifying their spontaneous

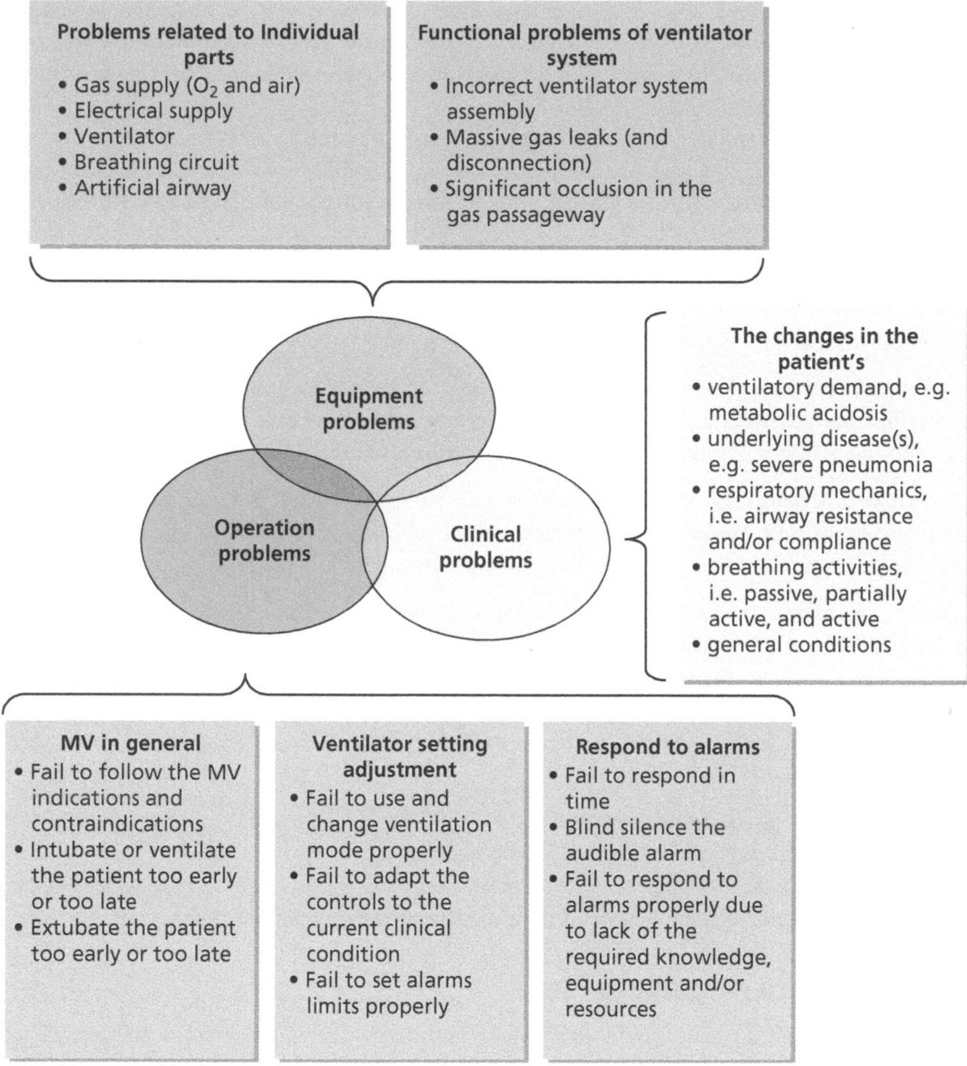

Fig. 13.3 Common problems associated with mechanical ventilation.

breathing activity to compensate. This is the pathophysiological basis of SSRD. Its signs are listed in Table 13.1.

Note that a passive patient does not display these signs, which are associated with intensification of spontaneous breathing activities. For passive patients, we must pay special attention to monitoring abnormalities, including SpO_2, heart rate, and $P_{et}CO_2$.

Deciding whether the ventilated patient suffers from SSRD is critical, because it determines which route to take in managing the emergency.

4. **Disconnect the patient from the ventilator**: If you confirm the diagnosis of SSRD but you cannot identify the root cause quickly, disconnect the patient from the ventilator at the airway. The ETT (endotracheal tube) or TT (tracheal tube) should stay in place.

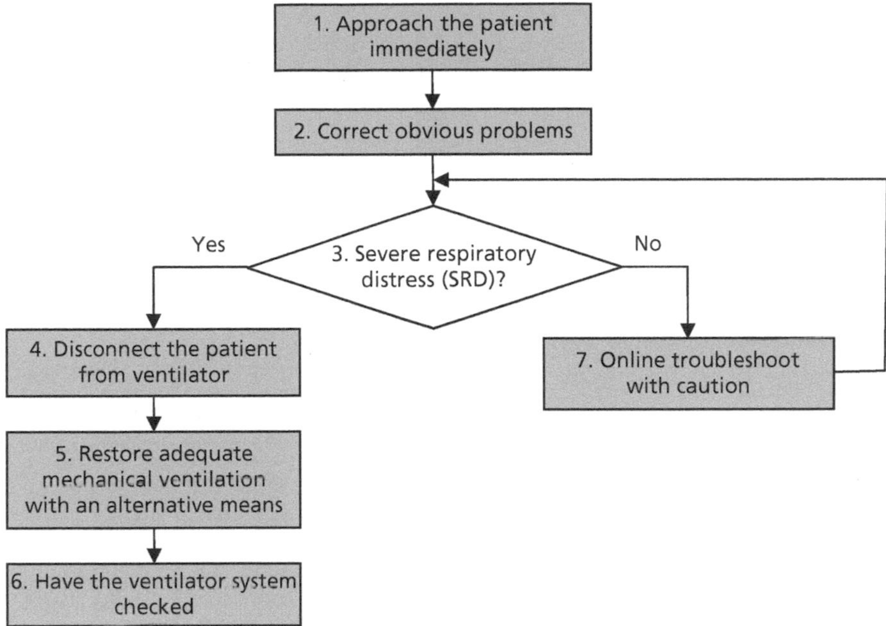

Fig. 13.4 General rules of emergency management.

The disconnection itself is diagnostic. If the disconnection improves the patient's clinical situation immediately, a ventilator system fault or operator error is the most likely culprit. If the disconnection does not improve the clinical situation, the problem involves the patient's airway, lungs, or chest wall. A typical example is ETT kinking.

5. **Restore adequate mechanical ventilation:** Immediately after the disconnection, restore ventilation with a resuscitator or another ventilator system. Do not spend precious time troubleshooting the ventilator system now.
6. **Have the ventilator system checked:** After the emergency is successfully resolved, have the ventilator system checked by a qualified staff member. Document the incident objectively and in detail. The affected ventilator should not be clinically used for the next patient until the investigation is completed.
7. **Troubleshoot the ventilator system with the patient attached:** If the root cause is not obvious, but the patient shows no strong and/or obvious signs of SSRD, try troubleshooting the problem in steps with the patient connected; refer to Box 13.1. The listed items are required

Table 13.1 Clinical signs of SSRD

Primary signs	Frequent accompanying signs
◆ Tachypnoea ◆ Nasal flaring ◆ Diaphoresis ◆ Use of accessory muscles, causing retraction of suprasternal, supraclavicular, and intercostal spaces	◆ Abnormal movement of the thorax and abdomen ◆ Cyanosis ◆ Abnormal findings on auscultation ◆ Tachycardia ◆ Arrhythmia ◆ Hypotension

Box 13.1 Troubleshooting checks

- All required parts are present and properly functioning
- The entire system is set up correctly and all parts are securely connected
- The air and oxygen supplies are continuous and stable within their specified pressure ranges
- The AC power supply is continuous and stable within the specified voltage range
- The system has no noticeable gas leak
- The gas passageway has no noticeable obstruction
- The patient's lungs are inflatable
- The ventilator settings (mode, controls, and alarm limits) are appropriate.

for the ventilator system to function properly. They can be regarded as the top-level guidelines for ventilator troubleshooting.

While troubleshooting, always keep an eye on the patient and react quickly if the patient's condition deteriorates.

Any alarm messages provide useful hints about possible root causes. It is a good idea to get help from nearby co-workers. Do not hesitate to call a specialist.

13.4 Troubleshooting common equipment problems

This subsection focuses on the five most common MV equipment problems: (a) gas supply failure, (b) electrical supply failure, (c) gas leak, (d) occlusion, and (e) circuit rainout (Box 13-1).

13.4.1 Gas supply problems

Gas supplies are an essential part of a ventilator system. Most positive-pressure ventilator systems require continuous supplies of compressed air and oxygen. Refer to section 5.3.1 for more information. Box 13.2 lists common gas supply problems.

Gas supply failure

Air or oxygen supplies can stop completely because of:

- Discontinuation of the central gas supply, malfunction of the air compressor, or empty gas cylinders.

Box 13.2 Common gas supply problems

- Complete failure of gas supply
- Inadequate gas supply
- Wet supply gas
- Questionable O_2 supply
- Supply gas contamination.

- Connection failure (i.e. the operator forgets to connect the ventilator to the gas supply or there is a sizeable leak at the gas connection line).

If one gas supply fails, a ventilator typically continues mechanical ventilation with the remaining gas supply and alarms to alert the clinician of the abnormal condition. Note: The patient is ventilated only with air or oxygen.

If both gas supplies fail, mechanical ventilation stops immediately, and the ventilator alarms. The ventilator switches to the ambient state (refer to section 12.6) and annunciates alarms. This is an emergency. The ventilated patient should be removed from the ventilator system and ventilated with an alternative means.

If a ventilator is supplied with cylinder gas, ensure continuation of the gas supply. It is a good idea to have spare, full gas cylinders always available.

Inadequate or restricted gas supply

In this case, the gas supply is available, but the supply pressure is too low or the supply gas flow is restricted. The common causes include:

- The gas cylinders are nearly empty;
- The compressor performs poorly;
- The supply gas pressure is too low;
- Gas consumption from the central gas supply pipeline network is abnormally high (e.g. due to a massive leak);
- The hospital gas supply pipeline is so thin that the gas flow is restricted.

These gas supply problems often trigger gas supply alarms, either continuously or intermittently. Hospital technical staff should fix the problem.

'Dancing flow meter'

This problem results from the thin diameter of the tubes in the central oxygen supply. The high resistance restricts gas flow, although the pressure may be normal.

Assume that a branch of the oxygen pipeline has several outlets. One outlet supplies a ventilator, and the others are used for oxygen therapy. To regulate the gas flow for oxygen therapy, a gravity flowmeter with an indicating metal ball is mounted at the outlet.

Some ventilators take in oxygen briefly at a high flow rate from time to time. At this time, the metal balls of the oxygen flowmeters fluctuate swiftly and make clicking sounds. This phenomenon is called the 'dancing flowmeter'. It confuses the clinicians on duty and disturbs the patients undergoing oxygen therapy, although it affects neither the ventilator performance nor the oxygen therapy.

The radical remedy for the dancing flowmeter is to replace the thin tubes with thick ones. This needs to be taken into consideration when the hospital oxygen pipeline is designed.

Wet supply gas

The air and oxygen supplied to ventilators should be cold (close to room temperature), dry, and clean. Wet supply gas is abnormal, typically resulting from an under-performing compressor or rarely, from moisture in the central supply pipeline. Here we are referring exclusively to the supply gas to the ventilator, but not the gas delivered from the ventilator to the patient.

As a preventive measure, a water trap may be installed at either gas inlet, as shown in Fig. 13.5. The water trap usually has a microfilter to capture any particles and droplets in the supply gases before entering the ventilator.

If the supply gas is dry, no or little water accumulates in the water trap. If the supply gas is wet, the trap can fill up quickly.

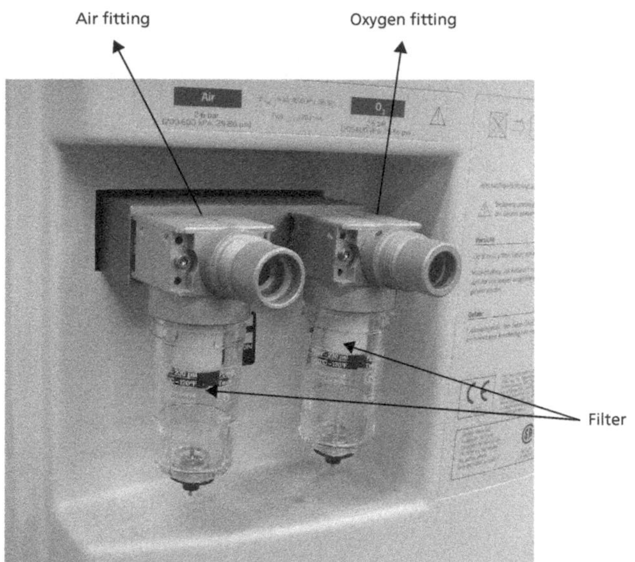

Fig. 13.5 Gas inlets with water traps (GALILEO ventilator).

As a routine practice, the clinician should periodically inspect the water traps of all running ventilators and empty them before they are nearly full. This is done either by pressing the pin at the trap bottom or unscrewing the screw-type mechanism. For optimal efficiency, the microfilter inside the water trap should be replaced periodically by the technical staff.

The consequences of wet supply gas vary, depending on the speed at which the water enters the ventilator and the peculiarities of the ventilator design. Some ventilators are more sensitive to unexpected water from the gas inlets. The worst scenario is that the affected ventilator cannot be clinically used due to technical failure.

Oxygen supply from an oxygen concentrator

Compressed oxygen is conventionally provided either from a central oxygen supply network or from an oxygen cylinder. The oxygen concentration of the oxygen supply should be at least 98%.

Recently a new type of oxygen supply was introduced and is being tested in hospitals. A special oxygen concentrator continuously produces compressed oxygen. This innovation could remove the hospital's dependency on oxygen cylinders. Use of oxygen cylinders brings with it not only safety concerns, but also the work and costs of cylinder exchange, transport, and storage.

These special concentrators are not always adequate for the job, however. The major drawback is that the supplied 'oxygen' has an unstable oxygen concentration, typically ranging between 85% and 95%, depending on the pattern of oxygen consumption.

A basic assumption of a ventilator design is that the oxygen supply is 100%. If the O_2 concentration in the source 'oxygen' is only 90%, the ventilator may alarm due to low oxygen. Furthermore, the questionable source of oxygen must not be used for oxygen cell calibration, otherwise, the oxygen monitoring will be systemically incorrect.

Supply gas contamination

Contamination of the central gas supply pipeline network is a nightmare in any hospital. It means that harmful bacteria or viruses can be disseminated through the network, threatening all patients connected.

Microfilters inside water traps at the ventilator gas inlets may protect the ventilator and the connected patient from this adverse event.

13.4.2 Electrical supply problems

The electrical supply is another essential part of a ventilator system. A ventilator cannot run without electrical power.

For almost all ventilator systems, AC power serves as the primary source of electricity. Many modern ventilators also have an internal battery as a secondary source to bridge temporary AC power loss. Transport ventilators can also be powered with DC power from ambulances or airplanes.

Generally speaking, electrical supply problems involve the AC supply itself, the connection between the AC supply and the ventilator, or the ventilator's internal battery (Box 13.3).

AC supply problems

AC power interruption The most common AC supply problem is blackout or the unexpected interruption of the local or regional AC power supply. Regardless of its cause, AC supply interruption is a nightmare for a hospital, as it affects not only ventilators, but all medical electrical equipment and hospital facilities. Therefore, it is mandatory that hospitals have an emergency electricity supply prepared even when AC power interruption seldom occurs.

A common preventive measure is an emergency diesel generator, which should start immediately when the local AC supply fails. However, use of a diesel generator may have two drawbacks.

First, it takes a few seconds for a diesel generator to start after an unexpected AC power interruption. If a ventilator does not have an internal battery, this time with no power may cause the ventilator to shut down. When AC power is later restored, it takes up to 40 seconds for the ventilator to complete its rebooting process. Caution: Mechanical ventilation is unavailable during the rebooting process! Clearly, an internal battery is the best fix for this problem.

The second drawback is that the generator may produce an initial power surge when it starts. An excessive surge can damage electrical devices, including the ventilator.

Unstable and/or insufficient AC voltage The quality of the AC power in some regions may be poor. The AC voltage may fluctuate considerably, and may be lower than the specified range when power consumption reaches its daily peak.

In general, a medical electrical device should tolerate voltage fluctuations as long as the voltage remains within ±10% of its nominal values. Although such fluctuations are an abnormal condition, some regard a device as 'good' if it continues to work under such conditions and 'bad' otherwise. Such a judgement is unfounded.

Where AC integrity is questionable, hospitals should strive to improve the quality of their AC power. Consult hospital technicians or the ventilator manufacturer for possible measures to take.

Box 13.3 Common electrical supply problems

- AC supply problems
- AC connection problems
- Internal battery problems.

AC voltage and frequency mismatch The voltage and frequency of the regional AC supply must match the specified requirements for the ventilator. A mismatch causes the ventilator to malfunction or become damaged. Hospital technical staff must pay attention to voltage and frequency matching when installing a ventilator.

AC connection problems

Even when both the AC power supply and the connected ventilator are technically in order, AC power may still be problematic due to faulty connection between the two. Possible connection issues include:

- Accidental unplugging of the power cord: AC may be interrupted by inadvertent unplugging (e.g. during routine room cleaning). Unplugging can occur at either side of the power cord, but more often it occurs at the wall side. When the power cord becomes unplugged, the ventilator annunciates an alarm. In such a case, the internal battery ensures continuous mechanical ventilation.
- Poor or loose connection: This can have multiple causes but a single common result: unreliable AC supply to the ventilator, causing intermittent ventilator functioning.
- Dead socket: The socket in use is not powered.
- Broken power cord: The power cord may appear intact, but an internal wire is faulty.
- Plug-socket mismatch: This can occur at either the wall or device side of a power cord.

Internal battery problems

Whenever the AC supply fails, the ventilator battery can serve as a temporary power source so that mechanical ventilation continues. However, internal battery capacity is limited. An alternative means of mechanical ventilation must be ready before the internal battery 'dies'.

The internal battery lets the ventilator run even when it is not connected to AC power. In this case, the ventilator should repeatedly annunciate an AC power failure alarm.

If the internal battery is not fully charged, the battery time will be noticeably shortened. For this reason all ventilators should be connected to AC power, even when not in clinical use.

Finally, a battery loses capacity as it ages, and it can't power the ventilator for as long as a new battery can. It is important to replace the battery periodically as per the manufacturer's recommendation.

13.4.3 Gas leakage

Pneumatically, the core of an intermittent positive pressure ventilator (IPPV) system is a gas tubing system in which the gas pressure changes regularly, driving the gas to move as designed. This system has to be gas tight. The gas should exit the ventilator system exclusively via the expiratory valve.

Typically the pressure inside a ventilator system is greater than atmospheric pressure, more positive during inspiration, and less positive during expiration. There are two exceptions: (a) PEEP is set to zero, which is not recommended, and (b) the patient is active, with a strong drive. This positive pressure will push gas out of any hole within the ventilator system. Gas flow from such a leak is determined by the resistance (i.e. the size of the hole, and the gradient between internal pressure and atmospheric pressure).

Gas leakage: where and how?

A ventilator system is assembled from multiple tubes, connectors, and designed openings. Clearly, gas leakage can also occur at multiple locations. Common locations for leaks are listed in Table 13.2 and shown in Fig. 13.6.

Table 13.2 Locations of leaks in the ventilator system

Leakage in breathing circuit	Leakage in airway	Leakage in lungs
Worn plastic or silicone rubber tubes	Airway disconnection, i.e. ETT or TT	Bronchopleural fistula or an abnormal gas exit via a chest tube
Disconnection	Leak around an ETT, e.g. uncuffed neonatal ETT, unintended deflated tube cuff	Leaking test lung
Unsealed part, e.g. water trap not tightly closed	Cracked item in artificial airway, e.g. proximal flow sensor, HME, CO_2 probe, flex tube, closed-suctioning device	
Cracked plastic items such as humidifier chamber, water trap, connectors, or nebulizer jar	Leaking airway interface for NIV, e.g. poorly fitting mask	
Open ports, e.g. water chamber refill port, temperature probe port, or side port of a filter	Gas leaking through open mouth during NIV	

In rare cases gas leakage may occur inside the ventilator or in the gas supply route. A ventilator exhibiting internal leakage should be removed from clinical use and serviced by the technical staff.

Gas leakage and the pneumatic system

Gas leakage disturbs the pneumatics of a ventilator system. The magnitude of disturbance varies greatly, depending on the following factors:

- Leak flow: The size of a leak is often expressed either in leak flow or in leak volume for a single breath. In truth, ventilator systems are not absolutely gas tight. Most IPPV ventilator systems can tolerate a tiny amount of leakage well. However, a noticeable leak can impair the functioning of a ventilator system, because the ventilator cannot establish the required pressure gradients. No ventilator system can function if the gas passageway is disconnected—the greatest leak possible.
- Mechanical breath type: Pressure or adaptive breaths can tolerate moderate gas leakage, while volume breaths cannot tolerate any.
- Patient triggering: Both flow triggering and pressure triggering are sensitive to leakage. Auto-triggering is a common consequence. Time triggering is not affected by gas leakage, however.
- Flow cycling: A large leak can cause flow cycling to fail, resulting in an endless inspiration.
- Pressure baseline: A noticeable gas leak causes the baseline to drop below the set PEEP/CPAP. This directly affects pressure triggering.

How to recognize a gas leak A significant gas leak (e.g. airway disconnection) is very easy to recognize. It may be more difficult, however, to recognize a small leak, but one that nevertheless interferes with ventilator performance. The following phenomena are often associated with, and even caused exclusively by, a gas leak.

A. Auto-triggering:

Auto-triggering is the phenomenon where a ventilator is triggered by pneumatic artefacts rather than the patient's inspiratory efforts. The ventilator itself is unable to differentiate the two and delivers a mechanical breath in either case.

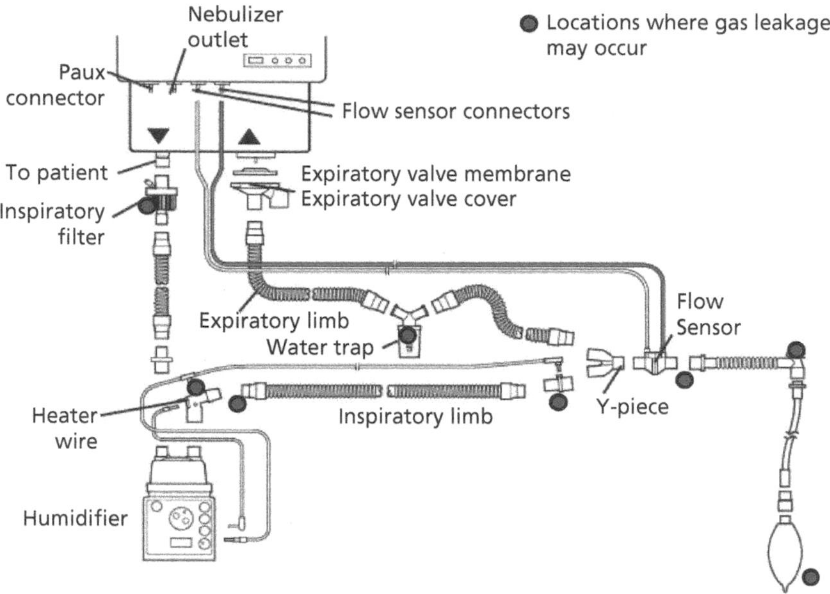

Fig. 13.6 Possible locations for gas leakage at breathing circuit, airway, and lungs.

Typically, auto-triggering presents as a series of quick rhythmic mechanical breaths with an expiratory time (T_e) much shorter than expected.

Auto-triggering is often associated with gas leakage. But this phenomenon can also appear when the circuit has accumulated condensed water or when patient triggering is set at an overly sensitive level.

Figures 13.7, 13.8 and 13.9 show waveforms associated with auto-triggering and leakage.

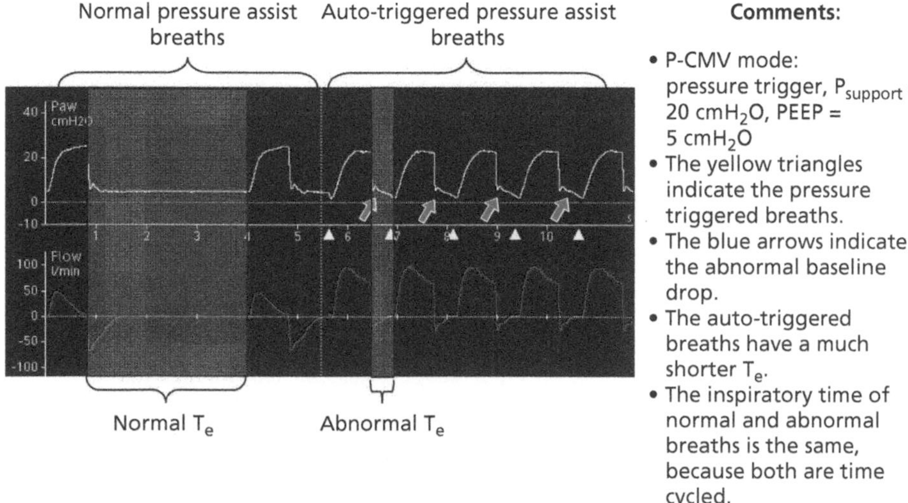

Fig. 13.7 Auto-triggering with a pressure trigger.

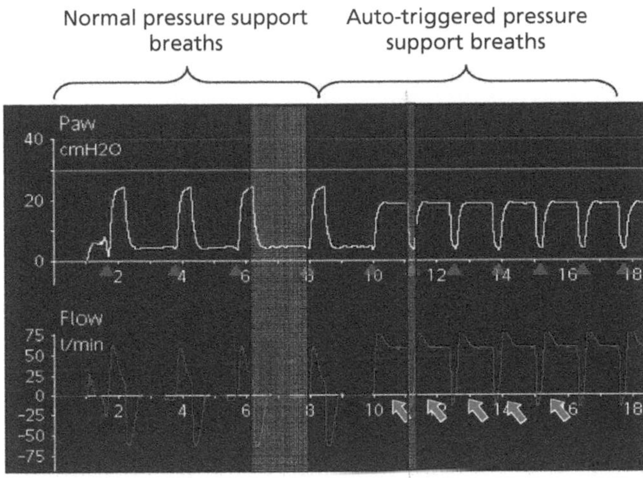

Comments:

- SPONT/PSV mode: flow trigger, $P_{support}$ = 20 cmH_2O, PEEP = 5 cmH_2O, flow cycling = 25%
- The pink triangles indicate the flow-triggered breaths.
- The blue arrows indicate abnormal inspiratory flow (hardly visible) at the end of expiration.
- The auto-triggered breaths have a much shorter T_e.
- A sizeable gas leak causes the peak pressure to be lower than expected.

Fig. 13.8 Auto-triggering with a flow trigger.

B. Abnormal flow waveform:

In a flow-time graph, a mechanical breath has an inspiratory flow area and an expiratory flow area. The inspiratory flow area is between the inspiratory flow waveform and the zero line, representing the inspiratory tidal volume of the breath. The expiratory flow area is the area between the expiratory flow waveform and the zero line, representing the expiratory tidal volume of the breath. Under normal conditions, both areas (and tidal volumes) are roughly equal in size.

A gas leak at the airway or lungs causes the inspiratory flow area to be considerably larger than the expiratory flow area. The greater the gas leak, the greater the difference. Disconnection, the largest leak possible, causes the expiratory area to disappear completely. See Fig. 13.9.

An abnormal flow waveform always points to leakage.

C. Abnormal volume waveform:

For a normal volume or pressure breath, the volume waveform rises from zero to the peak, representing the inspiratory tidal volume. Then it returns from the peak to zero, representing the expiratory tidal volume.

A leak at the airway or lungs causes the volume waveform to stay high during expiration, and then to end with a sharp drop to zero. The drop represents the reset of volume monitoring. Figs 13.10, 13.11 and 13.12 show waveforms of pressure and volume breaths with gas leakage present.

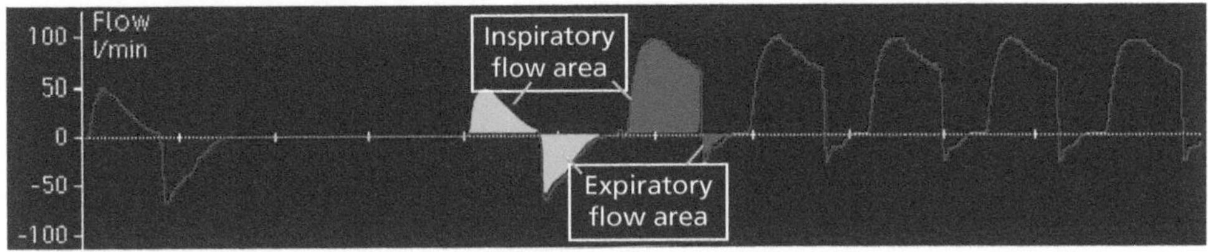

Fig. 13.9 A gas leak can be easily recognized by comparing inspiratory and expiratory areas. Normally, the two areas are roughly equal (the green areas). A gas leak causes the inspiratory area to be considerably larger than the expiratory area (the blue areas).

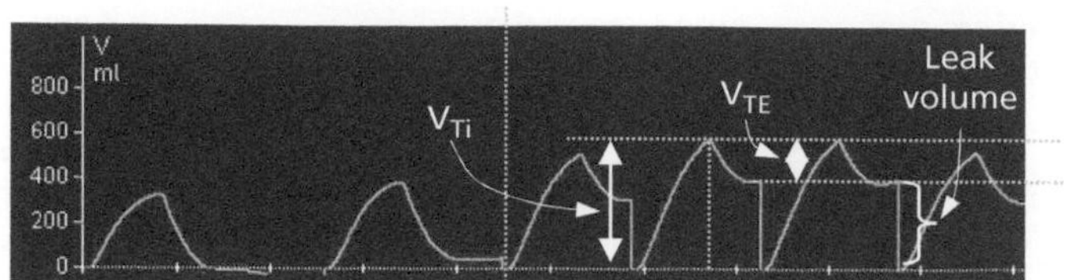

Fig. 13.10 Normal and abnormal volume waveform in pressure breaths. Abnormalities include: (a) the volume waveform fails to return to zero, (b) the volume peak increases (this is not so in volume breaths), and (c) the monitored VTE is considerably smaller than the VTI.
VTE: expiratory tidal volume; VTI: inspiratory tidal volume.

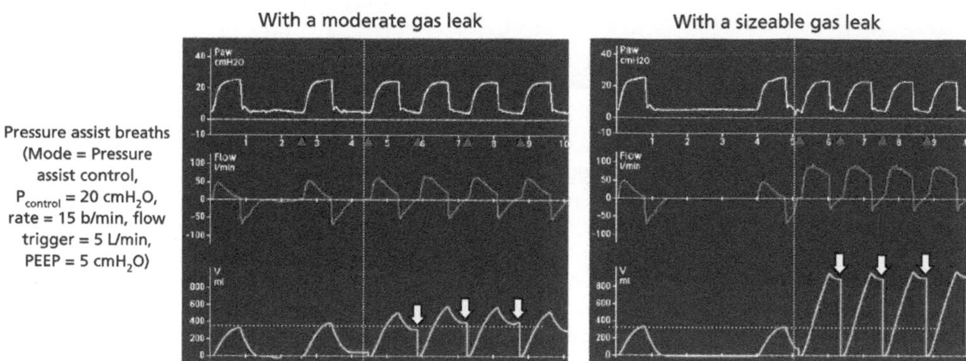

Fig. 13.11 Waveforms of pressure breaths with gas leakage. Both graphs have three waveforms: from top down, pressure (white), flow (pink), and volume (green). The breaths on the left of each graph are normal (leak free), and the breaths on the right are abnormal due to a moderate or sizeable gas leak. The yellow arrows indicate the reset of volume monitoring. Abnormalities include: (a) auto-triggering, (b) a difference in size of flow area, (c) a higher-than-normal peak of the volume waveform, and (d) a sharp drop in volume at end expiration.

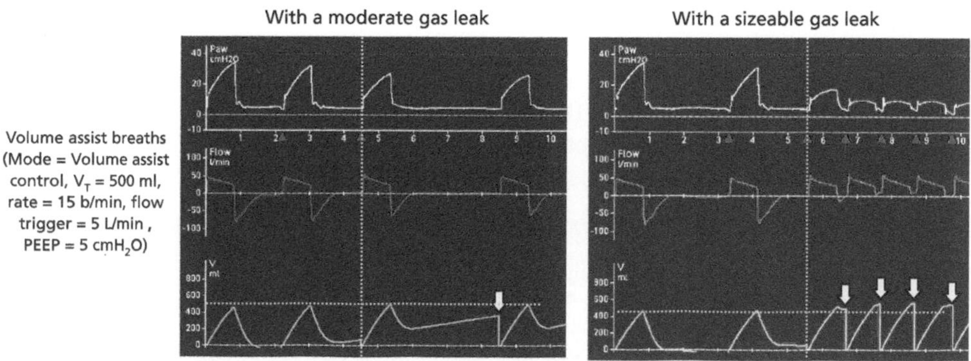

Fig. 13.12 Waveforms of volume breaths with gas leakage. Abnormalities include: (a) auto-triggering, (b) a difference in size of flow areas, (c) a lower-than-normal peak pressure, and (d) a sharp drop in volume at end expiration.

Thus, during the expiratory phase, the height of the volume waveform has two parts. The first part is monitored expiratory tidal volume (VTE). The second part is the height of the sharp drop, which is a good indicator of the leak volume.

Pressure breaths have an inherent ability to compensate leaks: the ventilator increases the inspiratory flow, causing a greater inspiratory tidal volume (VTI). This explains why gas leakage causes the peak of the volume waveform to be higher than normal, a phenomenon that does not occur in volume breaths.

D. Reduction in monitored expiratory tidal volume:

Ventilators calculate monitored volume from flow measurements taken over time. As we saw above, a gas leak causes the expiratory flow area to decrease, resulting in a significantly reduced expiratory tidal volume (VTE).

This reduced VTE does not necessarily mean that ventilator monitoring is malfunctioning. It means that most of the expired tidal volume exited the system through the abnormal opening (i.e. without being 'seen' by the flow sensor).

The VTE represents the minimum tidal volume that the patient actually received. In other words, the patient may have received more, but not less, than the displayed VTE. This is why a patient can still survive with an unbelievably small VTE.

When the displayed VTE is abnormally low, you need to consider the possibility of a gas leak.

E. Flow cycling failure:

In pressure support and adaptive support modes, a sizeable gas leak can cause a failure of the flow cycling mechanism.

As we saw in Chapter 7, flow cycling is based on inspiratory flow measurements in its descending part. The ventilator switches from inspiration to expiration when the inspiratory flow drops to a preset threshold. An excessive leak may cause the inspiratory flow to stay higher than the cycling threshold so that inspiration does not end. Such an endless inspiration is clinically unacceptable.

To prevent this possible abnormality, some ventilators implement an additional time cycling mechanism as a backup. For instance, Hamilton Medical ventilators have a Timax control. When the operator-set maximum inspiratory time ends, the ventilator terminates inspiration and starts expiration regardless of the inspiratory flow rate (Fig. 13.13).

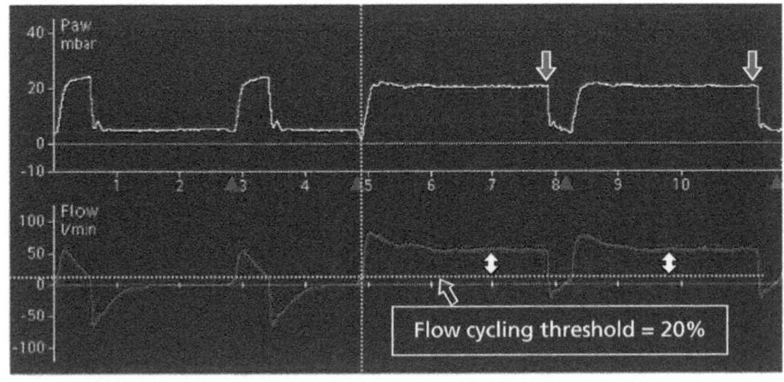

Comments:

- The gas leak is sizeable.
- The set flow cycling is 20%, indicated by the horizontal dotted line in the flow-time graph.
- Auto-triggering is present.
- The T_i of the abnormal breaths is much longer than the T_e.
- The inspiration in abnormal breaths is terminated by Timax, indicated by a blue arrow. Timax is set to 3 seconds.

Fig. 13.13 Normal and abnormal pressure support breaths. In the two breaths on the right, flow cycling fails due to a sizeable gas leak. The ventilator does not switch from inspiration to expiration as expected, causing the inspiration to be much longer than expected. Finally, the inspiration is terminated by the backup time cycling mechanism.

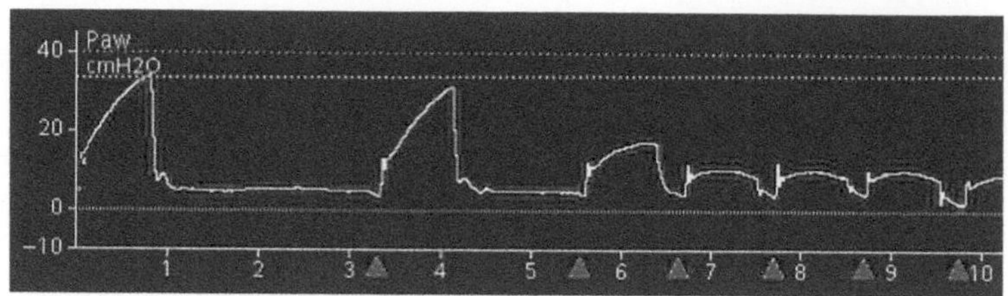

Fig. 13.14 A sizeable gas leak causes abnormally low peak pressure in a volume mode, indicating failure of positive-pressure ventilation.

F. Abnormally low peak pressure:

In volume modes, a sizeable gas leak causes the peak pressure to decrease (Fig. 13.14). In a volume breath, the tidal volume and inspiratory flow are predefined. When there is a leak, the ventilator does not deliver more gas into the circuit to compensate. The consequence is decreased peak pressure.

Pressure breaths are much less affected unless the leak is massive.

Common alarms associated with gas leakage

The following alarms are typically activated when a ventilator system has a moderate or sizeable leak, provided that the alarms are set properly:

- Low tidal volume;
- Low minute volume;
- High respiratory rate, if auto-triggering is present;
- Low airway pressure, particularly in a volume mode;
- Low PEEP or loss of PEEP, if the leak is sizeable.

Note that none of these alarms is specific to gas leakage alone. They may be activated by a gas leak or by other causes.

Remedies for gas leakage

The key to remedying gas leakage is to recognize and identify its cause. Once the leak is identified, the remedy is simple and straightforward:

- Reconnect the system;
- Replace the broken or cracked items;
- Close the open port;
- Reinflate the ETT cuff;
- Use optimally fitting masks for non-invasive ventilation.

The ventilator system should function normally after the true root cause is successfully eliminated. Leak-related alarms should disappear.

Leak compensation

The term *leak compensation* is widely used by ventilator manufacturers. It may be misleading, leading one to believe that sufficiently strong leak compensation can offset any level of leak.

Leak compensation is a technical feature derived from the pressure controlling mechanism described in section 7.2.3. In short, a gas leak decreases the internal pressure of the ventilator. The ventilator in turn increases the inspiratory flow, delivering more gas into the circuit during inspiration. If the gas leak is small, this leak compensation mechanism enables the ventilator system to maintain the expected peak and baseline pressures, as shown in Fig. 13.11.

Leak compensation has several drawbacks. First, leak compensation is limited: it does not work if the leak is massive. Second, it alone cannot prevent auto-triggering or a flow cycling failure: the corresponding settings (trigger sensitivity and flow cycle) must be appropriately adjusted. Third, leak compensation causes (much) higher gas consumption. To address the second issue, Philips Respironics introduced a software algorithm called *Auto-Trak*, which enables the ventilator to automatically adjust flow trigger sensitivity and flow cycle settings based on the monitored leak flow. Auto-Trak does not work with pressure triggering.

The best solution is always to identify and stop a gas leak rather than relying on so-called 'leak compensation.'

13.4.4 Occlusion of the gas passageway

As we learned earlier, a ventilator system functions properly only when (a) it is gas tight, and (b) it is not occluded, so that gas can move freely according to the pressure gradient. *Occlusion* is an unexpected increase in resistance to flow of passing gas, impairing the system performance.

A ventilator system can become occluded at various locations for a number of reasons. The clinical consequences of the occlusion vary from being negligible to mortal, depending on the size of the occlusion. Most occlusions are partial or incomplete, which can, however make them difficult to recognize. A complete occlusion occurs less frequently. It is an emergency, as the patient cannot breathe, and it requires immediate correction.

Common causes of occlusion

Occlusions of the gas passageway can be classified according to their characteristics, as follows:

- Size: minor, noticeable, complete;
- Location: airway, inspiratory limb, expiratory limb;
- Type: internal tube occlusion, external tube compression.

Possible locations of occlusions are shown in Fig. 13.15. The common causes of occlusion are listed in Table 13.3.

Circuit rainout (excessive condensed water in the circuit) is a special form of partial occlusion. Refer to section 6.3.2 for details.

Pneumatic disturbances

An occlusion means increased resistance. According to Ohm's law, flow is equal to the pressure difference divided by resistance:

$$Flow = \frac{\Delta P}{R}$$

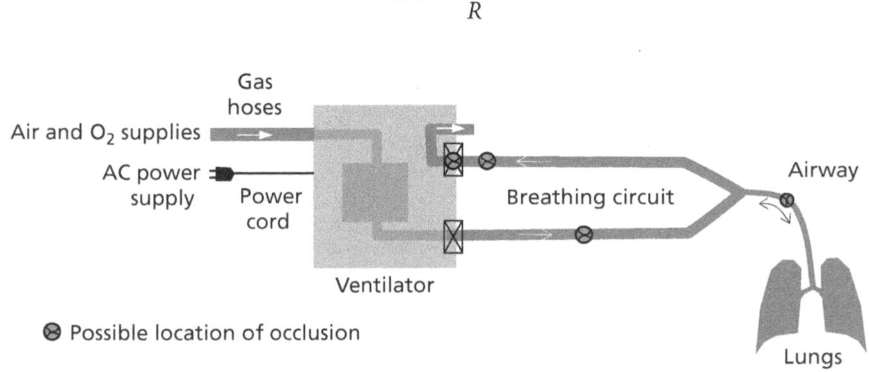

Fig. 13.15 An occlusion of the gas passageway can occur at the airway or in the inspiratory or expiratory limb of the patient circuit.

Table 13.3 Common causes of occlusion

Airway occlusion	Inspiratory limb occlusion	Expiratory limb occlusion
◆ Kinked ETT ◆ ETT or TT too thin ◆ Excessive tracheal secretions ◆ Clogged HME filter	◆ Neonatal circuit used for an adult ◆ Bent or kinked tube ◆ Compressed tube ◆ Inner diameter of connector too small ◆ Overly long heating wire bunched inside inspiratory limb	◆ Neonatal circuit used for an adult ◆ Bent or kinked tube ◆ Compressed tube ◆ Inner diameter of connector too small ◆ Occluded expiratory filter ◆ Blocked expiratory valve

ETT: endotracheal tube; HME: heat and moisture exchanger; TT: tracheal tube.

Therefore, for a given pressure gradient, increased resistance causes decreased gas flow. In a pressure mode, a significant occlusion results in a sharp decrease in the generated tidal volume. In a volume breath where the tidal volume is predefined and controlled, a significant occlusion causes a sharp increase in peak pressure.

Consequences of an occlusion

In theory, the ventilated patient cannot:

- Inhale if the inspiratory limb is completely occluded;
- Exhale if the expiratory limb is completely occluded;
- Inhale and exhale if the airway is completely occluded.

Obviously, none of these situations is clinically tolerable. The clinical consequences of gas passageway occlusion are determined by the size of occlusion and the clinician's response.

Hypoventilation is the inevitable consequence of all types of occlusion. An active patient will fight frantically for life. Multiple alarms will be annunciated. If the occlusion is close to complete, clinical signs of sudden and serious respiratory distress syndrome appear, requiring immediate correction.

How to recognize an occlusion

An occlusion can happen to any ventilated patient at any time. Compared to a gas leak, a partial occlusion is typically more difficult to recognize, even for experienced clinicians. In an emergency, therefore, the general rules of emergency management apply; refer to section 13.3.

Most manifestations of occlusion are non-specific. Ventilator alarms are indeed a help, but only when they are set sensitively. If hypoventilation and patient-ventilator asynchrony do not respond to corrective measures as expected, the clinician in charge should consider the possibility of occlusion and conduct the investigation as explained in Tables 13.4, 13.5 and 13.6.

As you apply the information above, note the following:

- It assumes a passive patient and use of a proximal flow sensor at the Y-piece;
- Typical changes in waveforms and monitoring parameters appear only when the occlusion is severe but incomplete;
- The alarms mentioned may be activated only when alarm limits are set properly;
- Trending these parameters, if available, may help to identify small and progressive changes.

You can relieve all three types of occlusion, with the exception of ETT kinking, by disconnecting the patient from the ventilator. If you suspect ETT kinking, pass a suction catheter through the ETT for verification. If the tube is occluded, the catheter cannot pass through.

Table 13.4 How to recognize a partial occlusion of the inspiratory limb

Indication	Volume breaths	Pressure breaths
	P_{ao} / Time / Airway flow	P_{ao} / Time / Airway flow
Waveforms	Partial occlusion causes no noticeable change in pressure and flow waveforms.	Inspiratory occlusion slows the pressure rise and lowers the peak inspiratory flow during inspiration. The waveforms are unaffected during expiration.
Monitoring	No noticeable change.	Inspiratory peak flow drops, while expiratory peak flow remains unchanged.
Alarms	Most likely no alarm is active.	Most likely no alarm is activate.

Table 13.5 How to recognize a partial occlusion of the expiratory limb

Indication	Volume breaths	Pressure breaths
	P_{ao} / Time / Airway flow	P_{ao} / Time / Airway flow
Waveforms	Expiratory occlusion slows the pressure drop during expiration and lowers the peak expiratory flow.	Same as for volume breaths, because the expiratory process is the same for both pressure and volume breaths.
Monitoring	Expiratory peak flow drops, while peak inspiratory flow remains unchanged.	Same as for volume breaths.
Alarms	If the occlusion is nearly total, an "Expiration occluded" alarm is annunciated if available.	Same as for volume breaths.

Table 13.6 How to recognize a partial occlusion of the airway

Indication	Volume breaths	Pressure breaths
	P_{ao} Time Airway flow	P_{ao} Time Airway flow
Waveform	• Inspiratory peak pressure rises sharply • Pressure drops sharply at the beginning of expiration • Peak inspiratory flow decreases slightly • Peak expiratory flow decreases	• A square pressure profile appears, i.e., sharp pressure rise and sharp pressure drop • Peak inspiratory flow decreases • Peak expiratory flow decreases
Monitoring	• Peak pressure increases • Peak inspiratory flow decreases • Peak expiratory flow decreases • Inspiratory resistance increases • Expiratory resistance increases	• Tidal volume decreases • Peak inspiratory flow decreases • Peak expiratory flow decreases • Inspiratory resistance increases • Expiratory resistance increases
Alarms	• High peak pressure	• Low tidal volume • Low minute volume

How to remedy an occlusion

Recognizing a partial occlusion of the ventilator system and identifying its root cause can be challenging. Once the root cause is identified, the remedy is typically easy, such as replacing a blocked filter or kinked tube, removing the compression from a tube, or suctioning the trachea.

The following recommendations may help to prevent the incidence of occlusion:

- Make sure all clinicians involved in mechanical ventilation maintain keen vigilance at all times.
- If the patient shows signs of severe respiratory distress syndrome and you cannot find the root cause quickly, disconnect the patient from ventilator system without delay.
- Periodically clear tracheal secretions, shortening the interval between clearings as needed.
- Inspect the running ventilator system periodically. Immediately replace worn or ageing components, such as tubes, flow sensors, or filters.
- Check the heat and moisture exchanger (HME) and expiratory filter periodically. Replace them immediately if you suspect occlusion.
- Remove the HME for in-line nebulization.
- Replace the expiratory filter or expiratory valve after each in-line nebulization treatment.
- Do not reuse items intended for single (patient) use.
- Do not use an HME with a ventilated patient who has excessive tracheal secretions.

13.4.5 Circuit rainout

Refer to section 6.2.3, which details the causes, manifestations, and diagnosis of and remedy for circuit rainout.

13.4.6 Ventilator 'inoperative'

Modern ventilators continuously monitor their internal functional status as well as that of the entire ventilator system. If the status has seriously deteriorated, the ventilator alarms and automatically enters a special 'ambient' state; refer to section 12.6. A typical accompanying alarm message might be 'Ventilator Inoperative' or 'Technical fault/failure (TF).'

If such a condition occurs, the recommended actions, in sequence, are (a) remove the ventilator from clinical use, (b) continue mechanical ventilation with a spare ventilator or a resuscitator, and (c) have the affected ventilator serviced. Do not try to resolve the problem while the patient is still connected.

13.5 Error reporting

During mechanical ventilation therapy, adverse events can occur at any time. As we learned earlier in this chapter, they can be classified as equipment problems, operation problems, or patient problems. There are numerous possible combinations of these.

Whenever such an event occurs, the highest priority is the patient's safety. Afterwards, the event must be documented concretely and objectively. The clinician in charge has another task: error reporting. It is often intentionally or unintentionally ignored.

The objective of such reporting is not, and should never be, to identify or punish the individuals who were involved in or responsible for the event. Instead, it may be the best way for the public to learn from the mistakes of others.

Error reporting provides a good starting point for authorities at all levels to take necessary actions and modify policies or regulations. For instance, if the event was caused by a technical fault in a ventilator, it is likely that all ventilators of this model potentially have the same issue. The informed authority can require the ventilator manufacturer to take necessary corrective actions to prevent the same event from affecting additional patients.

Error reporting must be objective, complete, concrete, and sequenced. Below is an example of a poor report:

> Three days ago, xxx ventilator was used to ventilate a patient. The ventilator gave a number of alarms constantly and the patient was in very bad situation. We tried, unsuccessfully, to change the settings. We were really upset at the performance of this ventilator.

Such a report contains little useful information to provide others a clear picture of the problem. Refer to Table 13.7 for guidance on how to write an adverse event report.

Table 13.7 Guidance for error reporting

	Necessary facts to provide	Remark
Reporter	◆ Full name ◆ Title, such as physician, intensive nurse, or respiratory therapist ◆ Telephone number and email address	This is the contact information for the adverse event reporter
Healthcare institution	◆ Full name of department/division ◆ Full name of institution ◆ Detailed address of institution, including street number, street, postal code, city, and country ◆ Telephone number of institution ◆ Web address of institution	A large hospital can have several ICUs. Do identify your ICU or department. Do not forget city and country
Date and time	◆ Exact time and date when the incident began ◆ Exact time and date when the incident ended	Modern ventilators may chronologically record selected events (event log). The information may help pinpoint all events during the time period
Patient	◆ Patient ID ◆ Age ◆ Gender ◆ Body weight (gestation weeks for neonates) ◆ Primary diagnosis ◆ Reason for intubation and mechanical ventilation	
Affected ventilator system	◆ Ventilator brand and model ◆ Serial number or unit ID number ◆ Hardware and software versions ◆ Service history ◆ Details about any similar previous event ◆ Composition of the ventilator system at time of event, i.e. type of circuit, humidifier/HME, proximal flow sensor, CO_2 sensor, etc.	Ask for help from the technical staff. Take photos with a digital camera or mobile phone to show: ◆ the entire system composition, ◆ the mode and control settings, ◆ the alarm limit settings, and ◆ the waveforms. Attach the photos to the report
Event	◆ Describe the event chronologically ◆ List the names of those directly involved ◆ Describe what happened to the patient because of the incident, i.e. injured (not at all, slightly, or seriously) or died ◆ State whether the ventilator completely stopped operating ◆ State whether any audible and/or visual alarms were annunciated before and during the incident, and provide any associated alarm messages ◆ State whether there were any problems related to AC power and gas supplies before and during the incident ◆ Describe the actions taken to handle the event	
Previous investigations	If the event was already investigated, attach the investigation report	

Glossary

absolute humidity The amount of water vapour present in a unit volume of air, usually expressed in kg/m^3 or mg/L. Absolute humidity does not fluctuate with the temperature of the air.

A/C Assist/control, which is a standard ventilation mode.

accuracy The deviation between the truth and the monitored results. If the deviation is sufficiently small, the monitoring is considered to be accurate.

active exhalation valve A mechanism to regulate the expiratory valve, with which the patient can exhale even during inspiration. It is the basis of biphasic modes.

active humidifier A medical device used to warm and humidify the gas that an intubated and mechanically ventilated patient inhales. An active humidifier is integrated into the breathing circuit of a ventilator system.

acute respiratory distress syndrome (ARDS) A rapidly developing, life-threatening condition in which the lung is injured to the point where it prevents sufficient oxygen from getting to the lungs and into the blood.

adaptive assist/control mode An adaptive ventilation mode with two mechanical breath types: adaptive control breath and adaptive assist breath. This mode is suitable for passive and partially active patients.

adaptive control breath A type of mechanical breath that is time triggered, adaptive controlled, and time cycled.

adaptive controlling A controlling mechanism by which a ventilator automatically regulates inspiratory pressure to achieve a preset target tidal volume.

adaptive pressure ventilation (APV) mode Another name for adaptive assist/control mode.

adaptive ventilation mode Any ventilation mode with adaptive breaths, such as adaptive A/C mode, adaptive SIMV mode, and volume support mode.

aerosol Extremely fine liquid droplets or solid particles that remain suspended in air as fog or smoke.

airway The passage by which air reaches a person's lungs. It begins at the nose and mouth and ends at the alveoli. Also called *pulmonary airway* or *respiratory tract*.

airway pressure release ventilation (APRV) A biphasic ventilation mode with alternating baseline pressures. It typically has a relatively long high PEEP period and a very short low PEEP period for pressure relief. Spontaneous breaths occur at the high PEEP.

airway resistance The force that tends to oppose gas movement through the airway. Airway resistance is a key property of respiratory mechanics.

alarm A mechanism to audibly or visually warn of danger.

alarm priority The estimated severity of an alarm condition.

alarm setting An operator-set alarm limit to define a non-alarm zone.

alarm signal Audible and/or visual signals to indicate that one or more defined alarm conditions are detected.

alarm silence A ventilator function with which one can temporarily stop an audible alarm while the alarm condition is still present.

ALI Acute lung injury.

alveolar dead space The volume of those alveoli that are ventilated but not perfused, and where, as a result, no gas exchange can occur.

alveolar minute volume/ alveolar ventilation The sum of the alveolar tidal volume (inspiratory or expiratory) of all breaths occurring per minute.

alveolar pressure (Palv) Pressure in the alveoli or on the lung side of the ventilator system.

alveolar tidal volume The part of tidal volume that participates in alveolar gas exchange.

alveoli (alveolus) Tiny air sacs of the lungs where gas exchange takes place.

ambient state An automatic safety mechanism that enables the ventilated patient to breathe unassisted if the ventilator system can no longer function as specified. Mechanical ventilation is discontinued during the ambient state.

ambient valve See *safety valve.*

anatomical dead space The volume of gas to fill the respiratory tract except for gas exchange areas.

Apnoea In mechanical ventilation, the situation where no patient breathing activity is detected during the set apnoea time.

apnoea alarm A warning that apnoea is detected.

apnoea time The maximum acceptable interval between two consecutive mechanical breaths. It is set by the operator.

apnoea ventilation/apnoea backup ventilation A safety mechanism that enables the ventilator to automatically switch from a support mode to a backup control mode when apnoea is detected.

application alarm A warning about a functional abnormality of a ventilator system or improper ventilator settings. Also known as a clinical alarm. An application alarm typically does not indicate a technical issue of the ventilator.

APRV See *airway pressure release ventilation.*

ARDS Acute respiratory distress syndrome.

artificial airway A device that connects the Y-piece and the natural airway in various ways, such as an endotracheal tube or a face mask.

artificial humidification The technique of artificially warming and humidifying the inspiratory gas.

assist breath/assisted breath Any mechanical breath that is patient (pressure or flow) triggered and time cycled.

asynchrony See *patient-ventilator asynchrony.*

automatic tube compensation (ATC) Also called tube resistance compensation (TRC). See *tube resistance compensation.*

autoPEEP Abnormally high alveolar pressure at end expiration due to incomplete expiration. Also called *intrinsic PEEP.*

auto-triggering A triggering abnormality where a ventilator is triggered by pneumatic artefacts but not the expected patient inhaling effort. Auto-triggering is associated with patient triggering.

barotrauma A complication of mechanical ventilation. Lung injury caused by continuous and excessively high positive pressures applied.

base flow/bias flow A constant gas flow from the inspiratory valve to the expiratory valve during late expiration. Base flow is required for flow triggering.

baseline pressure The pressure baseline above which positive pressure is applied intermittently. Also called *PEEP*.

bilevel positive airway pressure (BiPAP) A biphasic ventilation mode where the baseline pressure automatically alternates between two preset levels and the patient can breathe freely at either level.

biphasic ventilation mode A ventilation mode where the baseline pressure automatically alternates between two preset levels according to the settings. BiPAP and APRV are typical biphasic ventilation modes.

breath cycle time (BCT) The duration of a mechanical breath. It counts from a valid triggering to the next valid triggering and contains two portions, inspiratory time (T_i) and expiratory time (T_e). BCT is also known as total cycle time (TCT).

breathing circuit The flexible tubing set connecting a ventilator to an artificial airway. Typically it contains an inspiratory limb, an expiratory limb, and a Y-piece. A breathing circuit is a required part of a ventilator system and is where the active humidifier, in-line nebulizer, and gas filter are installed. Also called a *patient circuit*.

bronchiole The terminal part of bronchial tree, just before alveoli.

bronchus One of the two divisions of the trachea, which go to each of the two lungs.

calibration The act of checking or adjusting the accuracy of a measuring instrument.

capillary The smallest blood vessels in tissues for microcirculation.

capnography The measurement of inhaled and exhaled CO_2.

capnogram The graphical representation of a CO_2 measurement.

chest Part of the human trunk between the neck and the abdomen. Also called the *thorax*.

chest wall The bony and muscular structures that form the outer framework of the thorax. It moves during breathing. It protects the vital organs such as heart and lungs and is involved in natural lung ventilation.

circuit compliance The phenomenon where the gas volume changes when passing through a breathing circuit because of gas compression and circuit elasticity. In a volume mode, circuit compliance causes a difference between the tidal volume delivered by a ventilator and the tidal volume received by the patient.

circuit compliance compensation An automatic mechanism that automatically compensates the volume lost due to circuit compliance.

circuit rainout Accumulation of condensed water in a breathing circuit. It can seriously affect the normal pneumatics of a ventilator system.

closed-loop control A controlling mechanism that enables a system to automatically adjust its performance or operation according to the operator set target and the monitoring feedback.

CMV See *continuous mandatory ventilation.*

CO2 production The generation of the major waste product of metabolism.

communication interface A function by which a ventilator transmits monitored data and alarms to another device, such as a patient monitor or a patient data management system (PDMS).

compliance A parameter that indicates a pressure-volume relationship in a balloon-like elastic structure.

condensation A process by which water is converted from its vapour form to its liquid form (droplets). Condensation is the consequence of air or gas oversaturation.

configuration A function used to adjust default settings so that the ventilator always starts up in a desired manner.

continuous mandatory ventilation (CMV) A classical ventilation mode, which delivers breaths based on set variables, independent from patient breathing effort.

continuous positive airway pressure (CPAP) A respiratory therapy where a patient breathes spontaneously at an elevated baseline pressure, which is generated by continuous inspiratory flow.

control breath A mechanical breath that is time triggered and time cycled

controlling or control variable The mechanism by which a ventilator controls or regulates delivery of inspiratory gas. An essential property of a mechanical breath.

conventional ventilation mode A mature or standard IPPV (intermittent positive pressure ventilation) mode typically characterized by a constant baseline pressure and manually adjusted controls.

CPAP See *continuous positive airway pressure.*

cycling/cycle variable The mechanism by which a ventilator ends inspiration. An essential property of a mechanical breath.

dead space An inevitable part of tidal volume, which does not participate in gas exchange. There are three types of dead space: (a) anatomic dead space, (b) alveolar dead space, and (c) instrumental dead space (associated exclusively with mechanical ventilation).

dead space ventilation Ineffective lung ventilation, because the tidal volume is equal to or below the dead space volume.

deflation The process to decrease the total volume of the lungs, from the inflated position to the resting position.

dew point The temperature at which air becomes 100% vapour saturated.

diaphragm The soft tissue that separates the chest and abdomen, which permits thoracic pressure to be easily transmitted to the abdomen, and vice versa.

DISS Diameter indexed safety system—a standard for gas cylinder fittings.

double-limb circuit A classic breathing circuit with an inspiratory limb, an expiratory limb, and a Y-piece.

dynamic loop A graphical presentation of monitoring data. A two-dimensional graph that plots one monitoring parameter against another in a closed figure. As the monitoring data continuously becomes available, the loop is dynamically displayed in real time.

elastic recoil force The elastic force to revert the stretched lung and chest wall to its original or resting shape or position. This reversion does not consume energy.

endotracheal tube (ETT) A tube inserted (as through the nose or mouth) into the trachea to maintain an unobstructed passageway for delivery of oxygen or anaesthesia to the lungs.

EPAP See *expiratory positive airway pressure.*

evaporation The process by which water is converted from liquid to vapour.

event log A function designed to chronologically record all ventilator 'events', such as alarm activations or setting changes.

exhalation See *expiration.*

expiration A process of lung deflation, i.e. the lung volume decreases from the inflated position to the resting position.

expiratory channel The gas passageway inside the ventilator on the expiratory side.

expiratory flow The flow at which the gas is moved away from the patient.

expiratory minute volume The sum of expiratory tidal volume per minute.

expiratory occlusion An abnormality resulting from excessive expiratory resistance. Typical causes are a clogged expiratory filter or a blocked expiratory valve.

expiratory positive airway pressure (EPAP) The lower level of PEEP in the BiPAP non-invasive ventilation mode.

expiratory tidal volume (VTE) The monitored volume of gas expelled during a mechanical breath.

expiratory time (Te) The duration of expiration.

expiratory trigger sensitivity (ETS) A control parameter of flow cycling.

expiratory valve The valve that controls gas exiting from the ventilator system.

Explanation TRC compensates at most the resistance imposed by ETT or TT. Airway resistance in a ventilated patient = airway resistance + tube resistance. So, airway resistance compensation is not appropriate.

extracorporeal membrane oxygenation (ECMO) A technique that provides both cardiac and respiratory support to persons whose heart and lungs cannot provide sufficient gas exchange to sustain life.

factory default Factory-set ventilator settings.

false negative alarm An abnormality where a ventilator does not alarm when an alarm condition is present.

false positive alarm An abnormality where a ventilator alarms when no alarm condition is present.

filtering The removal of particles from respiratory gas.

flex tube A flexible tube added to the artificial airway. It allows the patient to move their head easily and facilitates open tracheal suctioning.

flow The motion of gas volume over time.

flow cycling A cycling mechanism with which a ventilator ends inspiration, based on inspiratory flow. It is used in support breaths for active patients only.

flow pattern The inspiratory flow profile of volume breaths. The constant flow (square) pattern is the most common pattern.

flow sensor A device to detect the flow and pressure of the passing gas.

flow triggering A patient triggering mechanism. It enables a ventilator to initiate inspiration based on airway flow monitoring.

FRC See *functional residual capacity.*

freeze function A function with which an operator can temporarily stop the running waveforms or loops on the screen while mechanical ventilation continues in the background.

fTotal See *total breath rate.*

functional residual capacity (FRC) The total amount of gas left in the lungs after a normal, quiet exhalation. It plays a critical role in alveolar gas exchange.

gas diffusion A natural process in which gas molecules move from an area of high concentration to one of lower concentration.

gas hose A flexible pipe to convey gas.

gas inlet A part of a ventilator through which source gas enters the ventilator.

gas passageway A channel or duct inside a ventilator system through which gas moves based on local pressure gradients.

haemoglobin (Hb) A globular protein, which is the primary vehicle for oxygen transport in blood.

heat and moisture exchanger (HME) A passive, disposable device that humidifies and warms inspiratory gases in a ventilated patient.

heated (wire) circuit A breathing circuit in which the inspiratory limb is actively heated to reduce water condensation. In some cases, the expiratory limb may also be heated.

heating wire A special, isolated metal wire that becomes hot when an electrical current passes through it.

heliox A mixture of helium and oxygen, which is sometimes used as a supply gas in mechanical ventilation.

high-frequency ventilation (HFV) A principle of mechanical ventilation where the respiratory rate is much higher than the physiological one. HFV is typically used in neonatal ventilation and where intermittent positive pressure ventilation (IPPV) is not applicable.

HME See *heat and moisture exchanger.*

humidity The measure of moisture per unit volume of gas.

hybrid controlling A mechanism that employs both volume controlling and pressure controlling sequentially within the same mechanical breath.

hypercapnic respiratory failure See *type 2 respiratory failure.*

hypoxic respiratory failure See *type 1 respiratory failure.*

I:E ratio The ratio between inspiratory time and expiratory time of a mechanical breath. As a control, the I:E ratio is used to define inspiratory time.

in-line nebulization The application of nebulization to administer a drug to the respiratory passages of a ventilated patient. Because a ventilator system is gas tight, the application may cause unwanted problems that do not appear in conventional aerosol therapy (open nebulization).

inflation The process of lung expansion or increase in lung volume.

inhalation See *inspiration.*

INPV See *intermittent negative pressure ventilation.*

inspiration The action to draw air into the lungs.

inspiratory channel The passageway within the ventilator on the inspiratory side.

inspiratory flow The flow at which the gas is inhaled by the patient.

inspiratory valve The valve that controls gas that enters into breathing circuit.

inspiratory positive airway pressure (IPAP) The high level of PEEP in the BiPAP non-invasive ventilation mode.

inspiratory pressure The airway pressure that a ventilator applies above PEEP during inspiration.

inspiratory time (T_i) The duration of inspiration.

instrumental dead space The extra dead space introduced by the items between the Y-piece and the opening of the natural upper airway.

intermittent negative pressure ventilation (INPV) An operating principle of mechanical ventilation that is applied in negative pressure ventilators, such as the iron lung.

intermittent positive pressure ventilation (IPPV) An operating principle of mechanical ventilation that is the common foundation of most of modern ventilators.

intrinsic PEEP See *autoPEEP.*

intubation The placement of a breathing tube into the trachea. Also called tracheal intubation.

IPAP See *inspiratory positive airway pressure.*

IPPV See *intermittent positive pressure ventilation.*

iron lung A ventilator that was widely used to treat polio patients in the mid-1900s. A patient's body, except for the head, is placed in a sealed gas container with rigid walls, and an intermittent negative pressure inside the container results in inspiration and expiration.

jet nebulizer A device that generates medication aerosols for a patient to inhale.

leak compensation A ventilator function used to maintain the desired PEEP and inspiratory pressure in the presence of a moderate gas leak. Leak compensation is associated with pressure or adaptive breaths.

limiting/limit variable The mechanism that defines the size of a mechanical breath. It is also called *targeting.* An essential property of a mechanical breath.

lower airway The part of the respiratory tract that extends from the trachea to the terminal bronchioles.

lung Either of two sponge-like organs in the rib cage, which are used in respiration.

lung compliance A measure of the lungs' elasticity and a key property of lung mechanics.

lung failure See *type 1 respiratory failure.*

lung ventilation Gas movement in and out of the lungs. This essential part of respiration is responsible for the gas exchange between alveoli and the atmospheric air. It involves regularly replacing stale gases in the lungs with fresh gases from the atmosphere.

mandatory breath A category of mechanical breath that includes control breaths and assist breaths.

mandatory rate The set rate in assist/control and SIMV modes. It serves as the minimum rate or backup rate. In active patients, the actual rate can be higher than the mandatory rate.

manual triggering A mechanism by which an operator initiates an additional mechanical breath.

mechanical breath A breath that is realized through a ventilator system.

minute ventilation/ minute volume The sum of the tidal volumes of all mechanical breaths within one minute.

mode of ventilation See *ventilation mode.*

monitoring A ventilator function to sense pneumatic or non-pneumatic signals within a ventilator system.

natural breath A normal or physiological breath. The opposite of a mechanical breath.

nebulization volume The inevitable gas volume generated by use of a pneumatic nebulizer. The extra volume may be harmful in the neonatal population.

nebulizer A device to generate medication aerosols for a patient to inhale.

NIST Non-interchangeable screw thread—a standard for gas cylinder fittings.

non-invasive interface The non-invasive connection of a breathing circuit to a patient's airway. It may be a mask, nasal prongs, a mouthpiece, or a special helmet.

nose air conditioning A physiological function of the nose to warm, humidify, and filter the inhaled air.

numerical parameter Monitored data that is expressed numerically.

operation problem A problem related to improper operation of a ventilator system, such as improper intubation, mechanical ventilation, and extubation; improper ventilator settings and adjustment, etc. Typically, the ventilator does not have technical issues. Also called a use error.

oxygen concentrator A device that concentrates the oxygen typically from ambient air to produce an oxygen-enriched gas stream.

oxygen enrichment A ventilator function that allows the operator to increase the F_iO_2 temporarily.

oxygen sensor/oxygen cell An electronic device that measures the proportion of oxygen in inspiratory gas.

P_{alv} Alveolar pressure.

P_{ao} Airway opening pressure. Also known as airway pressure or P_{aw}.

patient circuit See *breathing circuit.*

patient triggering The common term for flow triggering and pressure triggering. Note that patient triggering may be associated with auto-triggering.

patient-ventilator asynchrony The mismatch between a patient's breathing efforts and ventilator operation in timing, phasing, and intensity. Also known as patient-ventilator dyssynchrony.

Paw Airway pressure. Also known as airway opening pressure or P_{ao}.

peak expiratory flow The most negative value of monitored expiratory flow in a mechanical breath.

peak flow The highest value of monitored inspiratory or expiratory flow in a mechanical breath. A control setting to define the desired inspiratory flow rate in a volume breath.

peak inspiratory flow The most positive value of monitored inspiratory flow in a mechanical breath.

peak inspiratory pressure (PIP) The highest level of monitored airway opening pressure in a mechanical breath.

PEEP See *positive end expiratory pressure.*

PEEP-high The control to define the high level of PEEP in a biphasic mode.

PEEP-low The control to define the low level of PEEP in a biphasic mode.

phrenic nerve The phrenic nerves originate in the neck (C3 – C5) and pass down between the lung and heart to reach the diaphragm. This nerve is important for breathing as it passes motor information to the diaphragm and receives sensory information from it. There are two phrenic nerves, a left one and a right one.

piezoelectric nebulizer A type of ultrasonic nebulizer that employs vibrating mesh technology.

plateau pressure (Pplateau) A monitored end-inspiratory pressure at zero flow, if available. It represents the alveolar pressure.

pneumatic nebulizer A device to generate pneumatically medication aerosols for a patient to inhale.

positive end expiratory pressure (PEEP) The baseline pressure above which a positive inspiratory pressure is applied intermittently.

positive pressure ventilator A ventilator based on intermittent positive pressure ventilation (IPPV).

Pplateau See *plateau pressure.*

precision An indicator of monitoring quality. It is generally synonymous with reproducibility.

pressure A force exerted against resistance or a force applied uniformly over a unit of surface area.

pressure assist/control (A/C) mode A ventilation mode with two breath types: pressure control breaths and pressure assist breaths. It is suitable for passive and partially active patients.

pressure assist breath A mechanical breath that is patient triggered, pressure controlled, and time cycled.

pressure control A control setting to define inspiratory pressure.

pressure control breath A mechanical breath that is time triggered, pressure controlled, and time cycled.

pressure controlling A mechanism by which a ventilator regulates the inspiratory gas flow based on the monitored airway pressure.

pressure cycling A mechanism by which a ventilator ends inspiration if the monitored airway pressure reaches a preset level.

pressure gradient The pressure difference between two connected areas.

pressure regulated volume control (PRVC) Another name for adaptive assist/control mode.

pressure SIMV mode A ventilation mode with three breath types: pressure control breaths, pressure assist breaths, and pressure support breaths. It is suitable for all ventilated patients if the mandatory rate is set appropriately.

pressure support A control setting to define inspiratory pressure.

pressure support breath A mechanical breath that is patient triggered, pressure controlled, and flow cycled.

pressure support ventilation (PSV) mode A ventilation mode with one breath type: pressure support. It is suitable for active patients only.

pressure triggering A patient triggering mechanism by which a ventilator initiates inspiration based on the detected pressure drop below PEEP.

PRVC See *pressure regulated volume control.*

PSV See *pressure support ventilation.*

pulmonary airway See *airway.*

pump failure See *type 2 respiratory failure.*

RC See *time constant.*

RDS Respiratory distress syndrome.

relative humidity The ratio of the amount of water vapour in the air at a specific temperature to the maximum amount that the air can hold at that temperature, expressed as a percentage.

reproducibility The variability of results when the same object is measured multiple times.

resistance A force that tends to oppose or retard gas movement.

resolution The ability to 'resolve' the differences of measurement results. A measurement device with higher resolution uses more gradations to report its measured results.

respiratory centre A group of nerve cells in the medulla oblongata and pons that regulates breathing activities including rate, site, and flow according to the sensed O_2, CO_2, and pH of blood and cerebrospinal fluid.

respiratory compliance A parameter to describe the pressure-volume relationship in a person's respiratory system. By nature, it is a static property. Respiratory compliance is the sum of lung compliance and chest wall compliance.

respiratory failure The syndrome where the respiratory system fails to maintain PaO_2 or $PaCO_2$ within normal ranges due to various clinical causes.

respiratory muscles The muscles that produce volume changes of the thorax during breathing.

respiratory nerves The nerves that supply the respiratory muscles, particularly the phrenic nerves.

respiratory rate The number of breaths per minute.

respiratory system The functional parts required to complete the process of gas exchange, including the airway, lungs, chest wall, respiratory muscles, phrenic nerve, and respiratory centre.

respiratory tract See *airway.*

rise time A control setting to define the speed at which the circuit or airway is pressurized in a pressure mode.

risk A potential problem or disaster that has not occurred yet, but that may occur at any time.

root cause The initiating cause of a causal chain that leads to an unwanted or disastrous consequence.

safety mechanism A function that is automatically activated to minimize potential harm.

safety valve A normally closed valve that opens when the ventilator is in the ambient state, allowing the patient to inhale room air. Also called *ambient valve.*

sensor A device that detects and converts a signal of interest into measurable form.

sigh A natural deep breath. Also a ventilator feature that periodically delivers larger-than-normal breaths.

single-limb circuit A special breathing circuit with an inspiratory limb only. In a single-limb circuit, the expiratory valve is positioned directly at the beginning of the artificial airway.

soft lung The situation where lung compliance is abnormally high.

spontaneous breath A natural breath in a normal, healthy human being. Also, a mechanical breath for which both the timing and size are controlled or influenced by the patient, i.e. patient triggered and flow cycled and with full, partial, or no pressure support.

standby A function that allows an operator to intentionally suspend mechanical ventilation.

stiff lung The situation where the lung compliance is abnormally low.

sudden and severe respiratory distress syndrome (SSRD) A serious respiratory disorder marked by such nonspecific signs as tachypnoea, nasal flaring, diaphoresis, and use of accessory muscles and causing retraction of suprasternal, supraclavicular, and intercostal spaces.

support breath A mechanical breath that is patient (pressure or flow) triggered and flow cycled.

synchronized intermittent mandatory ventilation (SIMV) A conventional ventilation mode with mandatory breaths (i.e. control breath and assist breath) and pressure support breath. Mandatory breaths are delivered according to the set rate and synchronized with patient triggering. Spontaneous breath can be inserted between two consecutive mandatory breaths if possible.

targeting (variable) The mechanism by which a ventilator defines the size of a mechanical breath in terms of volume or pressure. It is also known as limiting. An essential property of a mechanical breath.

target tidal volume The desired tidal volume in an adaptive breath or mode.

T_e See *expiratory time.*

technical alarm An alarm related to a technical abnormality of the ventilator, the electrical supply, or the gas (air and oxygen) supply.

technical tolerance A range of values within which a measurement is considered accurate.

test lung A device that can be used to mimic human lungs to complete a ventilator system. Also known as a demonstration lung.

thorax The thorax is a part of human trunk between the neck and the abdomen. The thorax wall is made up of bones and muscles. The bones, primarily ribs, sternum, and vertebrae, form a protective cage for the internal structures, including the heart, major blood vessels, lungs, trachea, oesophagus, etc.

T_i See *inspiratory time.*

tidal volume The amount of air passing into or out of the lungs during one breath.

time constant An estimation of the time needed to complete the process of lung inflation or deflation. The product of resistance and compliance. Also called *RC*.

time cycling A mechanism with which a ventilator ends inspiration based on the set inspiratory time.

Time high The defined duration of PEEP high in a biphasic mode.

Time low The defined duration of PEEP low in a biphasic mode.

time triggering A triggering mechanism with which a ventilator initiates inspiration based on the set rate.

total breath rate (fTotal) The total number of spontaneous and mandatory breaths of monitored mechanical breaths in a minute.

trachea The air passage extending from the throat and larynx to the main bronchi.

tracheostomy tube (TT) A special tube inserted into the trachea through a surgical opening at the neck to facilitate breathing.

TRC See *tube resistance compensation.*

trending curve A graph that shows how a monitoring parameter changed over the last hours.

triggering The initiation of inspiration.

triggering (variable) The mechanism with which a ventilator starts inspiration. An essential property of a mechanical breath.

trigger sensitivity A control setting to define the level of spontaneous effort (pressure or flow) needed to trigger a machine inspiratory breath.

tube resistance The resistance imposed by a tube to the flow of passing gas.

tube resistance compensation (TRC) A ventilator function to automatically compensate for the resistance imposed by an ETT or TT. Also called *automatic tube compensation (ATC).*

type 1 respiratory failure A type of respiratory failure characterized by abnormally low PaO_2 but nearly normal $PaCO_2$. Also called *hypoxic respiratory failure* or *lung failure.*

type 2 respiratory failure A type of respiratory failure that is characterized by abnormally high $PaCO_2$ and abnormally low PaO_2. Also called *hypercapnic respiratory failure* or *pump failure.*

ultrasonic nebulizer A nebulizer that generates medication aerosols by employing the ultrasonic principle.

upper airway The part of the respiratory tract that includes the nose, nasal cavity, mouth, pharynx, and larynx.

user interface A device with which a human being may interact with a machine, such as a touch screen.

variable A factor, feature, or function that can vary. In the terminology of mechanical ventilation, a variable refers to an essential property of mechanical breaths that can be realized through multiple mechanisms.

ventilation The process of gas exchange between the lungs and environmental air.

ventilation mode A set of ventilator operations with one or more predefined mechanical breath types occurring in a predefined sequence.

ventilator A device that is an essential part of a ventilator system for mechanical ventilation therapy.

ventilator system A set of specialized medical equipment used to perform mechanical ventilation therapy.

volume A measure of the space occupied by an amount of gas at a given pressure.

volume A/C mode A conventional ventilation mode with two breath types: volume control breaths and volume assist breaths. This mode is suitable for passive or partially active patients.

volume assist breath A mechanical breath that is patient triggered, volume controlled, and time cycled.

volume control breath A mechanical breath that is time triggered, volume controlled, and time cycled.

volume controlling A mechanism by which a ventilator regulates inspiratory gas delivery based on the set inspiratory time, tidal volume, and/or inspiratory peak flow.

volume SIMV mode A conventional ventilation mode with three breath types: volume control breaths, volume assist breaths, and pressure support breaths. This mode is suitable for all patients if the mandatory rate is appropriately set.

volume support (VS) mode An adaptive ventilation mode with one breath type: adaptive support breaths. This mode is suitable for active patients only.

volutrauma A complication of mechanical ventilation. Lung injury caused by excessively large tidal volumes.

VTE See *expiratory tidal volume.*

water trap A device to drain condensed water from the breathing circuit.

waveform A graphical presentation of a monitored parameter over time. A typical example is a pressure waveform.

work of breathing The work that is required to overcome the mechanical impedance to respiration. It is the sum of work required to overcome both elastic and air flow resistance.

Wye/Y-piece A part of the breathing circuit that joins the inspiratory and expiratory limbs. Also called a *Y-piece.*

Index

Tables, figures, and boxes are indicated by an italic *t*, *f*, and *b* following the page number.